**PEARSON**

# EKG Technician Program
## Standard

Third Custom Edition for Condensed Curriculum International

Taken from:
*EKG: Plain and Simple,* Fourth Edition
by Karen M. Ellis

Cover Art: Courtesy of Chaikom, PeterPhoto123/Shutterstock.

Taken from:

*EKG: Plain and Simple,* Fourth Edition
by Karen M. Ellis
Copyright © 2017, 2012, 2007 by Pearson Education, Inc.
New York, New York 10013

This special edition published in cooperation with Pearson Education, Inc.

Pearson Education, Inc., 330 Hudson Street, New York, New York 10013
A Pearson Education Company
www.pearsoned.com

Printed in the United States of America

4 2020


000200010272214658

NF

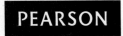

ISBN 10: 0-13-659564-2
ISBN 13: 978-0-13-659564-9

# Contents

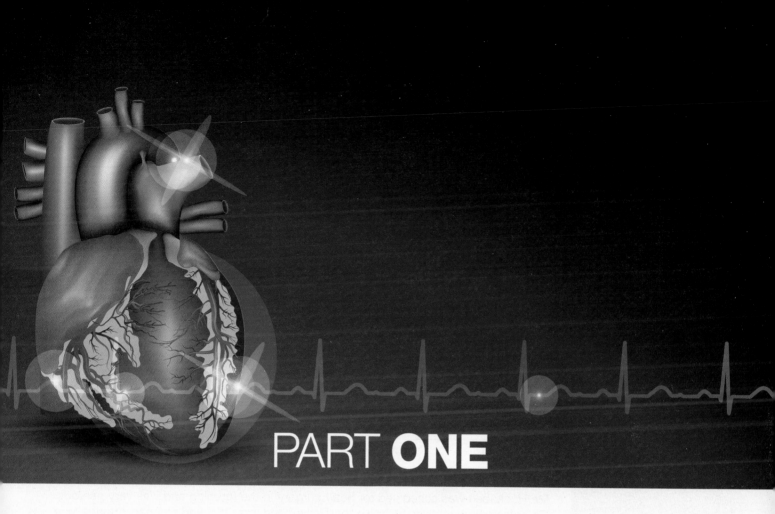

# PART **ONE**

# The Basics

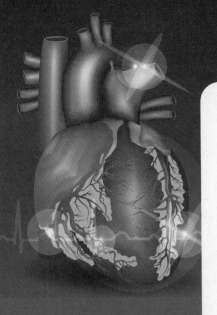

# Cardiac Anatomy and Physiology

## CHAPTER 1 OBJECTIVES

Upon completion of this chapter, the student will be able to

- State the location of the heart and its normal size.
- Name the walls and layers of the heart.
- Name all the structures of the heart.
- Track the flow of blood through the heart.
- State the oxygen saturation of the heart's chambers.
- Describe the function and location of the heart valves.
- Describe the relationship of the valves to heart sounds.
- List the great vessels and the chamber into which they empty or from which they arise.

- State what occurs in each phase of the cardiac cycle.
- Name and describe the function of the coronary arteries.
- Differentiate between the two kinds of cardiac cells.
- Describe the sympathetic and parasympathetic nervous systems.
- Describe the *fight-or-flight* and *rest-and-digest* responses.

## What It's All About

Mr. Huckabee was scheduled for heart surgery in the morning and was very nervous. His surgeon had told him he had a "bad valve" and three blocked coronary arteries, one of which was so bad it could cause a **myocardial infarction** (**MI**—a heart attack) any minute. All this had been discovered when Mr. Huckabee's heart rhythm became erratic, causing symptoms. The doctor did a cardiac workup on him and found the blockages and the valve problems. So now Mr. Huckabee is in the hospital, nervously awaiting his surgery. When his nurse asked him what exactly he was to have done in surgery the next morning, he replied the surgeon had "talked medicalese" and he hadn't really understood any of it. The nurse took out a model of the heart and pointed out the heart valves and coronary arteries, explaining what they do and how his symptoms were all related to his heart problems. She then explained how the surgery would correct the problems. Mr. Huckabee visibly relaxed afterward, saying he was grateful his nurse took the time to teach him about his heart.

## Introduction

The function of the heart, a muscular organ about the size of a man's closed fist, is to pump enough blood to meet the body's metabolic needs. To accomplish this, the heart beats 60 to 100 times per minute and circulates 4 to 8 liters of blood per minute. Thus, each day the average person's heart beats approximately 90,000 times and pumps out about 6,000 liters of blood. With stress, exertion, or certain pathological conditions, these numbers can quadruple.

The heart is located in the **thoracic (chest) cavity**, between the lungs in a cavity called the **mediastinum**, above the diaphragm, behind the **sternum** (breastbone), and in front of the spine. It is entirely surrounded by bony structures for protection. This bony cage also serves as a means to revive the stricken heart, as the external chest compressions of CPR compress the heart between the sternum and spine and squeeze blood out until the heart's function can be restored.

The top of the heart is the **base**, from which the great vessels emerge. The bottom of the heart is the **apex**, the pointy part that rests on the diaphragm. The heart lies at an angle in the chest, with the bottom pointing to the left. See Figure 1–1.

## Layers of the Heart

The heart has three layers:

- **Epicardium**   The outermost layer of the heart. The coronary arteries run along this layer.
- **Myocardium**   The middle and thickest layer. The myocardium is made of pure muscle and does the work of contracting. It is the part that is damaged during a heart attack.
- **Endocardium**   The thin innermost layer that lines the heart's chambers and folds back onto itself to form the heart valves. The endocardium is watertight to prevent leakage of blood into the other layers. The cardiac conduction system is found in this layer.

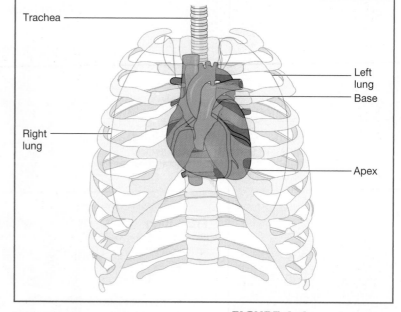

**FIGURE 1–1**

**Heart's location in thoracic cavity.**

Surrounding the heart is the **pericardium**, a double-walled sac that encloses the heart. Think of it as the film on a hard-boiled egg. The pericardium serves as support and protection and anchors the heart to the diaphragm and great vessels. A small amount of fluid is found between the layers of the pericardium. This **pericardial fluid** minimizes friction between these layers as they rub against each other with every heartbeat. See Figure 1–2 for an illustration of the heart's anatomy.

## Heart Chambers

The heart has four chambers (See Table 1–1):

- **Right atrium**   A receiving chamber for deoxygenated blood (blood that's had some oxygen removed by the body's tissues) returning to the heart from the body, the right atrium has an oxygen ($O_2$) saturation of only 60% to 75%. The blood in this chamber has so little oxygen, its color is dark maroon. Carbon dioxide ($CO_2$) concentration is high. The right atrium delivers its blood to the right ventricle.
- **Right ventricle**   The right ventricle pumps the blood to the lungs for a fresh supply of oxygen. $O_2$ saturation is 60% to 75%. Again, the blood is dark maroon in color. $CO_2$ concentration is high.
- **Left atrium**   This is a receiving chamber for the blood returning to the heart from the lungs. $O_2$ saturation is now about 100%. The blood is full of oxygen and is now bright red in color. $CO_2$ concentration is extremely low, as it was removed by the lungs. The left atrium delivers its blood to the left ventricle.
- **Left ventricle**   The left ventricle's job is to pump blood out to the entire body. It is the major pumping chamber of the heart. $O_2$ saturation is about 100%. Again, the blood is bright red in color. $CO_2$ concentration is minimal.

**TABLE 1–1   Heart Chambers**

| Chamber | $O_2$ Saturation | Receives Blood From | Delivers Blood To |
|---|---|---|---|
| Right atrium | 60–75% | Body | Right ventricle |
| Right ventricle | 60–75% | Right atrium | Lungs |
| Left atrium | ~100% | Lungs | Left ventricle |
| Left ventricle | ~100% | Left atrium | Body (systemic circulation) |

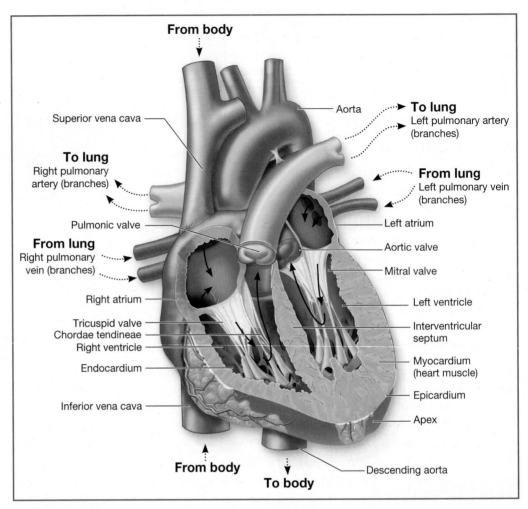

**FIGURE 1–2**

**The heart: Its layers, chambers, and blood flow.**

The atria's job is to deliver blood to the ventricles that lie directly below them. Because this is a short trip and minimal contraction is needed to transport this blood to the ventricles, the atria are thin-walled, low-pressure chambers.

The ventricles, on the other hand, are higher-pressure chambers because they must contract more forcefully to deliver their blood into the pulmonary system and the systemic circulation. Because the right ventricle must pump its blood only to the nearby lungs, and pulmonary pressures are normally low, the right ventricle's pressure is relatively low and its muscle bulk is relatively thin. The left ventricle generates the highest pressures, as it not only must pump the blood the farthest (throughout the entire body), it also must pump against great resistance—the blood pressure. Because of this heavy workload, the left ventricle has three times the muscle bulk of the right ventricle and plays the prominent role in the heart's function.

The heart is divided into right and left sides by the septum, a muscular band of tissue. The septum separating the atria is called the interatrial septum. The septum separating the ventricles is called the interventricular septum.

## Heart Valves

The heart has four valves to prevent backflow of blood. Two are semilunar valves and two are atrioventricular (AV) valves.

Semilunar valves separate a ventricle from an artery and have three half-moon-shaped cusps. The term *semilunar* means half moon. There are two *semilunar* valves.

- **Pulmonic valve**   This valve is located between the right ventricle and the pulmonary artery.
- **Aortic valve**   The aortic valve is located between the left ventricle and the aorta.

AV valves are located between an atrium and a ventricle. They are supported by chordae tendineae (tendonous cords), which are attached to papillary muscles (muscles that outpouch from the ventricular wall) and anchor the valve cusps to keep the closed AV valves from flopping backward and allowing backflow of blood. There are two AV valves.

- **Tricuspid**   This valve, located between the right atrium and ventricle, has three cusps.
- **Mitral**   The mitral valve, also called the *bicuspid valve,* is located between the left atrium and ventricle. It has two cusps.

Valves open and close based on changes in pressure. *And they open only in the direction of blood flow.* Blood flows down from atrium to ventricle, and up from ventricle to aorta and pulmonary artery. For example, the tricuspid and mitral valves are located between the right atrium and ventricle and the left atrium and ventricle, respectively. Because blood flows down from atrium to ventricle, these valves open only one way—down. Thus, when the atria's pressure is higher than the ventricles' pressure, the tricuspid and mitral valves open to allow blood to flow into the waiting ventricles. The aortic and pulmonic valves open upward only when the pressure in the ventricles exceeds that in the waiting aorta and pulmonary artery. Blood then flows up into those arteries. See Table 1–2.

Valve closure is responsible for the sounds made by the beating heart. The normal lub-dub of the heart is made not by blood flowing through the heart, but by the closing of the heart's valves. S1, the first heart sound, reflects closure of the mitral and tricuspid valves. S2, the second heart sound, reflects closure of the aortic and pulmonic valves. Between S1 and S2, the heart beats and expels its blood (called systole). Between S2 and the next S1, the heart rests and fills with blood (called diastole). Each heartbeat has an S1 and S2. Note the valves on Figure 1–2.

## Great Vessels

Attached to the heart at its base are the five great vessels.

- **Superior vena cava (SVC)**   The SVC is the large vein that returns deoxygenated blood to the right atrium from the head, neck, and upper chest and arms.
- **Inferior vena cava (IVC)**   The IVC is the large vein that returns deoxygenated blood to the right atrium from the lower chest, abdomen, and legs.
- **Pulmonary artery**   This is the large artery that takes deoxygenated blood from the right ventricle to the lungs to load up on oxygen and unload carbon dioxide. It is the *only* artery that carries deoxygenated blood.
- **Pulmonary veins**   These are four large veins that return the oxygenated blood from the lungs to the left atrium. They are the *only* veins that carry oxygenated blood.
- **Aorta**   The aorta is the largest artery in the body. It takes oxygenated blood from the left ventricle to the systemic circulation to feed all the organs of the body.

Note the great vessels on Figure 1–2. See Table 1–3.

**TABLE 1–2  Heart Valves**

| Valve | Location | Direction of Valve Opening |
|---|---|---|
| Pulmonic | Between right ventricle and pulmonary artery | Opens upward into pulmonary artery |
| Aortic | Between left ventricle and aorta | Opens upward into aorta |
| Tricuspid | Between right atrium and right ventricle | Opens downward into right ventricle |
| Mitral | Between left atrium and left ventricle | Opens downward into left ventricle |

**TABLE 1–3  Great Vessels**

| Vessel | Kind of Vessel | Oxygen Status of Transported Blood | Transports Blood from: | Transports Blood to: |
|---|---|---|---|---|
| Superior vena cava (SVC) | Vein | Deoxygenated | Head, neck, upper chest, arms | Right atrium |
| Inferior vena cava (IVC) | Vein | Deoxygenated | Lower chest, abdomen, legs | Right atrium |
| Pulmonary artery | Artery | Deoxygenated | Right ventricle | Lungs |
| Pulmonic veins | Veins | Oxygenated | Lungs | Left atrium |
| Aorta | Artery | Oxygenated | Left ventricle | Body |

## Blood Flow Through the Heart

Now let's track a single blood cell as it travels through the heart:

Superior or inferior vena cava → right atrium → tricuspid valve → right ventricle → pulmonic valve →→ pulmonary artery →→ lungs →→ pulmonary veins →→ left atrium →→ mitral valve →→ left ventricle →→ aortic valve →→ aorta →→ body (systemic circulation)

- The blood cell enters the heart via either the **superior** or **inferior vena cava**.
- It then enters the **right atrium**.
- Next it travels through the **tricuspid valve** into the **right ventricle**.
- Then it passes through the **pulmonic valve** into the **pulmonary artery**, then into the **lungs** for oxygen/carbon dioxide exchange.
- It is then sent through the **pulmonary veins** to the **left atrium**.
- Then it travels through the **mitral valve** into the **left ventricle**.
- It passes through the **aortic valve** into the **aorta** and out to the **body (systemic circulation)**.

**chapter** CHECKUP

We're about halfway through this chapter. To evaluate your understanding of the material thus far, answer the following questions. If you have trouble with them, review the material again before continuing.

1. Name the heart layers, chambers, valves, and great vessels. Describe the function of each.
2. Track the flow of blood through the heart.

Blood flow through the heart is accomplished by way of the cardiac cycle. Let's look at that now.

**Quick Tip**

Rapid-filling phase = atria pouring blood into ventricles

Diastasis = slowing blood flow

Atrial kick = atria contracting to squeeze remainder of blood into ventricles

## The Cardiac Cycle

The **cardiac cycle** refers to the mechanical events that occur to pump blood. There are two phases to the cardiac cycle—diastole and systole. During diastole, the ventricles relax and fill. During systole, the ventricles contract and expel their blood. Each of these phases has several phases of its own. See Figures 1–3 and 1–4 and Tables 1–4 and 1–5.

## Diastole

- **Rapid-filling phase**   This is the first phase of diastole. The atria, having received blood from the superior and inferior vena cava, are full of blood and therefore have high pressure. The ventricles, having just expelled their blood into the pulmonary artery and the aorta, are essentially empty and have lower pressure. This difference in pressure causes the AV valves to pop open and the atrial blood to flow down to the ventricles. To envision this, imagine two water balloons connected at their necks, one above the

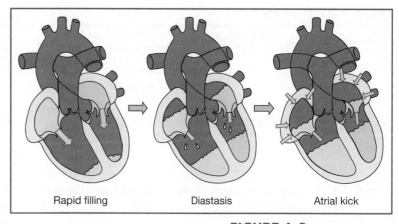

Rapid filling          Diastasis          Atrial kick

**FIGURE 1–3**

**Phases of diastole.**

other. The top balloon is full, representing the atrium; the empty bottom one is the ventricle. Imagine a pressure-sensitive valve separating the two balloons. Once this valve is popped open by the pressure difference, the water in the top full balloon will pour down into the empty bottom one. That's the rapid filling phase. The ventricles are filling with blood from the atria.

- **Diastasis**   Diastasis is the second phase of diastole. The pressure in the atria and ventricles starts to equalize as the ventricles fill and the atria empty, so blood flow slows. The fluid levels of the two balloons are equalizing, causing an equalization in pressure, so the flow from top to bottom slows until the top is almost empty and the bottom is almost full.

- **Atrial kick**   Atrial kick is the last phase of diastole. The atria are essentially empty, but there is still a little blood to deliver to the ventricle. Because the top balloon is almost empty of water, what must be done to get the last little bit of water out of it? Squeeze. The atria contract, squeezing in on themselves and propelling the remainder of the blood into the ventricles. The pressure in the ventricles at the end of this phase is high, as the ventricles are now full. Atrial pressure is low, as the atria are essentially empty. The AV valve leaflets, which have been hanging down in the ventricle in their open position, are pushed upward by the higher ventricular volume and its sharply rising pressure until they slam shut, ending diastole. S1 is heard at this time. Atrial kick provides 15% to 30% of ventricular filling and is an important phase.

Some heart rhythm abnormalities cause a loss of the atrial kick. This causes a decrease in **cardiac output** (amount of blood pumped by the heart every minute).

## Systole

- **Isovolumetric contraction**   This is the first phase of systole. All valves are closed. The ventricles are full, but the pressure in them is not yet high enough to exceed the blood pressure and pop the semilunar valves open. Because the ventricles cannot increase their pressure by adding more volume (they are as full as they are going to get with those valves closed),

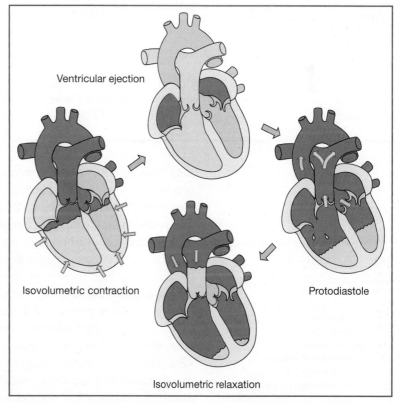

Ventricular ejection

Isovolumetric contraction

Protodiastole

Isovolumetric relaxation

**FIGURE 1–4**

**Phases of systole.**

**TABLE 1–4     Diastole**

| Phase | Atrial pressure at start of phase | Ventricular pressure at start of phase | Valve action during phase | Blood flow |
|---|---|---|---|---|
| Rapid filling | High (atria full of blood) | Low (ventricles essentially empty) | AV valves pop open | Strong flow of blood down from atria to ventricles |
| Diastasis | Equalizing | Equalizing | AV valves remain open | Flow from atria to ventricles slows, as pressure equalizes between atria and ventricles. |
| Atrial kick | Low (atria almost empty) | High (ventricles almost full) | AV valves are open at beginning of phase, then slam shut at end of phase. Diastole is complete once AV valves close. | Atrial contraction (kick) propels remainder of blood into ventricles. |

**TABLE 1–5     Systole**

| Phase | Ventricular pressure at start of phase | Aortic/Pulmonary artery pressures at start of phase | Valve action during phase | Blood flow |
|---|---|---|---|---|
| Isovolumetric contraction | High (ventricles full) | Low (aorta and pulmonary artery essentially empty) | All valves closed | No blood flow. Myocardial contraction occurring, sharply increasing ventricular pressures. |
| Ventricular ejection | High (ventricles full) | Low (aorta and pulmonary artery essentially empty) | Aortic and pulmonic valves pop open | Blood pours out into aorta and pulmonary artery. Half of blood empties very quickly. |
| Protodiastole | Equalizing | Equalizing | Aortic and pulmonic valves remain open. | Flow from ventricles into aorta and pulmonary artery slows as pressures equalize between them. |
| Isovolumetric relaxation | Low (ventricles essentially empty) | High (aorta and pulmonary artery full of blood) | Aortic and pulmonic valves slam shut at end of phase, concluding systole. | Flow out of ventricles stops. |

they squeeze down on themselves, forcing their muscular walls inward, putting pressure on the blood inside and causing the ventricular pressure to rise sharply. No blood flow occurs during this phase because all the valves are closed. *This is like squeezing a plastic cola bottle HARD with the cap still on.* This phase results in the greatest consumption of myocardial oxygen.

- **Ventricular ejection**   This is the second phase of systole. With the ventricular pressures now high enough, the semilunar valves pop open and blood pours out of the ventricles into the pulmonary artery and the aorta. *The cola bottle has been squeezed so hard, the cap now pops off.* Half the blood empties quickly and the rest a little slower.
- **Protodiastole**   Protodiastole is the third phase of systole. Ventricular contraction continues, but blood flow slows as the ventricular pressure drops (because the ventricles are becoming empty) and the aortic and pulmonary arterial pressures rise (because they are filling with blood from the ventricles). Pressures are equalizing between the ventricles and the aorta and pulmonary artery.
- **Isovolumetric relaxation**   This is the final phase of systole. Ventricular pressure is low because the blood has essentially been pumped out. The ventricles relax, causing the pressure to drop further. The aorta and pulmonary artery have

**Quick Tip**

- Isovolumetric contraction = ventricles squeezing but not pumping
- Ventricular ejection = pumping vigorously
- Protodiastole = pumping less
- Isovolumetric relaxation = relaxing, valves closing to end systole

higher pressures now, as they are full of blood. Because there is no longer any forward pressure from the ventricles to propel this blood further into the aorta and pulmonary artery, some of the blood in these arteries starts to flow back toward the aortic and pulmonic valves. This back pressure causes the valve leaflets, which had been pushed up into the aorta and pulmonary arteries in their open position, to slam shut, ending systole. S2 is heard now.

## Blood Flow Through the Systemic Circulation

We've tracked the flow of blood through the heart. Now let's track its course as it heads throughout the systemic circulation:

Aorta →→ arteries →→ arterioles →→ capillary bed →→ venules →→ veins →→ vena cava

- Oxygenated blood leaves the aorta and enters the arteries, which narrow into arterioles and empty into each organ's capillary bed, where nutrient and oxygen extraction occurs.
- Then, on the other side of the capillary bed, this now-deoxygenated blood enters narrow venules, which widen into veins, and then return to the vena cava for transport back to the heart. Then the cycle repeats.
  See Figure 1–5.

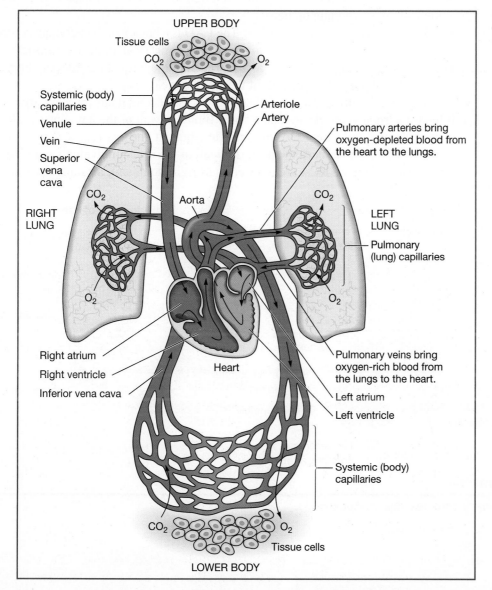

**FIGURE 1–5**

**Systemic circulation.**

## Coronary Arteries

The heart must not only meet the needs of the body, it has its own needs. With the endocardium being watertight, none of the blood in the chambers can reach the myocardium to nourish it. So the heart has its own circulation—the coronary arteries—to do that. Once the myocardium has extracted the nutrients and oxygen from the coronary arteries, the now-deoxygenated blood is returned to the right atrium by the coronary sinus, a large coronary vein. Let's look at the coronary arteries in more depth.

Coronary arteries arise from the base of the aorta and course along the epicardial surface of the heart, then dive into the myocardium to provide its blood supply. The myocardium, unlike the rest of the body, does not receive its blood supply during systole. Only in diastole is the heart able to feed itself. This is because during systole the heart muscle is contracting and essentially squeezing the coronary arteries shut. During diastole, this contraction stops and the blood can then enter the coronary arteries and feed the myocardium. Let's look at the two main coronary arteries. See Figure 1–6.

- **Left Main Coronary Artery (LMCA)**   The left main coronary artery and its two main branches provide blood flow to the anterior and lateral walls of the left ventricle, thus **perfusing** (providing blood flow to) about 60% of the myocardium. Blockage of the LMCA would knock out flow to both its branches and can produce a huge heart attack sometimes referred to as the *widow maker*. Let's look at the LMCA's two main branches.
  - **Left anterior descending (LAD)**   The LAD is a branch of the left main coronary artery. The LAD supplies blood to the anterior (front) wall of the left ventricle.
  - **Circumflex**   The circumflex, also a branch of the left main coronary artery, feeds the lateral (left side) wall of the left ventricle.
- **Right coronary artery (RCA)**   The RCA is the second main coronary artery. It feeds the right ventricle and the inferior (bottom) wall of the left ventricle. In about 70% of people, the RCA gives rise to a branch, the **posterior descending artery (PDA)**, which feeds the posterior wall of the heart. Individuals with the PDA arising from the RCA are referred to as right-dominant, meaning the right

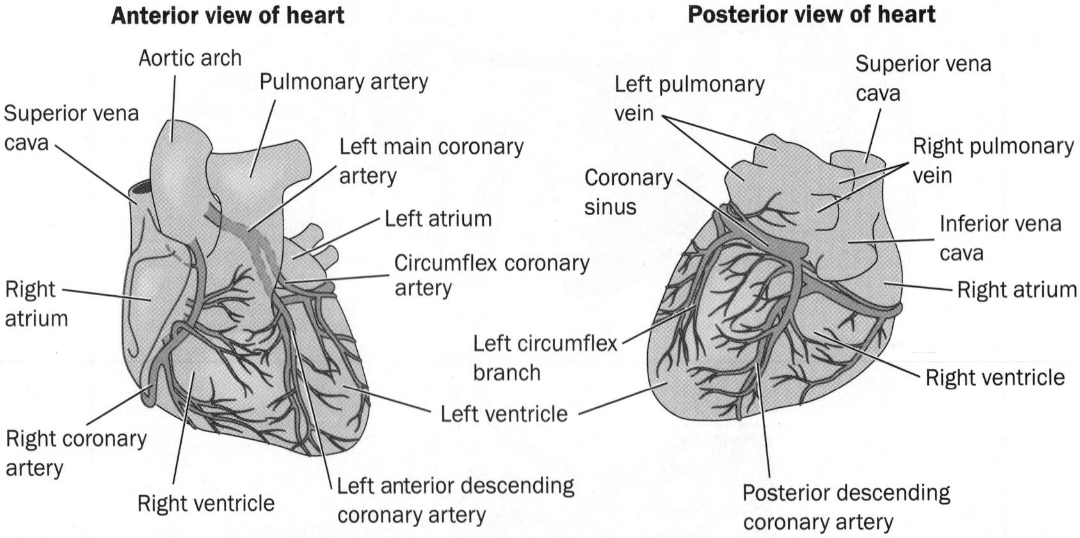

**FIGURE 1–6**

**Coronary arteries** (Blamb/Shutterstock).

coronary artery is dominant in perfusing the posterior wall of the heart. In the other 30% of people, the PDA arises from the circumflex coronary artery, which is part of the left coronary artery system. These individuals are referred to as left-dominant. Different coronary artery configurations are common and are not cause for concern, so long as the myocardium is perfused. See Table 1–6 for more info on the areas fed by the coronary arteries.

## Heart Cells

The heart has two kinds of cells:

- **Contractile cells**   The contractile cells cause the heart muscle to contract, resulting in a heartbeat.
- **Conduction system cells**   The conduction system cells create and conduct electrical signals to tell the heart when to beat. Without these electrical signals, the contractile cells would *never* contract.

## Nervous Control of the Heart

The heart is influenced by the autonomic nervous system (ANS), which controls involuntary biological functions. The ANS is subdivided into the sympathetic and parasympathetic nervous systems.

The sympathetic nervous system is mediated by norepinephrine, a chemical released by the adrenal gland. Norepinephrine increases heart rate and blood pressure, causes pupils to dilate, and slows digestion. This is the fight-or-flight response, and it is triggered by stress, exertion, or fear. Imagine you're walking to your car at night and a stranger runs toward you. Your fear triggers the adrenal gland to pour out norepinephrine. Your heart rate and blood pressure shoot up. Your pupils dilate to let in more light so you can see the danger and the escape path better. Digestion slows

**TABLE 1–6    Areas Supplied by the Coronary Arteries**

| Coronary artery | Areas supplied |
| --- | --- |
| Left anterior descending | Anterior two-thirds of septum |
| | Right bundle branch |
| | Anterior fascicle (branch) of the left bundle branch |
| | Anterior wall of left ventricle |
| | Lower segment of AV junction |
| Circumflex | Sinus node in 45% of people |
| | Posterior fascicle of the left bundle branch |
| | Lateral wall of left ventricle |
| Right coronary artery | Sinus node in 55% of people |
| | AN node in 90% of people |
| | Bundle of His |
| | Posterior fascicle of the left bundle branch |
| | Posterior third of the septum |
| | Right atrial and ventricular walls |
| | Inferior wall of the left ventricle |

down as the body shunts blood away from nonvital areas. (Is it essential to be digesting your pizza when your life is at stake? The pizza can wait.) Blood is shunted to vital organs, such as the brain, to help you think more clearly, and to the muscles to help you fight or flee.

The parasympathetic nervous system is mediated by acetylcholine, a chemical secreted as a result of stimulation of the vagus nerve, a nerve that travels from the brain to the heart, stomach, and other areas. It slows the heart rate, decreases blood pressure, and enhances digestion. This is the rest-and-digest response. Parasympathetic stimulation can be caused by any action that closes the glottis, the flap over the top of the trachea (the windpipe). Breath holding and straining to have a bowel movement are two actions that can cause the heart rate to slow down. It is not uncommon for paramedics to be summoned to the scene of a "person found down" in the bathroom. Straining at stool causes vagal stimulation, which causes the heart rate to slow down. If the heart rate slows enough, syncope (fainting) can result. In extreme cases, the heart can stop, requiring resuscitation. Although the heart is influenced by the autonomic nervous system, it can also, in certain extreme circumstances, function for a time without any input from this system. For example, a heart that is removed from a donor in preparation for transplant is no longer in communication with the body, yet it continues to beat on its own for a while. This is possible because of the heart's conduction system cells, which create and conduct electrical impulses to tell the heart to beat.

In a nutshell, the sympathetic nervous system hits the accelerator and the parasympathetic nervous system puts on the brakes.

## chapter one notes TO SUM IT ALL UP . . .

- **Heart's function**—Pump enough blood to meet the body's metabolic needs.
- Heart has three layers:
  - *Epicardium*—Outermost layer—where coronary arteries lie.
  - *Myocardium*—Middle muscular layer—does the work of contracting—damaged during a heart attack.
  - *Endocardium*—Innermost layer—watertight—lines the chambers and forms the heart valves. The conduction system is in this layer.
- **Heart has four chambers:**
  - *Right atrium*—Receiving chamber for deoxygenated blood returning to heart from body. Oxygen saturation is 60% to 75%. Blood is dark maroon.
  - *Right ventricle*—Pumps deoxygenated blood to lungs so it can be oxygenated. Oxygen saturation is 60% to 75%. Blood is dark maroon.
  - *Left atrium*—Receiving chamber for oxygenated blood coming from lungs. Oxygen saturation is 100%. Blood is bright red.
  - *Left ventricle*—Major pumping chamber of heart—pumps oxygenated blood to systemic circulation. Oxygen saturation is 100%. Blood is bright red.
- **Interventricular septum**—Band of tissue that separates right and left ventricles.
- **Interatrial septum**—Separates right and left atria.
- **Four heart valves**—Job is to prevent back flow of blood. Valves open in direction of blood flow—AV valves open downward, semilunar valves open upward.

- *Pulmonic valve*—Semilunar valve between right ventricle and pulmonary artery.
- *Aortic valve*—Semilunar valve between left ventricle and aorta.
- *Tricuspid valve*—AV valve between right atrium and right ventricle.
- *Mitral valve*—AV valve between left atrium and left ventricle.
- **Five great vessels:**
  - *Superior vena cava (SVC)*—Large vein—returns deoxygenated blood from upper body to the heart.
  - *Inferior vena cava (IVC)*—Large vein—returns deoxygenated blood from lower body to the heart.
  - *Pulmonary artery (PA)*—Takes deoxygenated blood from right ventricle to lungs—only artery in the body that carries deoxygenated blood.
  - *Pulmonary veins*—Take oxygenated blood from lungs to left atrium—only veins that carry oxygenated blood.
  - *Aorta (Ao)*—Main artery of the body—carries oxygenated blood to the body.
- **Blood flow through heart:**
  - Superior/inferior vena cava → right atrium → tricuspid valve → right ventricle → pulmonic valve → pulmonary artery → lungs → pulmonary veins → left atrium → mitral valve → left ventricle → aortic valve → aorta → body

- **Cardiac cycle**—Mechanical events that occur to pump blood. Two phases—diastole and systole. **Diastole**—ventricles relax and fill with blood. **Systole**—ventricles contract and expel blood.
- **Diastole**—three phases
  - *Rapid filling*—Atria full of blood, ventricles empty. Pressure differential causes AV valves to pop open—blood rapidly fills ventricles.
  - *Diastasis*—Pressures equalize between atria and ventricles—flow into ventricles slows.
  - *Atrial kick*—Atria contract to squeeze remainder of blood into the ventricles.
- **Systole**—four phases
  - *Isovolumetric contraction*—Ventricles contracting, no blood flow occurring because the aortic and pulmonic valves are still closed. Huge expenditure of myocardial oxygen consumption.
  - *Ventricular ejection*—Valves open—blood pours out of ventricles into pulmonary artery and aorta.
  - *Protodiastole*—Pressures equalize between ventricles and pulmonary artery and aorta—blood flow slows.
  - *Isovolumetric relaxation*—Ventricles relax—pulmonic and aortic valves close.
- **Blood flow through the systemic circulation:**
  - Aorta → arteries → arterioles → capillary bed → venules → veins → vena cava
- **Coronary arteries**—Supply blood flow to myocardium. Two major coronary arteries:
  - **Left main coronary artery**—Has two main branches:
    - *Left anterior descending (LAD)*—provides blood flow to anterior wall of left ventricle.
    - *Circumflex*—provides blood flow to lateral wall of left ventricle.
  - **Right coronary artery**—Provides blood flow to right ventricle and inferior wall of left ventricle. Has one major branch in 70% of people—the posterior descending coronary artery. (In the other 30%, the PDA arises from the circumflex coronary artery).
- **Two kinds of heart cells:**
  - *Contractile cells*—Cause the heart to contract, resulting in a heartbeat.
  - *Conduction system cells*—Create and conduct electrical impulses to tell the heart when to beat.
- **Heart influenced by the autonomic nervous system (ANS), which controls involuntary biological functions.** ANS subdivided into sympathetic (SNS) and parasympathetic nervous systems (PNS). Sympathetic nervous system hits the accelerator; parasympathetic puts on the brakes.
  - *SNS*—Mediated by hormone norepinephrine—causes fight-or-flight response—speeds up heart rate, increases blood pressure, dilates pupils, and slows digestion.
  - *PNS*—Mediated by acetylcholine—causes rest-and-digest response. Slows heart rate, lowers blood pressure, enhances digestion.

## Practice Quiz

1. The function of the heart is to _____ _____

2. Name the three layers of the heart. _____ _____ _____ _____

3. Name the four chambers of the heart. _____ _____ _____ _____

4. Name the four heart valves. _____ _____

5. The purpose of the heart valves is to _____ _____

6. Name the five great vessels of the heart. _____ _____

7. List the phases of diastole. _____ _____ _____

8. List the phases of systole. _____ _____ _____

9. Name the two divisions of the autonomic nervous system. _____ _____

10. The two main coronary arteries are _____ _____

# Putting It All Together—Critical Thinking Exercises

These exercises may consist of diagrams to label, scenarios to analyze, brain-stumping questions to ponder, or other challenging exercises to boost your understanding of the chapter material.

**1.** Label the heart diagram.

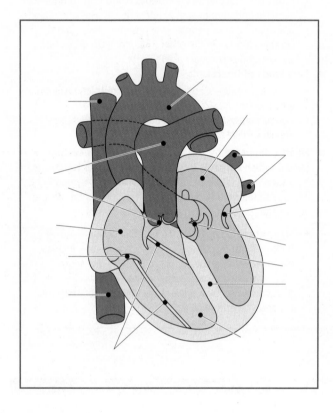

**2.** Number the following structures 1–14 in the order of blood flow through the heart:

_____ superior and inferior vena cava

_____ pulmonary artery

_____ tricuspid valve

_____ lungs

_____ mitral valve

_____ pulmonary veins

_____ aortic valve

_____ right atrium

_____ pulmonic valve

_____ left atrium

_____ body

_____ right ventricle

_____ aorta

_____ left ventricle

**3.** What would happen to the tricuspid and mitral valves if their chordae tendineae "snapped" loose?

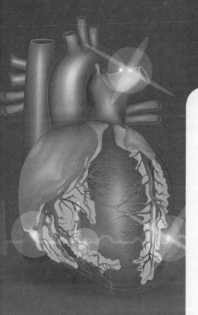

# Electrophysiology

## 2

## CHAPTER 2 OBJECTIVES

Upon completion of this chapter, the student will be able to

- Define the terms *polarized, depolarization,* and *repolarization* and relate them to contraction and relaxation.
- Describe and label the phases of the action potential.
- Define *transmembrane potential*.
- Draw and explain the P wave, QRS complex, T wave, and U wave.
- Explain where the PR and ST segments are located.
- Define the *absolute* and *relative refractory periods* and the implications of each.
- Be able to label, on a rhythm strip, all the waves and complexes.
- Explain the delineations of EKG paper.
- On a rhythm strip, determine if the PR, QRS, and QT intervals are normal or abnormal.

- Name the waves in a variety of QRS complexes.
- Define *pacemaker*.
- List the different pacemakers of the heart and their inherent rates.
- Track the cardiac impulse from the sinus node through the conduction system.
- Define the four characteristics of cardiac cells.
- Describe the difference between *escape* and *usurpation*.
- Define *arrhythmia*.
- Tell what happens:
  When the sinus node fails
  When the sinus node and atria both fail
  When the sinus node, atria, and AV node all fail

## What It's All About

Mrs. Mahoney was admitted to the hospital because her physician wanted to watch her closely while he adjusted her heart rhythm medications. Mrs. Mahoney had an extensive cardiac history, including two heart attacks and cardiac arrest. On admission her PR interval was 0.16 seconds, QRS interval was 0.08 secs, QT interval 0.36 secs, heart rate was 88, sinus rhythm—all normal. Mrs. Mahoney's rhythm, intervals, and heart rate were checked every 4 hours per hospital protocol. Sixteen hours after being started on her new medication, her PR and QT intervals had increased. The physician was notified, and he decreased her medication dose. The staff's close assessment of Mrs. Mahoney's intervals allowed the physician to adjust her medication safely.

## Introduction

Cardiac cells at rest are electrically negative on the inside compared with the outside. Movement of charged particles (**ions**) of sodium and potassium into and out of the cell causes changes that can be picked up by sensors on the skin and printed out as an EKG.

## Depolarization and Repolarization

The negatively charged resting cardiac cell is **polarized**. There are sodium ions primarily outside the cell (extracellular) and potassium ions primarily inside the cell (intracellular). Though both these ions carry a positive electrical charge, the intracellular potassium has a much weaker positive charge than the extracellular sodium. Thus, the inside of the cell is electrically negative compared with the outside. The polarized state is a state of readiness—the cardiac cell is ready for electrical action. When the cardiac cell is stimulated by an electrical impulse, a large amount of sodium rushes into the

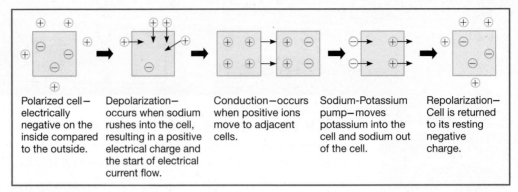

**FIGURE 2–1**

**Depolarization and repolarization.**

cell and a small amount of potassium leaks out, causing a discharge of electricity. The cell then becomes positively charged. This is called depolarization. An electrical wave then courses from cell to cell like a wave emanating from a pebble tossed into the water. This electrical charge spreads throughout the heart. During cell recovery, sodium and potassium ions are shifted back to their original places by way of the sodium-potassium pump, an active transport system that returns the cell to its negative charge. This is called repolarization. See Figure 2–1.

Depolarization and repolarization are the myocardium's electrical stimuli. Myocardial contraction and relaxation should be the mechanical response. Depolarization should result in muscle contraction; repolarization should result in muscle relaxation. *Electrical stimulus precedes mechanical response. There can be no heartbeat (a mechanical event) without first having had depolarization (the electrical stimulus).* To illustrate this principle, let's look at a vacuum cleaner. Its mechanical function is to suck up dirt, but it can't do its job without being plugged into an electrical source first. So if your power goes out, your vacuum cleaner won't work, will it? Likewise, if the heart's electrical system "goes out," the heart's pumping will stop. *Electrical stimulus precedes mechanical response.*

What happens if you plug in your vacuum and it still doesn't work? There could be a mechanical malfunction that prevents it from working. Likewise with the heart: The electrical stimulus may be there, but if there is a bad enough mechanical problem with the heart itself, it won't be able to respond to that stimulus by pumping.

The heart's electrical and mechanical systems are two separate systems. They can malfunction separately or together. Electrical malfunctions show up on the EKG. Mechanical malfunctions show up clinically.

Imagine this scenario: A man has a massive heart attack that damages a large portion of his myocardium. His heart's electrical system has not been damaged, so it sends out its impulses as usual. The heart muscle cells, however, have been so damaged that they are unable to respond to those impulses by contracting. Consequently, the EKG shows the electrical system is still working, but the patient's heart is not beating. He has no pulse and is not breathing. The vacuum was plugged in, but it was broken and couldn't do its job. *Electrical stimulus precedes—but does not guarantee—mechanical response.*

## The Action Potential

**Quick Tip**

Depolarization *should* result in muscle contraction. Repolarization *should* result in muscle relaxation.

Let's look at what happens to a ventricular muscle cell when it's stimulated. See Figure 2–2. There are five phases to the action potential:

- *In phase 4.* The cardiac cell is at rest. It is negatively charged with a resting transmembrane potential (the electrical charge at the cell membrane) of

−90 millivolts. Electrically, nothing is happening. (Note phase 4 is a flat line. *Flat lines indicate electrical silence.*)

- **In phase 0.**    The cardiac cell is stimulated. Sodium rushes into the cell, and potassium leaks out, resulting in a positive charge within the cell. This is called depolarization. You can see that at the top of phase 0, the cell's charge is above the zero mark, and the cell is thus positively charged. Phase 0 corresponds with the QRS complex on the EKG. The QRS complex is a spiked waveform that represents depolarization of the ventricular myocardium.

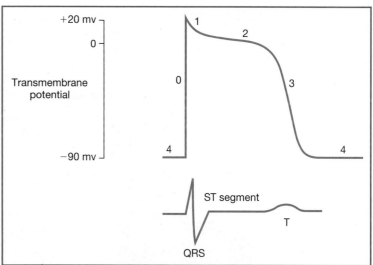

**FIGURE 2–2**

**Action potential.**

- **Phases 1 and 2 are *early repolarization*.** Calcium is released in these two phases, resulting in ventricular contraction. Phases 1 and 2 correspond with the ST segment of the EKG. The ST segment is a flat line on the EKG that follows the QRS complex and represents a period of electrical silence. But the heart is not physically at rest—it is contracting. Phase 2 is called the plateau phase because the waveform levels off here.

- **Phase 3 is *rapid repolarization*.**    Sodium and potassium return to their normal places via the sodium-potassium pump, thus returning the cell to its resting negative charge. Phase 3 corresponds with the T wave of the EKG. The T wave is a broad rounded wave that follows the ST segment and represents ventricular repolarization. The cardiac cell then relaxes.

## Refractory Periods

The word refractory means "resistant to." Let's look at the periods when the cardiac cell resists responding to an impulse. See Figure 2–3.

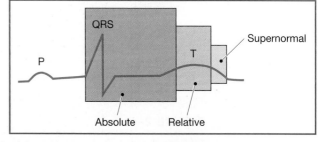

**FIGURE 2–3**

**Refractory periods.**

- Absolute   The cell cannot accept another impulse because it's still dealing with the last one. Absolutely no stimulus, no matter how strong, will result in another depolarization. This is like trying to flush your toilet again immediately after flushing it. No matter how hard you try to flush again right away, the toilet won't flush. It's not ready.

- Relative   A strong stimulus will result in depolarization. The toilet tank has filled up some, so now it will flush, but not with the same vigor as when the tank is completely full.

- Supernormal period   Even a weak stimulus will cause depolarization. The cardiac cell is "hyper." Stimulation at this time can result in very fast, dangerous rhythms. The toilet flushes fully again.

## EKG Waves and Complexes

Depolarization and repolarization of the atria and ventricles result in waves and complexes on the EKG paper. Let's examine these waveforms. See Figure 2–4.

- P wave   Represents atrial depolarization. The normal P is small, rounded, and upright, but many things can alter the P wave shape.

- $T_a$ wave   Represents atrial repolarization—usually not seen, as it occurs at the same time as the QRS complex.

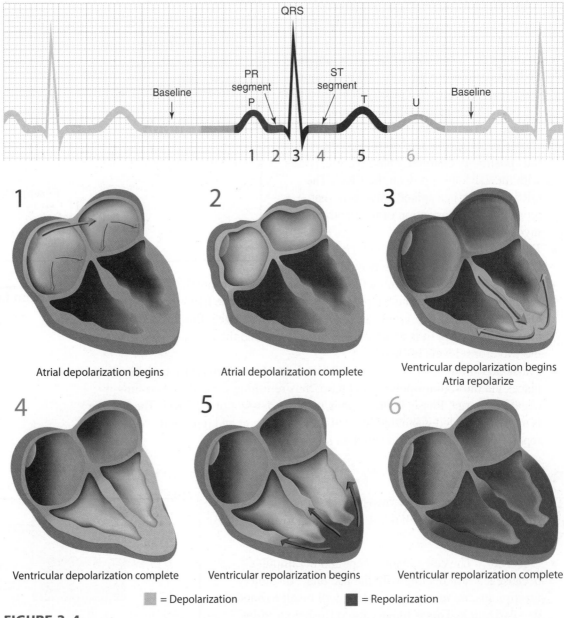

**FIGURE 2–4**

**EKG and electrical activity of the myocardium** (Alila Medical Media/Shutterstock).

- **QRS complex**  Represents ventricular depolarization. The normal QRS is spiked in appearance, consisting of one or more deflections from the baseline. The QRS complex is the most easily identified structure on the EKG tracing. Its shape can vary.
- **T wave**  Represents ventricular repolarization. The normal T wave is broad and rounded. If the QRS is upright, the T wave usually is also. If there is a QRS complex, there *must* be a T wave after it. *Any tissue that depolarizes must repolarize.* Many things can alter the T wave shape.
- **U wave**  Represents late ventricular repolarization and is not normally seen. If present, the U wave follows the T wave. It should be shallow and rounded, the same deflection as the T wave (i.e., if the T wave is upright, the U wave should be also).

See Table 2–1 for a summary of the waves and complexes.

**TABLE 2–1    Waves and Complexes Summary**

| Wave | Represents | Normal Shape |
|---|---|---|
| P wave | Atrial depolarization | Small, rounded, upright in most leads |
| $T_a$ wave | Atrial repolarization | Usually not seen as it's inside QRS |
| QRS complex | Ventricular depolarization | Spiked upward and/or downward deflections |
| T wave | Ventricular repolarization | Broad, rounded, upright if the QRS is upright |
| U wave | Late ventricular repolarization | Shallow, broad, rounded, same deflection as T wave |

Each P-QRS-T sequence is one heartbeat. The flat lines between the P wave and the QRS and between the QRS and T wave are called the **PR segment** and the **ST segment**, respectively. During these segments, no electrical activity is occurring. (Flat lines indicate electrical silence.) The flat line between the T wave of one beat and the P wave of the next beat is called the **baseline** or **isoelectric line**. The baseline is the line from which the waves and complexes take off.

Atrial contraction occurs during the P wave and the PR segment. Ventricular contraction occurs during the QRS and the ST segment. When the atria depolarize, a P wave is written on the EKG paper. Following this, the atria contract, filling the ventricles with blood. Then the ventricles depolarize, causing a QRS complex on the EKG paper. The ventricles then contract.

## Waves and Complexes Identification Practice

Following are strips on which to practice identifying P waves, QRS complexes, and T waves. You'll recall that P waves are normally upright, but they can also be inverted (upside down) or biphasic (up *and* down). P waves usually precede the QRS complex, so find the QRS and then look for the P wave. Some rhythms have more than one P wave and others have no P at all. Write the letter *P* over each P wave you see.

The QRS complex is the most easily identified structure on the strip because of its spiked appearance. Write *QRS* over each QRS complex.

T waves are normally upright but can also be inverted or biphasic. Wherever there is a QRS complex, there must be a T wave. Write a *T* over each T wave.

1.

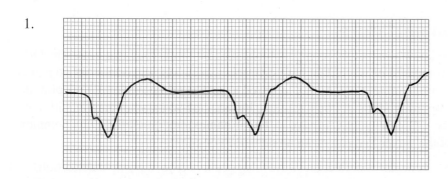

2.

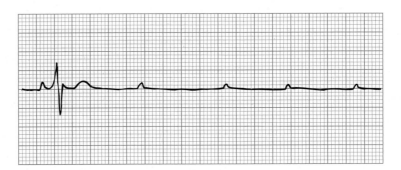

3.

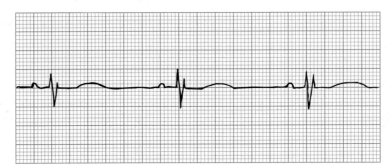

4.

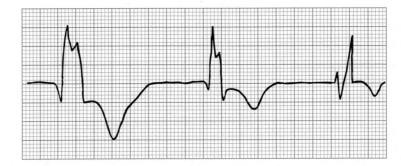

5.

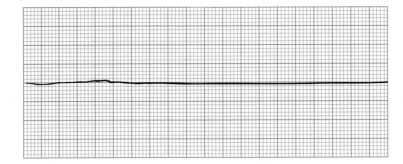

## QRS Nomenclature

Now that we know what a QRS complex looks like, let's fine-tune that a bit. The QRS complex is composed of waves that have different names—Q, R, and S—but no matter which waves it is composed of, it's still referred to as the **QRS complex**. Think of it like this: There are many kinds of dogs—collies, boxers, and so on—but they're still dogs. Likewise, the QRS complex can have different names, but it's still a QRS complex. Let's look at the waves that can make up the QRS complex.

- **Q wave**   A negative deflection (wave) that occurs before a positive deflection. There can be only one Q wave. If present, it must always be the first wave of the QRS complex.
- **R wave**   Any positive deflection. There can be more than one R wave. A second R wave is called **R prime**, written **R'**.

- **S wave**   A negative deflection that follows an R wave.
- **QS wave**   A negative deflection with no positive deflection at all.

As in the alphabet, Q comes before R and S comes after R. See Figure 2–5. The dotted line indicates the baseline. Any wave in the QRS complex that goes above the baseline is an R wave; any wave going below the baseline is either a Q or an S wave.

See Table 2–2 for a summary of the QRS waves.

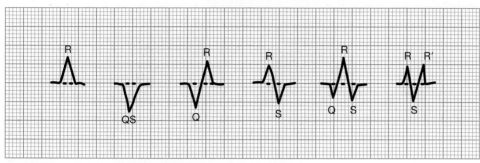

**FIGURE 2–5**

**Examples of QRS complexes.**

**TABLE 2–2   Summary of QRS Waves**

| Wave | Deflection | Location | Comments |
|---|---|---|---|
| Q wave | Negative | Precedes R wave | If present, Q wave is *always* first wave of QRS complex |
| R wave | Positive | Can stand alone or be preceded or followed by Q and/or S | Can have more than one; second R wave is called R prime, written R' |
| S wave | Negative | Follows R wave | |
| QS wave | Negative | Stands alone | |

## QRS Nomenclature Practice

Name the waves in the following QRS complexes:

1. _____      2. _____      3. _____

4. _____      5. _____      6. _____

Now draw the following:

1. RSR'              2. QRS              3. QS


4. QR               5. RS               6. R

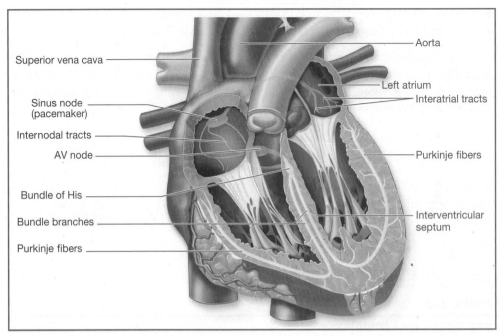

**FIGURE 2–6**

**Cardiac conduction system.**

## Cardiac Conduction System

The **conduction system** is a pathway of specialized cells whose job is to create and conduct the electrical impulses that tell the heart when to pump. The area of the conduction system that initiates the impulses is called the **pacemaker**. See Figure 2–6.

### Conduction Pathway

Let's look at the conduction pathway through the heart

Sinus node ➡➡ interatrial tracts ➡➡ atrium ➡➡ internodal tracts ➡➡ AV node➡➡ bundle of His ➡➡ bundle branches ➡➡ Purkinje fibers➡➡ ventricle

- The impulse originates in the **sinus node**, located in the upper right atrium just beneath the opening of the superior vena cava. The sinus node is the heart's normal pacemaker.
- From here it travels through the **interatrial tracts**. These special conductive highways carry the impulses through the atria to the **atrial tissue**. The atria then depolarize, and a P wave is written on the EKG.
- The impulse travels through the **internodal tracts** to the **AV node**, a specialized group of cells located just to the right of the septum in the lower right atrium. The AV node slows impulse transmission a little, allowing the newly depolarized atria to propel their blood into the ventricles.
- Then the impulse travels through the **bundle of His**, located just beneath the AV node, to the left and right **bundle branches**, the main highways to the ventricles.
- Then the impulse is propelled through the **Purkinje fibers**.
- Finally, the impulse arrives at the **ventricle** itself, causing it to depolarize. A QRS complex is written on the EKG paper.

## Cardiac Cells

Cardiac cells have several characteristics:

- **Automaticity**   The ability to create an impulse without outside stimulation.
- **Conductivity**   The ability to pass this impulse along to neighboring cells.

- **Excitability**   The ability to respond to this stimulus by depolarizing.
- **Contractility**   The ability to contract and do work.

The first three characteristics are electrical. The last is mechanical.

Though the sinus node is the normal pacemaker of the heart, other cardiac cells can become the pacemaker if the sinus node fails. Let's look at that a little more closely. But first let's see how well you understand the material we've covered so far.

---

**chapter** CHECKUP

We're about halfway through this chapter. To evaluate your understanding of the material thus far, answer the following questions. If you have trouble with them, review the material again before continuing.

1. Explain *depolarization* and *repolarization*.
2. Name the EKG waves and complexes and state what each represents.
3. Track the electrical current through the conduction system.

---

## Inherent (Escape) Rates of the Pacemaker Cells

- Sinus node: 60 to 100 beats per minute
- AV junction: 40 to 60 beats per minute
- Ventricle: 20 to 40 beats per minute

The sinus node, you will note, has the fastest inherent rate of all the potential pacemaker cells. This means that barring any outside stimuli that speed it up or slow it down, the sinus node will fire regularly at its rate of 60 to 100 beats per minute. The lower pacemakers (AV junction and ventricle) have slower inherent rates, each one having a slower rate than the one above it.

*The fastest pacemaker at any given moment is the one in control.* The lower pacemakers serve as a backup in case of conduction failure from above, and are inhibited from firing as long as some other pacemaker is faster.

What if the sinus node doesn't create an impulse? The AV junction should then create the impulse and send it down to the ventricle.

What if neither the sinus node nor the AV junction creates the impulse? The ventricle should then create the impulse and conduct it through the ventricular tissue.

## Conduction Variations

Normal conduction of cardiac impulses is dependent on the health of each part of the conduction system. Failure of any part of the system necessitates a variation in conduction. Let's look at several conductive possibilities. In the following figures, the large heart represents the pacemaker in control. See Figure 2–7.

In Figure 2–7, the sinus node fires out its impulse. When the impulse depolarizes the atrium, a P wave is written. The impulse then travels to the AV node, and on to the ventricle. A QRS is written when the ventricle is depolarized.

If the sinus node fails, however, one of the lower pacemakers will escape its restraints and take over at its slower inherent rate, thus becoming the heart's new pacemaker. If the

> **Quick Tip**
>
> Unlike the sinus node and the ventricle, the AV node itself has no pacemaker cells. The tissue between the atria and the AV node, however—an area called the AV junction—does have pacemaking capabilities. Thus, the term AV node is an anatomical term and AV junction refers to a pacemaking area.

> **Quick Tip**
>
> Once a lower pacemaker (the AV junction or the ventricle) has received an impulse from above, all it has to do is conduct that impulse down the conduction pathway.

**FIGURE 2–7**

**Normal conduction.**

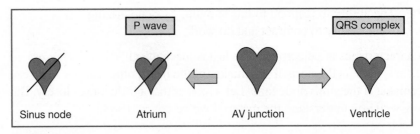

**FIGURE 2–8**

**Sinus fails; AV junction escapes.**

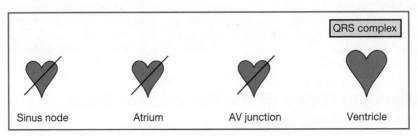

**FIGURE 2–9**

**All higher pacemakers fail; ventricle escapes.**

AV junction escapes (takes over as the pacemaker at its slower inherent rate) it will fire at a rate of 40 to 60 beats per minute. If the ventricle takes over, the rate will be 20 to 40 beats per minute. Needless to say, if the ventricle has to kick in as the pacemaker, it is a grave situation, as it means that all the pacemakers above it have failed. Remember—no pacemaker can escape unless it is the fastest at that particular time.

In Figure 2–8, the sinus node has failed. The AV junction is now the fastest escape pacemaker. It creates an impulse and sends it forward toward the ventricle and backward toward the atria, providing the P and the QRS.

In Figure 2–9, both the sinus node and AV junction have failed. The only remaining pacemaker is the ventricle, so it takes over as the pacemaker, providing the QRS. There is no P wave when the ventricle escapes.

What if the sinus node fires its impulse out but the impulse is blocked at some point along the conduction pathway? The first pacemaker below the block should escape and become the new pacemaker.

In Figure 2–10, the sinus node fires out its impulse, which depolarizes the atrium and writes a P wave. The impulse is then blocked between the atrium and the AV node. Because the faster sinus impulse never reaches the AV node, the AV junction assumes the sinus node has failed. So it escapes, creates its own new impulse, and becomes the new pacemaker, sending the impulse down to the ventricle and backward to the atria. (Backward conduction can work even when forward conduction is blocked.)

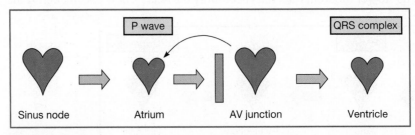

**FIGURE 2–10**

**Block in conduction; AV junction escapes.**

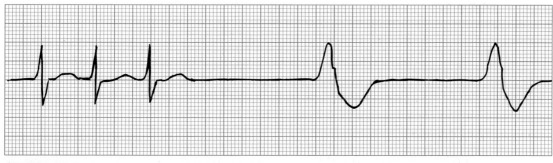

**FIGURE 2–11**

**Escape.**

If the impulse were blocked between the AV node and the ventricle, the ventricle should become the new pacemaker.

Each of the pacemakers can fire at rates faster or slower than their inherent rates if there are outside stimuli. We've talked briefly about escape. Let's look at an example of escape compared with usurpation.

Escape occurs when the predominant pacemaker slows dramatically (or fails completely) and a lower pacemaker takes over at its inherent rate, providing a new rhythm that is slower than the previous rhythm. *An escape beat is any beat that comes in after a pause that's longer than the normal heartbeat-to-heartbeat cycle* (R-R interval). Escape beats are lifesavers. An **escape rhythm** is a series of escape beats.

In Figure 2–11, the normal pacemaker stops suddenly and there is a long pause, at the end of which is a beat from a lower pacemaker and then a new rhythm with a heart rate slower than before. This is escape.

Usurpation, also called irritability, means "to take control away from" and occurs when one of the lower pacemakers becomes irritable and fires in at an accelerated rate, stealing control away from the predominant pacemaker. Usurpation results in a faster rhythm than before, and it starts with a beat that comes in earlier than expected.

In Figure 2–12, the controlling pacemaker is cruising along and suddenly an impulse from a lower pacemaker (the third beat) fires in early, takes control, and is off and running with a new, faster rhythm. This is usurpation.

Proper function of the conduction system results in a heart rhythm, a pattern of successive depolarizations, that originates in the sinus node. Abnormalities of the conduction system can produce arrhythmias, abnormal heart rhythms. Although these conduction system problems are often related to heart disease, there are also diseases that affect the conduction system outright. Whatever the cause, conduction system abnormalities can prove harmful or fatal if not treated appropriately.

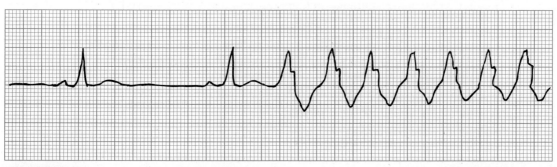

**FIGURE 2–12**

**Usurpation.**

**TABLE 2–3    EKG Paper Delineations**

| EKG Feature | Equals |
| --- | --- |
| Each small block | 0.04 secs (from one small line to the next) |
| Five small blocks | One big block |
| One big block | 0.20 secs |
| 25 small blocks | 1 sec |
| Five big blocks | 1 sec |
| 1,500 small blocks | 1 minute |
| 300 big blocks | 1 minute |
| One small block in amplitude | A millimeter |

## EKG Paper

EKG paper is graph paper divided into small blocks that are 1 millimeter (mm) in height and width. Dark lines are present every fifth block to subdivide the paper vertically and horizontally. Measurements of the EKG waves and complexes are done by counting these blocks. Counting horizontally measures time, or **intervals**. Intervals are measured in seconds. Counting vertically measures **amplitude**, or the height of the complexes. Amplitude is measured in millimeters.

A **12-lead EKG** is a printout of the heart's electrical activity viewed from 12 different angles as seen in 12 different leads. A **lead** is simply an electrocardiographic picture of the heart's electrical activity. A 12-lead EKG is typically done on special paper, using a digital recorder that prints a simultaneous view of three leads at a time in sequence until all 12 leads are recorded.

A **rhythm strip** is a printout of one or two leads at a time and is done to assess the patient's heart rhythm. Rhythm strips are recorded on special paper about 3 to 5 inches wide. A 6- to 12-second strip is usually obtained and interpreted. Rhythm strip paper often has lines at the top of the paper at 1- to 3-second intervals. Let's look at the EKG paper delineations. See Table 2–3. All of these measurements are assuming normal EKG settings.

No matter whether the EKG paper is 12-lead size or rhythm strip size, the delineations will be the same.

Figure 2–13 is an example of EKG paper. **Identifying data**, such as name, date, time, and room number, and **interpretive data**, such as heart rate, are printed at the top

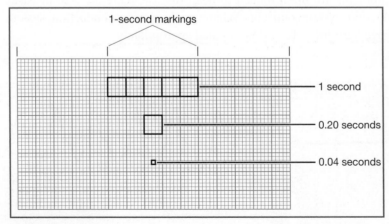

**FIGURE 2–13**

EKG paper.

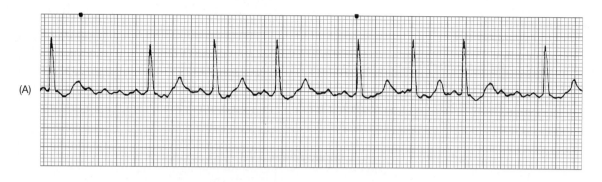

(A)

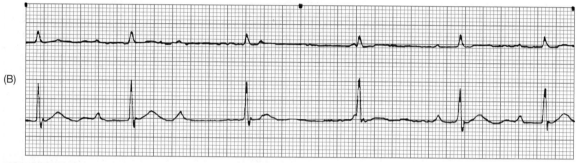

(B)

**FIGURE 2–14**

**(A) Single- and (B) double-lead rhythm strips.**

of the paper. Figure 2–14 shows single- and double-lead rhythm strips. Note that on the double-lead strip, one lead's waves and complexes show up much more clearly than on the other lead. This is typical.

See Figure 2–15 for a 12-lead EKG. Note the lead markings. Leads are arranged in four columns of three leads. Leads I, II, and III are in the first column, then aVR, aVL, and aVF in the second column, V1 to V3 in the third column, and V4 to V6 in the last column. At the bottom of the paper is a page-wide rhythm strip, usually of either Lead II or V1. Part II of this text covers 12-lead EKGs in more detail.

## Intervals

Now let's look at intervals, the measurement of time between the P-QRS-T waves and complexes. The heart's current normally starts in the right atrium and then spreads through both atria and down to the ventricles. Interval measurements enable a determination of the heart's efficiency at transmitting its impulses down the pathway. See Figure 2–16.

- **PR interval**   Measures the time it takes for the impulse to get from the atria to the ventricles. Normal PR interval is 0.12 to 0.20 seconds. It's measured from the beginning of the P wave to the beginning of the QRS and includes the P wave and the PR segment. The P wave itself should measure no more than 0.10 seconds wide and 2.5 mm high.
- **QRS interval**   Measures the time it takes to depolarize the ventricles. Normal QRS interval is less than 0.12 seconds, usually between 0.06 and 0.10 seconds. It's measured from the beginning of the QRS to the end of the QRS.
- **QT interval**   Measures depolarization and repolarization time of the ventricles. The QT interval is measured from the beginning of the QRS to the end of the T wave and includes the QRS complex and the T wave. At normal heart rates of

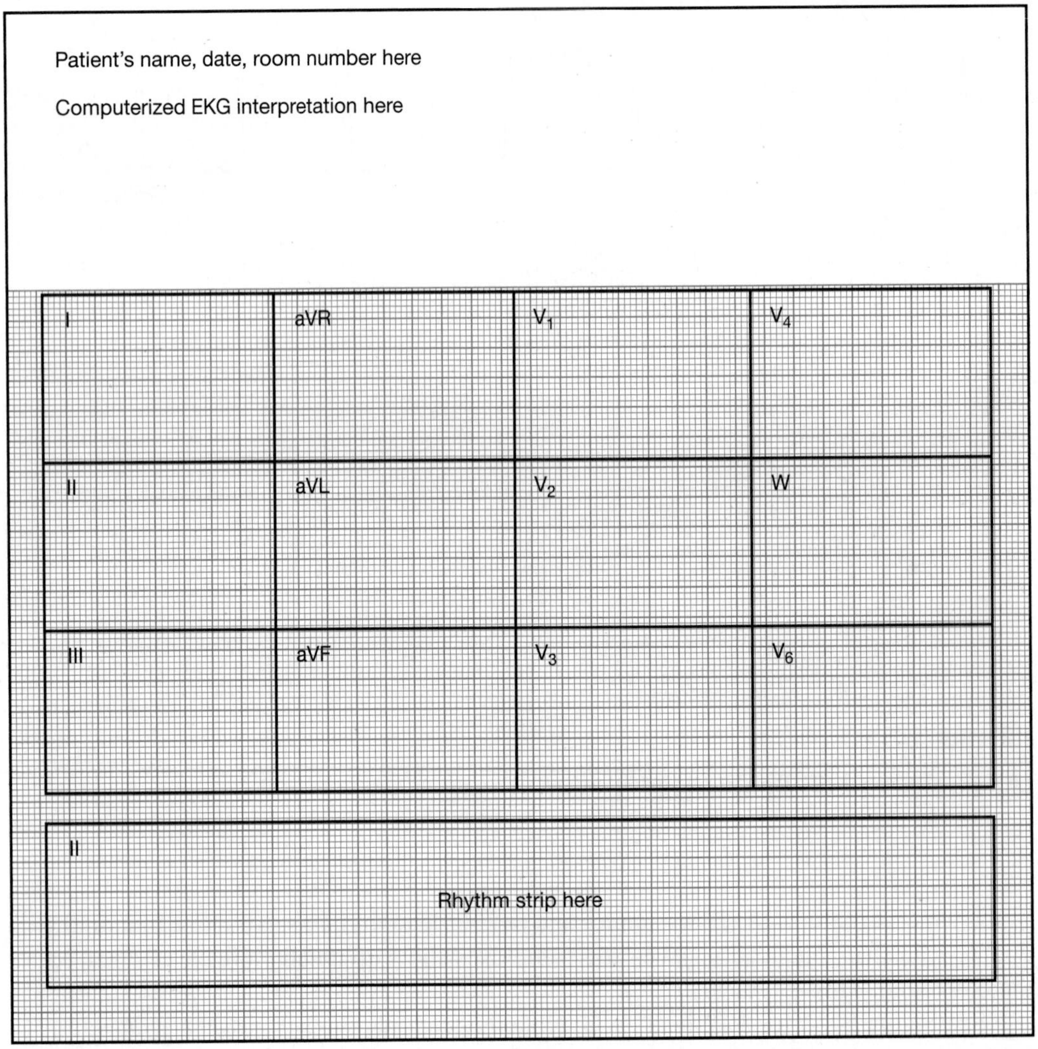

Patient's name, date, room number here

Computerized EKG interpretation here

| I | aVR | V₁ | V₄ |

| II | aVL | V₂ | W |

| III | aVF | V₃ | V₆ |

| II | | | |
Rhythm strip here

**FIGURE 2–15**

**12-lead EKG.**

60 to 100, the QT interval should be less than or equal to one-half the distance between successive QRS complexes (the R-R interval). To quickly determine if the QT is prolonged, draw a line midway between QRS complexes. If the T wave ends at or before this line, the QT is normal. If it ends after the line, it is prolonged and can lead to lethal arrhythmias. QTc is the QT interval corrected for heart rate, and is usually calculated by the EKG machine.

See Table 2–4 for an intervals summary.

**TABLE 2–4   Intervals Summary**

| INTERVAL | MEASURES | NORMAL VALUE |
|---|---|---|
| PR interval | Time traveling from atrium to ventricle | 0.12–0.20 seconds |
| QRS interval | Ventricular depolarization time | Less than 0.12 seconds (usually between 0.06 and 0.10 seconds) |
| QT interval | Ventricular depolarization and repolarization time | Varies with heart rate—should be less than half the R-R interval if heart rate 60–100 |

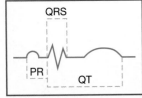

**FIGURE 2–16**

**Intervals.**

### Intervals Practice

Determine the intervals on the enlarged rhythm strips that follow.

      *PR interval.*    Count the number of small blocks between the beginning of the P and the beginning of the QRS. Multiply by 0.04 second.

      *QRS interval.*    Count the number of small blocks between the beginning and end of the QRS complex. Multiply by 0.04 second.

      *QT interval.*    Count the number of small blocks between the beginning of the QRS and the end of the T wave. Multiply by 0.04 second.

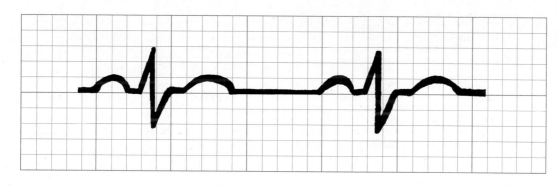

1. PR _____    QRS _____    QT _____

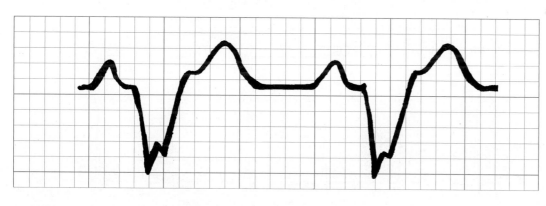

2. PR _____    QRS _____    QT _____

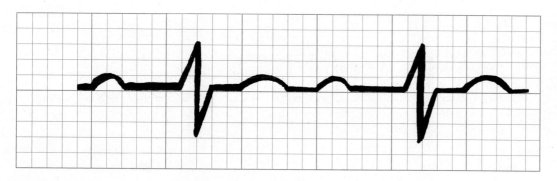

3. PR _____    QRS _____    QT _____

Now let's practice intervals on normal-size EKG paper. Allow plus or minus 0.02 seconds for your answers. For example, if the answer is listed as 0.28, acceptable answers would be anywhere from 0.26 to 0.30. You'll note that intervals can vary slightly from beat to beat. This implies normal functioning of the sympathetic and parasympathetic nervous systems.

Intervals Practice on normal-size EKG paper

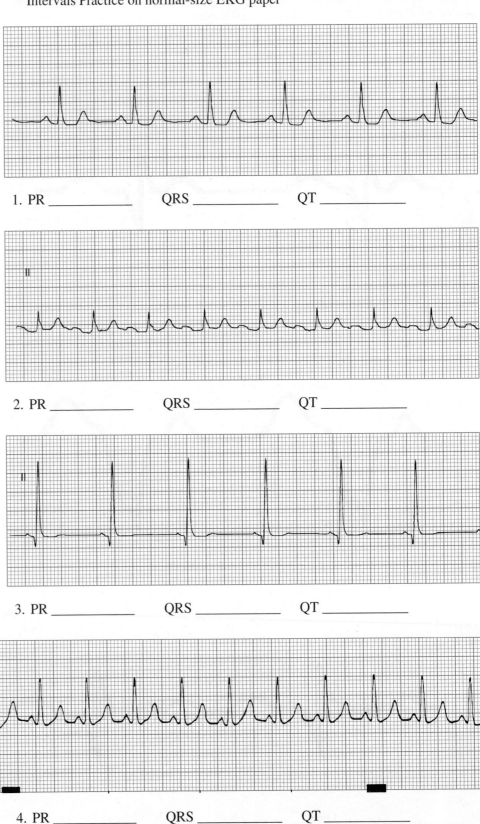

1. PR _____    QRS _____    QT _____

2. PR _____    QRS _____    QT _____

3. PR _____    QRS _____    QT _____

4. PR _____    QRS _____    QT _____

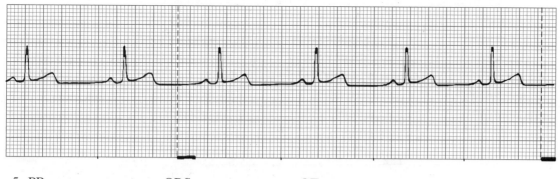

5. PR _____    QRS _____    QT _____

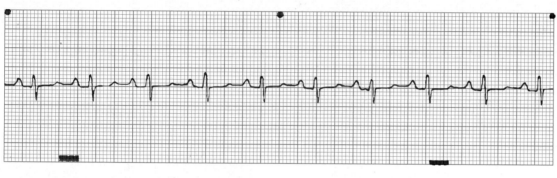

6. PR _____    QRS _____    QT _____

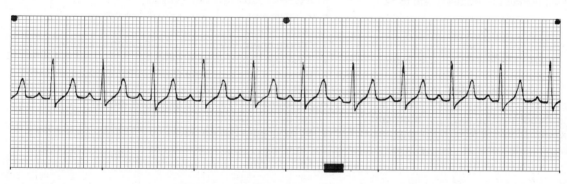

7. PR _____    QRS _____    QT _____

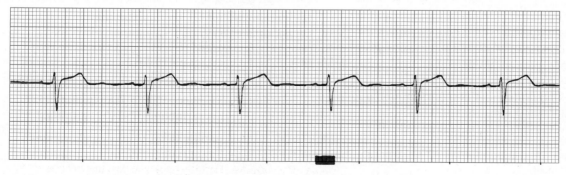

8. PR _____    QRS _____    QT _____

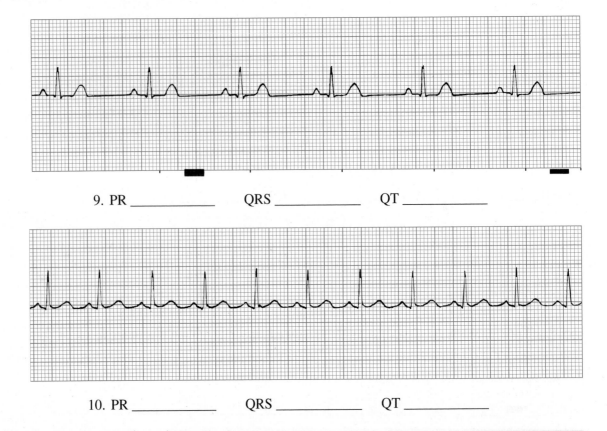

9. PR _____    QRS _____    QT _____

10. PR _____    QRS _____    QT _____

 CHAPTER TWO NOTES TO SUM IT ALL UP . . .

- **Negatively charged resting cardiac cell is said to be polarized.**
- **Depolarization**—Discharge of electricity—occurs when cardiac cell becomes positively charged.
- **Repolarization**—Return of the cardiac cell to its resting negative charge.
- **Electrical stimulus precedes mechanical response.** Cannot have myocardial contraction without first having had depolarization. **Depolarization and repolarization**—electrical events. **Contraction and relaxation**—mechanical.
- **Action potential**—What happens to cardiac cell when stimulated by electrical charge. Several phases:
  - *Phase 4*—Cardiac cell at rest. Corresponds with isoelectric line of EKG.
  - *Phase 0*—depolarization. Cell becomes positively charged. Corresponds with QRS complex on EKG.
  - *Phases 1 and 2*—Early repolarization. Calcium is released. Muscle contraction begins. Corresponds with ST segment of EKG.
  - *Phase 3*—Rapid repolarization. Cell is returning to electrically negative state. Corresponds with T wave of EKG.
- **Refractory periods**—Cardiac cell resists responding to/depolarizing from an impulse.
  - *Absolute refractory period*—Cardiac cell cannot respond to another impulse, no matter how strong.
  - *Relative refractory period*—Cell can respond only to very strong impulse.
  - *Supernormal period*—Cardiac cell is "hyper," will respond to very weak stimulus.
- **Each P-QRS-T sequence represents one heartbeat.**

- **P wave**— Atrial depolarization.
- **T$_a$ wave**— atrial repolarization—usually not seen, as it occurs simultaneous with QRS.
- **QRS complex**— Ventricular depolarization.
- **T wave**— Ventricular repolarization.
- **U wave**— Late ventricular repolarization—not usually seen.
- **PR segment**— Flat line between the P wave and the QRS complex.
- **ST segment**— Flat line between the QRS complex and the T wave.
- **QRS complex**— A series of spiky waves. Waves have names:
  - *Q wave*—Negative wave that precedes an R wave in the QRS complex. If present, it is always the first wave of the QRS.
  - *R wave*—Any positive wave in the QRS complex.
  - *S wave*—Negative wave that follows an R wave.
  - *R'*—A second R wave.
- **Cardiac conduction system**—pathway of specialized cells—job is to create and conduct impulses to tell the heart when to beat. Conduction pathway is as follows:
  - Sinus node → interatrial tracts → atrium → internodal tracts → AV node → bundle of His → bundle branches → Purkinje fibers → ventricle.
- **Characteristics of cardiac cells:**
  - *Automaticity*—Electrical—ability to create an impulse.
  - *Conductivity*— Electrical—ability to pass that impulse along to neighboring cells.

- • *Excitability*— Electrical—ability to respond to that impulse by depolarizing.
- • *Contractility*— Mechanical—ability to contract and do work.
- ■ **Inherent rates of pacemaker cells:**
  - • *Sinus node*— 60–100.
  - • *AV junction*— 40–60.
  - • *Ventricle*— 20–40.
- ■ **Sinus node—**Normal pacemaker of the heart.
- ■ Fastest pacemaker at any given moment is the one in control.
- ■ **Escape—**Predominant pacemaker slows down; lower pacemaker takes over at its slower inherent rate—results in a slower heart rate than before.
- ■ **Escape beat—**Beat that comes in after a pause longer than normal R-R interval.
- ■ **Escape rhythm—**Series of escape beats.
- ■ **Usurpation (irritability)—**Lower pacemaker becomes "hyper"; fires in at an accelerated rate, stealing control away from slower predominant pacemaker—results in a faster heart rate than before.
- ■ **Heart rhythm—**Pattern of successive heart beats.
- ■ **Arrhythmia—**Abnormal heart rhythm.
- ■ **12-lead EKG—**Printout of heart's electrical activity from 12 different angles.

- ■ **Lead—**Electrocardiographic picture of the heart's electricity.
- ■ **Rhythm strip—**Printout of 1 to 2 leads.
- ■ **EKG paper—**Graph paper divided into small vertical and horizontal blocks:
  - • One small block is 0.04 seconds wide.
  - • One big block is 0.20 seconds wide.
  - • Five small blocks equals one big block.
  - • Five big blocks equals one second.
  - • 25 small blocks equals one second.
  - • 300 big blocks equals one minute.
  - • 1,500 small blocks equals one minute.
- ■ **Intervals—**Measurements of time between EKG waves and complexes:
  - • *PR interval*—Measures time it takes impulse to get from atrium to ventricle—measured from beginning of P wave to beginning of QRS (even if QRS does not begin with an R wave!). Normal PR interval 0.12–0.20 seconds.
  - • *QRS interval*—Measures time it takes to depolarize the ventricle—measured from beginning of QRS to its end. Normal QRS interval is less than 0.12 seconds.
  - • *QT interval*—Measures depolarization/repolarization time in ventricle—measured from beginning of QRS to end of T wave. QT interval varies with heart rate but should be less than or equal to half the R-R interval.

## Practice Quiz

1. Cardiac cells at rest are electrically _____

2. Depolarization and repolarization are what kinds of events? _____

3. State what occurs in each of the following phases of the action potential:

   Phase 4. _____

   Phase 0. _____

   Phase 1. _____

   Phase 2. _____

   Phase 3. _____

4. State what each of the following waves/complexes represents:

   P wave. _____

   QRS complex. _____

   T wave. _____

5. What kind of impulse can result in depolarization during the absolute refractory period? _____

6. List the four characteristics of heart cells. _____

   _____

   _____

7. State the inherent rates of the pacemaker cells.

   Sinus node _____

   AV junction _____

   Ventricle _____

   _____

8. List, in order of conduction, the structures of the conduction pathway through the heart.

   _____

   _____

9. Define *escape*. _____

   _____

10. Define *usurpation*. _____

    _____

# Putting It All Together—Critical Thinking Exercises

These exercises may consist of diagrams to label, scenarios to analyze, brain-stumping questions to ponder, or other challenging exercises to boost your knowledge of the chapter material.

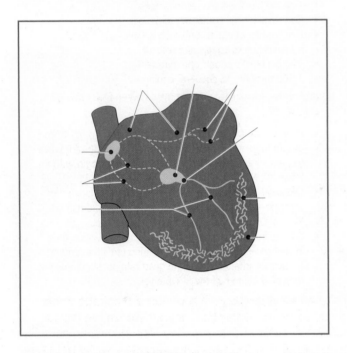

1. If the sinus node is firing at a rate of 65 and the AV junction kicks in at a rate of 70, what will happen? Which pacemaker will be in control? Explain your answer.

2. Your patient's PR interval last night was 0.16 seconds. This morning it is 0.22. Which part of the conduction system is responsible for this delay in impulse transmission?

3. Explain how it is possible for the heart's pumping ability to fail but its electrical conduction ability to remain intact.

4. Label the parts of the conduction system on the diagram.

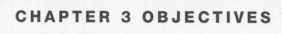

# Lead Morphology and Placement

**3**

## CHAPTER 3 OBJECTIVES

Upon completion of this chapter, the student will be able to

- Define *electrode*.
- Name the bipolar leads and state the limbs that comprise them.
- Name the unipolar augmented leads.
- Explain what augmentation does to the EKG.
- Explain Einthoven's law.
- Draw and label Einthoven's triangle.
- Name the leads comprising the hexiaxial diagram.

- Describe the location of the precordial leads.
- Name the two leads most commonly used for continuous monitoring in the hospital.
- Explain the electrocardiographic truths.
- Describe the normal QRS complex deflections in each of the 12 leads on an EKG.

## What It's All About

Mr. Hedges was admitted to the ICU after his angiogram revealed a blockage in his right coronary artery. He is scheduled to return to the cardiac catheterization lab for a procedure to open his blocked coronary artery in the morning. The physician asks nurse Becky to notify him of any inferior wall EKG changes overnight. Becky notes that the routine monitor leads used in that facility do not look at the inferior wall, so she turns the lead selector to monitor Lead II. At 3 A.M., Mr. Hedges complains of chest pain. The monitor strip shows ST segment changes in Lead II, so Becky does a 12-lead EKG, which confirms that Mr. Hedges is in the early stages of an inferior wall heart attack. Becky calls the physician and Mr. Hedges is taken to the cath lab immediately. His coronary artery is successfully opened up and his heart attack is aborted. Becky's knowledge of leads was important in Mr. Hedges's successful outcome.

## Introduction

**Electrocardiography** is the recording of the heart's electrical impulses by way of sensors, called **electrodes**, placed on the arms, legs, and chest. The right leg electrode is used as a ground electrode to minimize the hazard of electric shock to the patient and to stabilize the EKG. The electrodes on the other limbs and chest are used to create leads. A lead is simply an electrocardiographic picture of the heart. A 12-lead EKG provides 12 different views of the heart's electrical activity.

Why is it necessary to have 12 leads? Have you ever waved to someone you saw from a distance and then realized when you got a better look that it wasn't who you thought it was? Having more views of this person (say from the front, back, and side) might have increased your chance of recognizing this person. With the heart, the more views of the heart's electrical activity, the better the chance of recognizing its patterns and abnormalities. So we have leads that view the heart from top to bottom, right to left, and anterior to posterior (front to back).

The printed EKG is called an **electrocardiogram**.

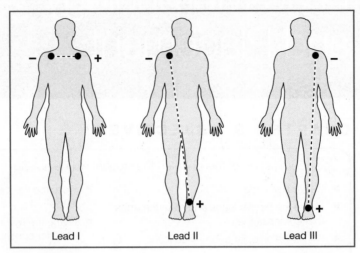

**FIGURE 3–1**

**The bipolar leads.**

**TABLE 3–1  Bipolar Leads**

| Lead | Measures Current Traveling From | Location Of Positive Pole |
|------|--------------------------------|---------------------------|
| I | Right arm to left arm | Left arm |
| II | Right arm to left leg | Left leg |
| III | Left arm to left leg | Left leg |

## Lead Types

Let's look at the three types of leads on the EKG. There are bipolar leads, which are limb leads that view the heart's current traveling between two limbs. One limb is designated the positive pole and the other is the negative pole. (Think of the positive pole as having a "seeing eye" that sees where the heart's current is traveling). Then there are three more limb leads called the augmented leads. These are unipolar leads (leads with only a positive pole) with the positive pole on one limb, and using the midway point between the other two limbs as the negative reference point. (The right leg is not utilized in making a lead—it holds the ground electrode). The augmented leads must have their printout augmented, or increased, to make it large enough to record on the EKG paper. Both the bipolar and augmented leads are also called frontal leads, as they view the heart's current from the frontal plane—top to bottom, right to left. They are called limb leads for obvious reasons. Finally, there are the precordial leads, which are six unipolar leads on the chest. These leads view the heart's current from the horizontal plane—anterior to posterior (front to back).

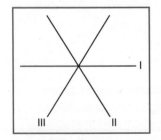

**FIGURE 3–2**

**The triaxial diagram.**

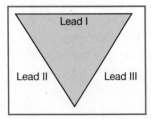

**FIGURE 3–3**

**Einthoven's triangle.**

## Bipolar Leads

See Table 3–1.

Look at Figure 3–1 now. You'll notice that in the bipolar leads, the right arm is always negative and the left leg is always positive. Also note that the left arm can be positive or negative depending on which lead it is a part of. If you join Leads I, II, and III at the middle, you get the triaxial diagram seen in Figure 3–2.

If you join Leads I, II, and III at their ends, you get a triangle called Einthoven's triangle, seen in Figure 3–3.

Cardiac research pioneer Willem Einthoven stated that Lead I + Lead III = Lead II. This is called Einthoven's law. It means that the height of the QRS in Lead I added to the height of the QRS in Lead III will equal the height of the QRS in Lead II. In other words, Lead II should have the tallest QRS of the bipolar leads. Einthoven's law can help determine if an EKG is truly abnormal or if the leads were inadvertently placed on the incorrect limb. See Figure 3–4.

## Augmented Leads

See Table 3–2 and Figure 3–5.

The letters aV stand for augmented voltage. The last letter refers to the location of the positive pole. R is right arm, L is left arm, F refers to left foot or leg. (Remember the right foot/leg holds the ground electrode only).

If you join leads aVR, aVL, and aVF in the middle, you get the triaxial diagram shown in Figure 3–6.

If all the frontal leads—I, II, III, aVR, aVL, and aVF—are joined at the center, the result looks like Figure 3–7. This hexiaxial diagram is used to help determine the direction of current flow in the heart. This diagram will be seen again in Part II of this text.

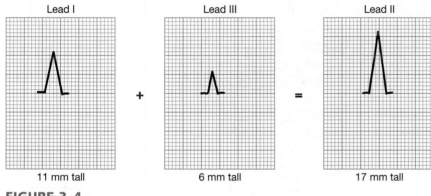

Lead I          +          Lead III          =          Lead II

11 mm tall          6 mm tall          17 mm tall

**FIGURE 3–4**

**Einthoven's law.**

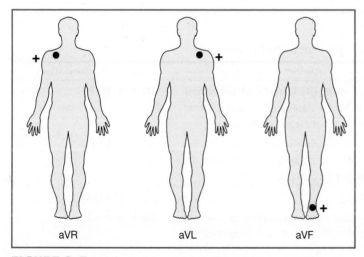

aVR          aVL          aVF

**FIGURE 3–5**

**The augmented leads.**

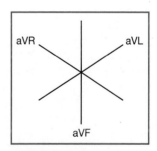

aVR          aVL

aVF

**FIGURE 3–6**

**Triaxial diagram with augmented leads.**

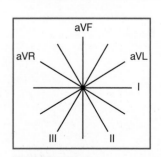

aVF

aVR          aVL

I

III          II

**FIGURE 3–7**

**Hexiaxial diagram.**

**TABLE 3–2    Augmented Leads**

| Lead | Measures Current Traveling Toward | Location of Positive Pole |
|------|-----------------------------------|---------------------------|
| aVR | Right arm | Right arm |
| aVL | Left arm | Left arm |
| aVF | Left leg | Left leg |

**chapter** CHECKUP

We're about halfway through this chapter. To evaluate your understanding of the material thus far, answer the following questions. If you have trouble with them, review the material again before continuing.

1. Name the bipolar leads and augmented leads and state where the positive pole of each lead is.
2. Define *electrocardiography, leads,* and *electrodes.*

## Precordial (Chest) Leads

These leads are located on the chest. They are also unipolar leads, and each one is a positive electrode. The precordial leads see a wraparound view of the heart from the horizontal plane. These leads are named $V_1$, $V_2$, $V_3$, $V_4$, $V_5$, and $V_6$. See Figure 3–8 and Table 3–3.

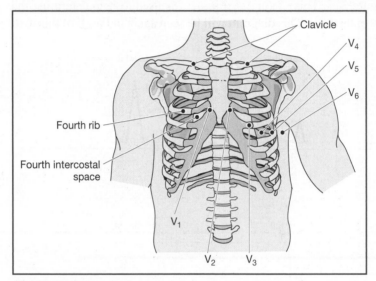

**FIGURE 3–8**

**The precordial leads.**

**TABLE 3–3  Location of the Precordial Leads**

| Lead | Location | Location Abbreviation |
|---|---|---|
| $V_1$ | Fourth intercostal space (ICS), right sternal border (RSB): The space below the 4th rib where it joins with the sternum on the patient's right side | 4th ICS, RSB |
| $V_2$ | Fourth intercostal space, left sternal border (LSB): The space below the 4th rib where it joins with the sternum on the patient's left side | 4th ICS, LSB |
| $V_3$ | Between $V_2$ and $V_4$ | 5th ICS, MCL |
| $V_4$ | Fifth intercostal space, midclavicular line (MCL): The space below the 5th rib where it joins with an imaginary line down from the middle of the clavicle on the patient's left side | 5th ICS, MCL |
| $V_5$ | Fifth intercostal space, anterior axillary line (AAL): The space below the 5th rib where it joins with an imaginary line down from the front of the patient's right armpit | 5th ICS, AAL |
| $V_6$ | Fifth intercostal space, midaxillary line (MAL): The space below the 5th rib where it joins with an imaginary line down from the middle of the patient's right armpit | 5th ICS, MAL |

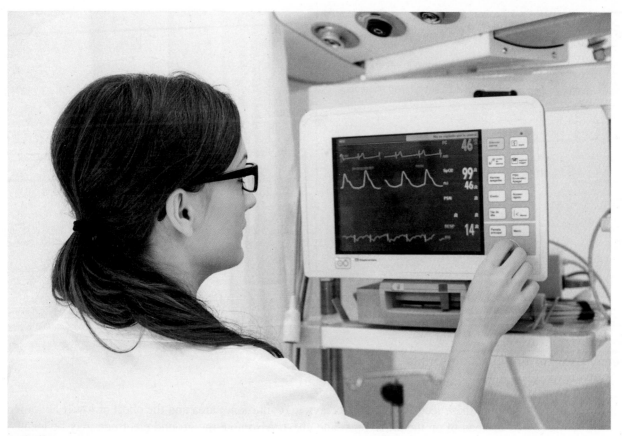

**FIGURE 3–9**

**Bedside monitor** (Santypan/Fotolia).

Intercostal spaces are the spaces between the ribs. The midclavicular line is an imaginary line down from the middle of the clavicle (collarbone). The anterior axillary line is an imaginary line down from the front of the axilla (armpit). The midaxillary line is an imaginary line down from the middle of the axilla.

## Continuous Monitoring

Hospitalized patients requiring continuous EKG monitoring are attached to either a 3-lead or a 5-lead cable connected to a remote receiver/transmitter (called telemetry) or to a monitor at the bedside (see Figure 3–9). Both of these setups send the EKG display to a central terminal where the rhythms are observed and identified.

Because these patients may be on the monitor for days or longer, it is necessary to alter the placement of lead electrodes to allow for freedom of movement and to minimize artifact (unwanted jitter or interference on the EKG tracing).

## The Most Commonly Used Leads for Continuous Monitoring

Figure 3–10 shows the two most commonly used leads for continuous monitoring—Leads II and $MCL_1$ or $V_1$ ( MCL means Modified Chest Lead. The 1 refers to the positive pole's location on the chest. It's at the $V_1$ location—fourth intercostal space, right sternal border). Lead II is by far the most commonly utilized lead for continuous monitoring, as it provides excellent views of atrial activity (P waves) as well as ventricular activity (QRS complexes). $MCL_1$ is useful for assessing rhythms with wide QRS complexes, as it can help pinpoint abnormalities in ventricular conduction. Note that placement for

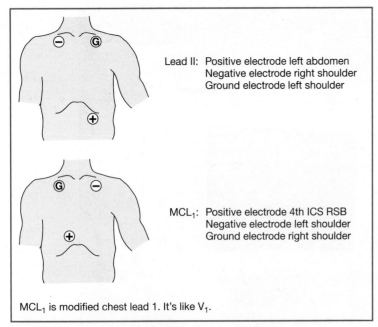

Lead II:  Positive electrode left abdomen
          Negative electrode right shoulder
          Ground electrode left shoulder

MCL₁:  Positive electrode 4th ICS RSB
       Negative electrode left shoulder
       Ground electrode right shoulder

MCL₁ is modified chest lead 1. It's like V₁.

**FIGURE 3–10**

**Lead placement for continuous monitoring.**

**FIGURE 3–11**

**Electrocardiographic truths.**

both these leads is on the subclavicle (collarbone) area and the chest or lower abdomen instead of on the arms, legs, and chest. Also note the ground electrode may be located somewhere other than the right leg.

## Electrocardiographic Truths

- An electrical impulse traveling toward (or parallel to) a positive electrode writes a positive (upward) QRS complex on the EKG.
- An impulse traveling away from a positive—or toward a negative—electrode writes a negative (downward) QRS complex.
- An impulse traveling at a right angle to the positive electrode writes an isoelectric complex (one that is as much positive as it is negative).
- If there is no impulse at all, there will be no complex—just a flat line.

See Figure 3–11. We can say what the QRS complexes in each lead should look like just by knowing the above truths. Let's look at that a bit more.

## Normal QRS Deflections

How should the QRS complexes in the normal EKG look? Let's look at the frontal leads:

Leads I , II, III, AVL, and AVF should have positive QRS complexes.

AVR's QRS complexes should be negative.

Why is this? Normal vector forces of the heart flow top to bottom, right to left. A vector is an arrow that points out the general direction of current flow. The current of the heart normally starts in the sinus node, which is in the top of the right atrium, and terminates in the left ventricle on the bottom left of the heart. (Though both ventricles are innervated simultaneously for the most part, the left ventricle finishes depolarizing last because of its larger muscle bulk). Figure 3–12 shows what the vector representing a normal heart current looks like.

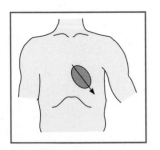

**FIGURE 3–12**

**Normal vector.**

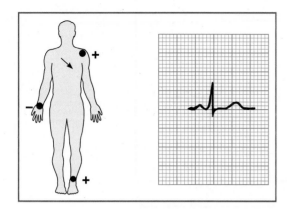

**FIGURE 3–13A**

**Normal QRS deflections in I, II, III, aVL, and aVF.**

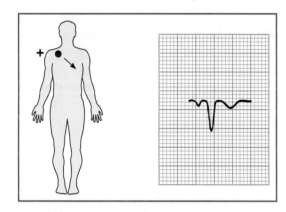

**FIGURE 3–13B**

**Normal QRS deflection in aVR.**

Think about the location of the positive pole in all of the frontal leads. See Figure 3–13A. All except AVR have their positive pole on the left arm or left leg. Because the heart's current normally travels top to bottom, right to left, it travels toward or parallel to those positive electrodes on the body's left side, recording a positive complex on the EKG. AVR's positive pole is on the right arm, however—completely opposite the normal direction of current flow. See Figure 3–13B. Poor AVR is very lonely, watching all that current moving away from it. Remember, a positive QRS complex is recorded when an impulse (wave of electrical flow) travels toward or parallel to the positive pole, and a negative QRS complex results from current traveling away from this positive electrode.

Now let's look at the normal QRS deflections in the precordial leads:

$V_1$ (or $MCL_1$ on continuous monitoring) and $V_2$ should be negative.

$V_3$ and $V_4$ should be about half up, half down (isoelectric).

$V_5$ and $V_6$ should be positive.

The precordial leads start out negative in $V_1$ and then go through a transition zone where they become isoelectric (half-and-half) by $V_3$ or $V_4$, then they become positive in $V_5$ or $V_6$. For the precordial leads, we look at current flow in the *horizontal plane*. The septum depolarizes from left to right and the ventricles from right to left.

See Figure 3–14. In $V_1$, septal and right ventricular depolarization send the current toward the positive electrode, resulting in an initial positive deflection. Then the current travels away from the positive electrode as it heads toward the left ventricle. Thus, $V_1$ should have a small R wave and a deep S wave. The complex is mostly negative, because most of the heart's current is traveling toward the left ventricle, away from the $V_1$ electrode.

> **Quick Tip**
>
> In the frontal leads, all QRS complexes should be upright except aVR.

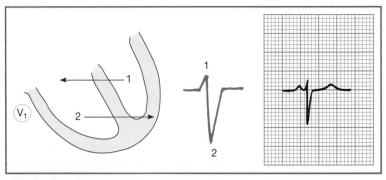

**FIGURE 3–14**

**Normal QRS deflection in $V_1$.**

In $V_6$, just the opposite occurs. Initially, the impulse is heading away from the positive electrode during septal and right ventricular depolarization; then it travels toward it during left ventricular activation. See Figure 3–15.

The other leads in between show a gradual transition from negative to positive complexes.

See Figure 3–16 for normal QRS deflections in the 12 leads.

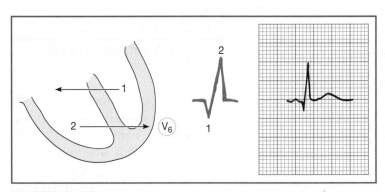

**FIGURE 3–15**

**Normal QRS deflection in $V_6$.**

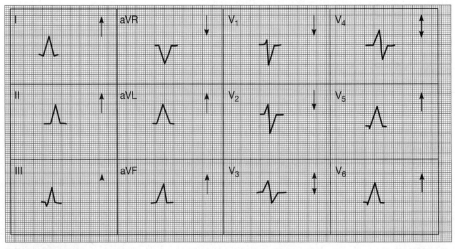

**FIGURE 3–16**

**Normal 12-Lead EKG.** The arrows indicate the correct deflection of the QRS complexes.

**chapter three notes** TO SUM IT ALL UP . . .

- **Electrocardiography**—Recording of heart's electrical impulses by way of electrodes placed at various locations on the body.
- **Electrocardiogram**—Printed EKG.
- **Bipolar leads**—Placed on the limbs—require positive and negative pole:
  - *Lead I*—Measures current traveling between right and left arms. Right arm is negative pole; left arm is positive pole. QRS should be positive.
  - *Lead II*—Measures current between right arm and left leg. Right arm is negative; left leg is positive pole. Lead II's QRS should be positive.
  - *Lead III*—Measures current between left arm and left leg. Left arm is negative pole; left leg is positive. QRS should be positive.
- **Einthoven's law**—Lead I + Lead III = Lead II. This means Lead II should have the tallest QRS of the bipolar leads.
- **Augmented leads**—Require EKG machine to augment (increase) voltage—otherwise waves and complexes are too small to see. Augmented leads are a kind of unipolar lead.
  - *aVR*—On right arm. Its QRS should be negative.
  - *aVL*—On left arm. Its QRS should be positive.
  - *aVF*—On left leg. Its QRS should be positive.
- Bipolar leads and augmented leads: also known as frontal leads, as they are located on the front of the body—and **limb leads**, as they are located on the limbs.

- **Triaxial diagram**—Made by joining either bipolar leads or augmented leads at the center.
- **Hexiaxial diagram**—Made by joining all frontal leads (I, II, III, aVR, aVL, and aVF) at the center.
- **Precordial leads**—Located on the chest—see the heart from the horizontal plane.
  - $V_1$—Located at 4th intercostal space, right sternal border. QRS should be negative.
  - $V_2$—4th intercostal space, left sternal border. QRS should be negative.
  - $V_3$—Between $V_2$ and $V_4$ QRS should be isoelectric (half up, half down).
  - $V_4$—5th intercostal space, midclavicular line. QRS isoelectric.
  - $V_5$—5th intercostal space, anterior axillary line. QRS positive.
  - $V_6$—5th intercostal space, midaxillary line. QRS positive.
- An impulse traveling toward a positive electrode ➜ positive QRS on EKG.
- An impulse traveling away from a positive—or toward a negative—electrode ➜ negative QRS.
- An impulse traveling at a right angle to a positive electrode ➜ isoelectric QRS.
- If there is no impulse at all ➜ flat line.

## Practice Quiz

1. Define electrocardiography. _____

2. List the three bipolar leads and the limbs they connect.

_____

_____

_____

3. List the three augmented leads and the location of their positive poles.

_____

_____

_____

4. The hexiaxial diagram consists of six leads joined at the center. List those six leads.

_____

5. The precordial leads see the heart from which plane?

_____

6. List the six precordial leads and state their locations.

_____

_____

_____

_____

_____

_____

7. Name the two leads most commonly used for continuous monitoring.

_____

8. An impulse traveling toward a positive electrode writes a(n) _____ complex on the EKG.

9. Should aVR have a positive or negative QRS complex?

_____

10. The QRS complexes in the precordial leads start out primarily

_____

# Putting It All Together—Critical Thinking Exercises

These exercises may consist of diagrams to label, scenarios to analyze, brain-stumping questions to ponder, or other challenging exercises to boost your understanding of the chapter material.

1. What can it imply if Lead I + Lead III does not equal Lead II?

   _____

   _____

2. If the QRS complex in Lead III is isoelectric, in which direction is the heart's current traveling?

   _____

   _____

   _____

3. If your patient has a heart rhythm in which the current starts in the left ventricle and travels upward toward the sinus node, what would you expect the frontal leads to look like (i.e., indicate lead by lead whether the QRS complex in those leads would be positive or negative)?

   _____

   _____

   _____

   _____

   _____

   _____

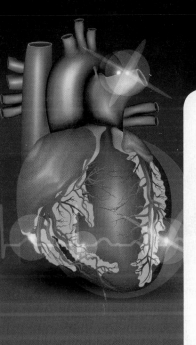

# Technical Aspects of the EKG

# 4

## CHAPTER 4 OBJECTIVES

Upon completion of this chapter, the student will be able to

- Identify the control features of an EKG machine and describe the functions of each.
- Describe what a digital converter does.
- Differentiate between *macroshock* and *microshock*.
- Describe and identify on a rhythm strip the different kinds of artifact.
- Correctly determine how to troubleshoot artifact.
- Tell how to differentiate between artifact and a real rhythm.
- Correctly identify artifact versus rhythm.

## What It's All About

The telemetry monitor technician on duty had no patient contact and thus no way to know if Mr. McCoy's "lethal" rhythm was a true rhythm or just artifact. So following hospital protocol, he paged a code (cardiac arrest alert). When the code team responded to his room, they expected Mr. McCoy to be unconscious and pulseless. Instead he was awake and reading the paper. His blood pressure was fine and he had no shortness of breath or pain. When the team examined the rhythm strip that had prompted the tech to call the code, they saw a flat line, which can indicate a lethal rhythm. Suspecting the gain setting had been inadvertently turned down, the code team increased it and the rhythm reappeared. The setting had been accidentally set so low that the waves and complexes had disappeared, making it seem as if Mr. McCoy was in cardiac arrest (cardiac standstill).

## Introduction

The heart, electrically speaking, is a transmitter, and the EKG machine is a receiver. Let's look at how the EKG machine works.

The electrical impulses generated by the heart course not only through the conduction system but also throughout the body. Electrodes, small adhesive patches with conductive gel on the skin side, are applied to the skin and pick up these impulses, sending them through lead wires (small wires attached to the electrodes) to a cable into the EKG machine. There an amplifier (an instrument that amplifies or magnifies a signal) turns up the signal and a digital converter converts the analog signal to a digital one so it can then be recorded on special paper. Most modern EKG machines are Bluetooth- and Wi-Fi-capable, allowing EMS responders to send a patient's EKG to the nearest hospital so that the physician can order treatment even before the patient arrives. See Figure 4–1.

## Control Features

EKG machines have various control features, including the following:

- Chart speed   This regulates the speed at which the paper records. Normal default speed is 25 mm/s. This means that the machine prints out 25 millimeters (25 little blocks) in one second. Changing the speed to 50 mm/s means it now takes 50 mm (50 little blocks) to equal one second. This doubles the width of the waves and

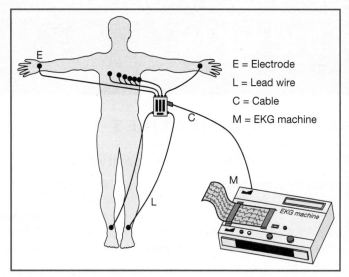
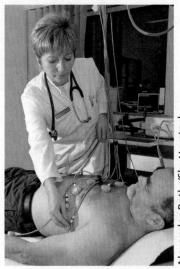

E = Electrode
L = Lead wire
C = Cable
M = EKG machine

Alexander Raths/Shutterstock

**FIGURE 4–1**

**Man attached to EKG machine.**

complexes. Changing the chart speed is useful when the patient has a very fast rhythm, as widening out the rhythm separates the waves and can aid in rhythm interpretation.

- **Gain**   This regulates the height of the complexes. The default gain setting is 10 millimeters/millivolt. This means that one millivolt of electricity causes the EKG recorder to deflect 10 millimeters (10 little blocks) upward. Increasing the gain is important if the rhythm printout is small and hard to read. *It is critical to check/ increase the gain setting if the patient appears to be in a flat-line rhythm.* It could be true cardiac arrest or it could be that the gain is set so low that the waves and complexes aren't even visible.
- **Frequency Response**   This filters out extraneous noise and artifact (unwanted jitter or interference) to provide a smoother EKG recording.

Whenever any setting is changed from the norm, document this change at the top of the EKG printout to prevent misinterpretation of any EKG changes caused by the setting change.

## Electrical Safety

There are two kinds of electrical shock that the patient can sustain from faulty equipment:

- **Macroshock**   A high-voltage shock resulting from inadequate grounding of electrical equipment. If there is a frayed or broken wire or cord, electrical outlet damage, or other electrical malfunction, the 110 volts of electricity running through the power line can go directly to the patient, causing burns, neurologic damage, or fatal heart rhythm disturbances. The patient's dry, intact skin will offer some resistance to the electricity, but not enough to prevent injury.
- **Microshock**   A smaller, but still dangerous, shock directly into the heart by means of a device such as a pacemaker. Normally a small leakage current (electrical current that escapes a device's insulation) is produced around the pacemaker and carried harmlessly away by the ground wire attaching the patient's bed to the electrical socket in the room. If the ground wire is frayed, however, a small amount of current could travel into the heart and shock it from the inside. Because the inside of the body is a wet environment, there is less protection against shock.

*Precaution: Check for frayed wires or components before doing an EKG.*

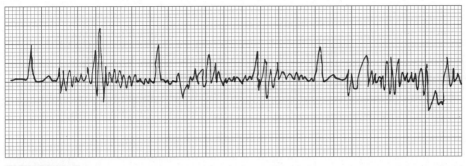

**FIGURE 4–2**

Somatic tremors artifact.

## Artifact

Artifact is unwanted interference or jitter on the EKG tracing. This makes reading the EKG difficult. There are four kinds of artifact:

- *Somatic tremors.*    The word somatic means "body." Somatic tremors artifact is a jittery pattern caused by the patient's tremors or by shaking wires. Try to help the patient relax. Cover him or her if cold. Make sure the wires are not tangled or loose. Sometimes this artifact cannot be corrected, as in a patient with tremors from Parkinson's disease. In that case, make a few attempts at a readable tracing and keep the best one. At the top of the EKG, write "best effort times three attempts" for example, so the physician will know this was not simply a poor tracing done by an inattentive technician. Note the shakiness of the tracing in Figure 4–2. Sometimes you can pick out the QRS complexes and sometimes not. Redo the EKG until the tracing is more easily readable.
- *Baseline sway.*    Here the baseline moves up and down on the EKG paper. It can be caused by the breathing pattern or by lotion or sweat on the skin interfering with the signal reaching the machine. Wipe off any lotion or sweat with a towel and replace the electrode patches. In Figure 4–3, the baseline looks as if someone snagged a finger under it and pulled it upward. As long as the waves and complexes are still clear, baseline sway is not a problem.
- *60-cycle interference.*    This results in a thick-looking pattern on the paper. It's caused by too many electrical devices close by. Unplug as many machines as you safely can until you finish doing the EKG. Don't forget portable phones, laptops, and pagers—they can cause interference also. (Modern EKG machines rarely display this interference, but older machines may, so it is useful to know how to troubleshoot it). In Figure 4–4, see how thick the baseline looks? It is as if someone used a thick highlighter to write it. Normally the baseline is much finer.

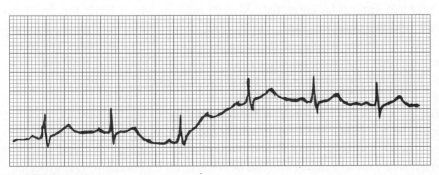

**FIGURE 4–3**

Baseline sway.

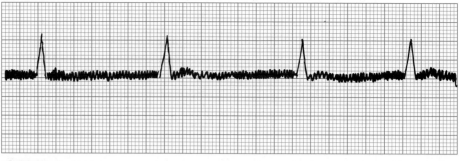

**FIGURE 4–4**

**60-cycle interference.**

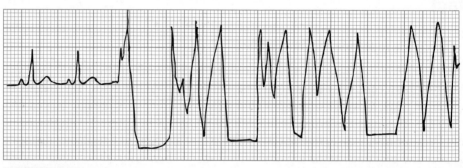

**FIGURE 4–5**

**Broken recording.**

- *Broken recording.* This can be caused by a frayed or fractured wire or by a loose electrode patch or cable. Check first for loose electrodes or cables. If those are OK, the artifact may be from a fractured wire. If so, use a different EKG machine. Never do an EKG with a faulty machine. In Figure 4–5, note that at first the QRS complexes are easily visible, then the pattern is all over the place, going up and down trying to find the signal.

## Troubleshooting

Troubleshooting involves determining and alleviating the cause of artifact and recording errors. For example, what if you saw baseline sway only in Leads I, II, and aVR? Lead I connects the right and left arms, Lead II is right arm and left leg, and aVR is right arm. The common limb is the right arm. Change that electrode, and the problem should be corrected. Always note in which leads the problem occurs and find the common limb. Direct your corrective efforts there. Though modern EKG machines display a message denoting which electrodes are loose or off (saving time searching for the culprit lead), older machines may not, so it is helpful to know how to troubleshoot. Check out Figure 4–6 to help recall lead locations.

If your patient is on a monitor in the hospital and is having artifact, another action could be to change the lead in which the patient is being monitored. For example, if he or she is in Lead II and having artifact, change the lead selector switch to a different lead without artifact, perhaps Lead I. (This is most appropriate when the patient is asleep, for example, and you don't want to awaken him or her for an electrode patch check.)

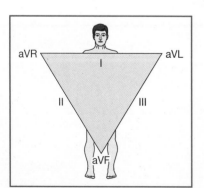

**FIGURE 4–6**

**Leads.**

## Artifact Troubleshooting Practice

On these EKGs, state in which leads the artifact is found, and the necessary corrective action.

**1.**

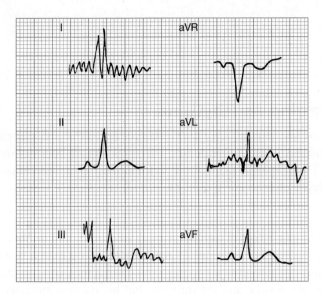

Artifact location _____

_____

Corrective action _____

_____

_____

_____

**2.**

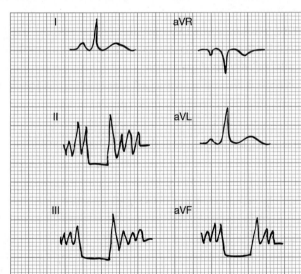

Artifact location _____

_____

Corrective action _____

_____

_____

_____

**3.**

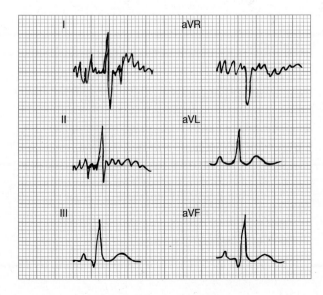

Artifact location _____

_____

Corrective action _____

_____

_____

_____

**chapter** CHECKUP

We're about halfway through this chapter. To evaluate your understanding of the material thus far, answer the following questions. If you have trouble with them, review the material again before continuing.

1. Explain the control features of an EKG machine.
2. Define *macroshock* and *microshock* and the cause of each.
3. Explain how to troubleshoot for the four types of artifact.

## Artifact Masquerading as Rhythms

Artifact can mimic rhythms so convincingly that emergency teams are sometimes summoned to deal with patients with "life-threatening" rhythms that are later discovered to be nothing but artifact. The scenarios that follow will emphasize the importance of assessing the patient who has a change in rhythm. *Do not always believe what you see on the rhythm strip. Check your patient.*

### Artifact Masquerading as Asystole (Flat Line)

Figure 4–7 is a strip from an elderly man who had had a myocardial infarction two days prior. The nurse at the monitoring station saw this rhythm on the screen and ran into the patient's room. The patient was awake and feeling fine, but his rhythm indicated that his heart had completely stopped beating. Because this obviously was not the case, the nurse checked the man's monitor patches and wires and discovered several were loose or disconnected. She reconnected them and his rhythm pattern returned to normal. Thus the rhythm in Figure 4–7 was artifact, *not* a real rhythm.

Now look at Figure 4–8. This is a strip of a heart that has indeed stopped beating. Notice the similarity between this strip and Figure 4–7.

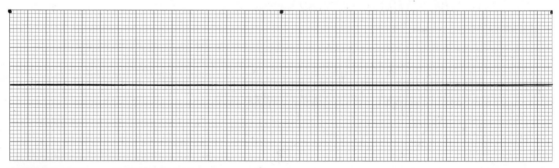

**FIGURE 4–7**

**Artifact masquerading as asystole (flat line).**

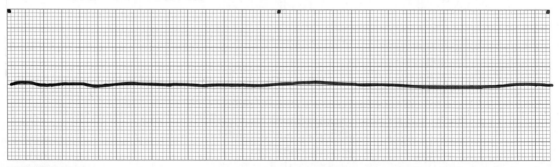

**FIGURE 4–8**

**True asystole.**

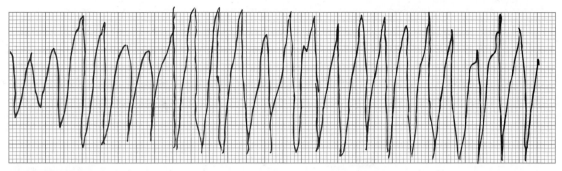

**FIGURE 4–9**

"Toothbrush tachycardia" masquerading as a lethal rhythm.

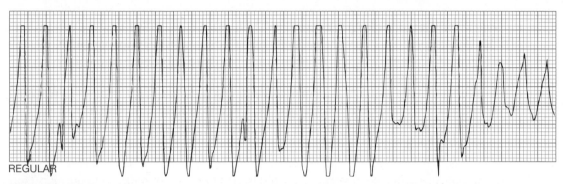

**FIGURE 4–10**

Ventricular tachycardia.

### "Toothbrush Tachycardia"

Mr. Johnson was brushing his teeth when his heart monitor alarmed and the strip in Figure 4–9 printed out at the nurses' station. His nurse, thinking Mr. Johnson was in a lethal rhythm, yelled for help and ran into his room to find him brushing his teeth and in no distress. The repetitive arm movements of his tooth brushing jiggled the EKG lead wires and caused a common type of artifact that health care workers sometimes refer to as "toothbrush tachycardia." When he stopped brushing his teeth, Mr. Johnson's rhythm strip returned to normal.

Now see Figure 4–10, this one of a patient in true lethal rhythm. Note the similarity.

### CPR Artifact

The chest compressions of CPR produce artifact that can resemble rhythms. See Figure 4–11, in which the pattern resembles a rhythm with abnormally wide QRS

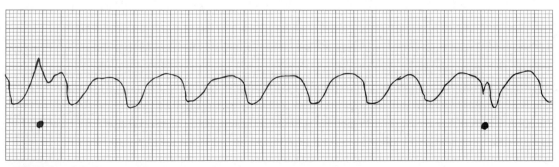

**FIGURE 4–11**

CPR artifact.

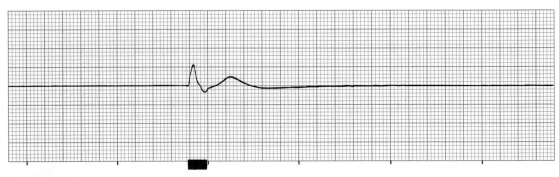

**FIGURE 4–12**

**Rhythm without CPR artifact.**

complexes. But look closer. See the dots? Look above them. See how the pattern gets a bit spiked here? Those are the patient's own QRS complexes popping out. Now look at Figure 4–12. Here CPR was stopped momentarily to allow evaluation of the rhythm without CPR artifact.

In Figure 4–12, there is one QRS complex and then a flat line. This is the patient's true rhythm. The two QRS complexes in the first strip were obviously the rhythm of a dying heart. The rest of the pattern in the first strip was simply pseudo-QRS complexes produced by CPR.

### Defibrillation/Cardioversion Artifact

Check out Figure 4–13. See the rhythm disappear and the baseline shoot down and up before the rhythm pattern comes back? That's the artifact produced when a patient is defibrillated or cardioverted (electrically shocked). You'll recall that the EKG records electrical current in the heart. Defibrillation and cardioversion introduce a sudden surge of electricity into the heart, causing the EKG pattern to go wild briefly. As that electricity is dispersed, the true rhythm reappears.

### Artifact in Three Leads Monitored Simultaneously

Figure 4–14 is a beautiful example of artifact masquerading as a rhythm. This patient was being monitored simultaneously in three leads—$V_1$, Lead II, and Lead I. *Because the three are recorded simultaneously, all three are the same rhythm, just seen in different leads.* Note that Leads II and I look alike, with multiple spiked waves scattered between the QRS complexes. But $V_1$ looks different, with the normal P waves preceding each QRS complex. How can that be? The strips all have to be the same rhythm. Think about this for a moment. Consider the location of the electrodes comprising each lead.

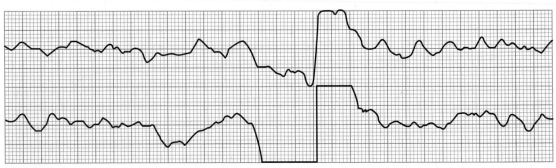

**FIGURE 4–13**

**Defibrillation/cardioversion artifact.**

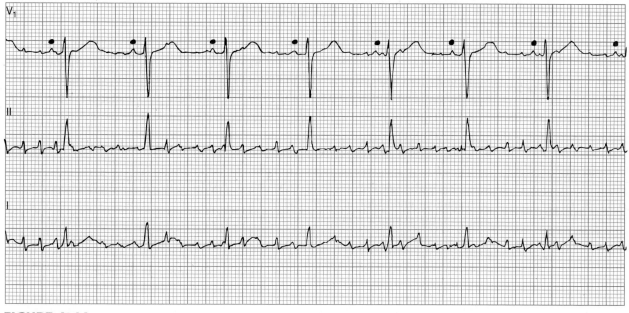

**FIGURE 4–14**

**Artifact in three leads monitored simultaneously.**

The true rhythm is seen in $V_1$. Leads II and I have artifact that obscures the P waves and provides what looks like spiked waves. Leads II and I are limb leads and are subject to artifact from muscle movement. Because $V_1$ is located on the chest, it picks up less artifact. This patient, it turns out, had Parkinson's disease and his tremors were causing the spiked artifact.

### Is it Real or is it Artifact?

What do you see in Figure 4–15?

If you say it's a regular rhythm with a funny-looking beat toward the end (the 8th beat), you'd be right. It looks like an extremely wide QRS, doesn't it? So is this a real QRS or is it artifact? Let's find out. See the dot on the strip? The normal QRS spike is right beneath it. The downward and upward blips that encompass it are artifact. Remember to follow the R-R intervals. Where should the next QRS be? You'll note this QRS spike is exactly where it is expected to be. The QRS complexes are all 14 to 15 small blocks apart, as is this QRS spike. If you see the normal QRS spike in the midst of what looks like another rhythm, the other rhythm is most likely artifact.

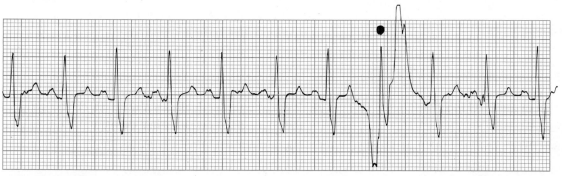

**FIGURE 4–15**

**Is it real or is it artifact?**

### Real or Artifact: How to Tell the Difference

- If the rhythm is different from the patient's previous rhythm, *put the rhythm strip down and immediately check your patient.* Ask how he or she feels and check vital signs (respiratory rate, heart rate, and blood pressure). This is especially important if the rhythm appears to be life-threatening. Patients with life-threatening arrhythmias will exhibit symptoms of **low cardiac output** (inadequate blood flow to meet the body's needs) and/or cardiovascular collapse. Artifact will not produce such symptoms.
- Observe the rhythm in another lead, preferably $V_1$ or $MCL_1$, which has less muscle artifact.
- Check to be sure the "rhythm" meets all its normal criteria. If it doesn't, be suspicious and check another lead.
- Check the patient's monitor wires and patches to see if they are loose or detached.
- See if the patient is having any muscle activity that could cause artifact.
- Follow the QRS complexes, if any are visible.
- The bottom line is this: *Always check your patient, not just the monitor!*

> **Quick Tip**
>
> Do not try to interpret a strip or EKG obscured by artifact! Redo the strip or EKG until you get a readable tracing. Remember the patient's treatment depends on accurate interpretation.

---

## chapter four notes TO SUM IT ALL UP . . .

- **Electrically speaking, the heart is a transmitter and an EKG machine is a receiver.**
- **Chart speed**—Controls speed of paper printout. Normal chart speed—25 millimeters per second.
- **Gain**—Controls height of EKG waves and complexes.
- **Frequency Response**—Filters out artifact.
- **Macroshock**—High-voltage electrical shock—caused by inadequate grounding of electrical equipment.
- **Microshock**—Low-voltage shock—involves a conduit directly into the heart, such as a pacemaker.
- **Death can occur from either macroshock or microshock.** Always check your equipment. Do not use an EKG machine with frayed wires or components.
- **Artifact**—Unwanted interference or jitter on EKG tracing. Artifact can make it impossible to interpret an EKG. Four kinds of artifact:
  - *Somatic tremors*—Jittery pattern—caused by patient tremors or shaking wires.
  - *Baseline sway*—Baseline swings up and down—related to breathing pattern or lotion on skin.

- *60-cycle interference*—Thickened pattern of waves and complexes—caused by electrical interference.
- *Broken recording*—Tracing varies between flat lines and wild scribbling—caused by a frayed or broken wire.
- **To troubleshoot artifact, find the limb common to the leads showing artifact.** For example: artifact in Leads II, III, and aVF—common limb is the left leg—check wires and patches on that limb.
- **Real or artifact?**
  - *Check your patient*—If rhythm looks lethal but patient is grinning at you with a blood pressure better than yours, that "lethal rhythm" is probably artifact.
  - *Check rhythm in another lead*—Preferably $V_1$ or $MCL_1$, as those leads pick up less artifact than limb leads.
  - *See if the "rhythm" meets its normal criteria*—If it doesn't, check another lead.
  - *Check the wires and patches*—to see if any are loose.
  - *Assess the patient for muscle activity*—such as tremors that could cause artifact.
  - *Follow the QRS complexes*—if any are visible.

---

## Practice Quiz

1. What is the function of the EKG machine? _____
   _____

2. Normal chart speed for running a 12-lead EKG is _____ millimeters per second.

3. What does the gain do? _____

4. What should the technician do if he or she changes the chart speed or gain when doing an EKG? _____
   _____

5. Define *macroshock*. _____

6. Define *microshock*. _____

7. Define *artifact*. _____
_____

8. Name the four kinds of artifact. _____
_____
_____
_____

9. If there is artifact in Leads I, aVR, and II, toward which limb would you direct your troubleshooting efforts? _____

10. List three ways to determine if a rhythm is real or artifact. _____
_____

## Putting It All Together—Critical Thinking Exercises

1. Your patient, who is on telemetry monitoring, is noted to have two electrodes that have fallen off—the right arm and left leg. In which leads would you expect to see artifact?

_____
_____
_____

2. Explain how you would know that your patient is having artifact and not a life-threatening arrhythmia (abnormal heart rhythm)?

_____
_____
_____

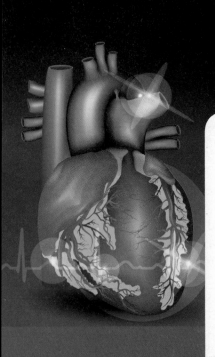

# Calculating Heart Rate

## CHAPTER 5 OBJECTIVES

Upon completion of this chapter, the student will be able to

- Define *heart rate.*
- Calculate the heart rate on a variety of strips, using different methods.
- Differentiate among the three types of rhythm regularity.
- Tell which kind of heart rate to calculate for the different kinds of rhythm regularities.

## What It's All About

Hattie Jefferson had a long history of an irregular heart rhythm that caused her heart rate to vary from 30s to the 160s. She'd been on the same medication for years, but now that she was on dialysis, her doctor wanted her on a different medication. Hattie had been on this new medication for about a week when she began to feel faint. She called 911 and was taken to the emergency department. Her physician met her there and found Hattie's heart rate to vary from 60 to 120 with a mean rate of 90. Her blood pressure was fine. "Your heart is responding well to the new medication," her physician told a relieved Hattie. "In fact, this is the best control over your heart rate we've ever achieved. Based on your heart rate, I'm convinced it's not the medication causing the faintness. So now we just have to figure out what else could be the problem."

## Introduction

Calculating heart rate involves counting the number of QRS complexes in one minute and it is recorded in beats per minute. Heart rate is the same as ventricular rate. We can also determine the **atrial rate** by counting P waves, but the bottom line is this: *When we calculate heart rate, we count QRS complexes.*

## Methods for Calculating Heart Rate

- *The 6-second strip method.* This is the least accurate of all the methods. Although it is considered by many experts to be the method of choice for irregular rhythms, it does not give much information and can be misleading. To use this method, count the number of QRS complexes on a 6-second rhythm strip and multiply by 10. This tells the **mean rate**, or ballpark heart rate. If there are 3 QRS complexes on a 6-second strip, for example, the rate would be 30 beats per minute. (If there are 3 QRS complexes in 6 secs, there would be 30 in 60 secs, or 1 minute.) See Figure 5–1.

  In Figure 5–1, both strips have 5 QRS complexes in 6 secs, so both have a mean rate of 50. Although both rhythms are irregular, with QRS complexes unevenly spaced throughout the strip, strip B shows wild swings in heart rate compared to strip A. Because treatment for rhythm disturbances depends in large part on the heart rate, it makes more sense to provide a *range* of heart rates from the slowest to the fastest, in addition to the mean rate. If a person is being treated with medication to slow down a fast heart rate, for example, it's important to know how slow and how fast the heart rate is in order to determine the effectiveness of treatment. A mean rate alone simply does not provide this

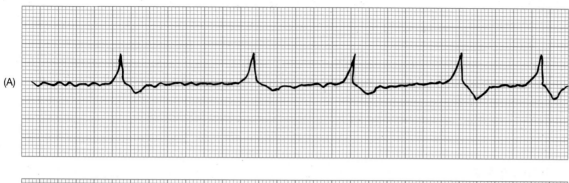

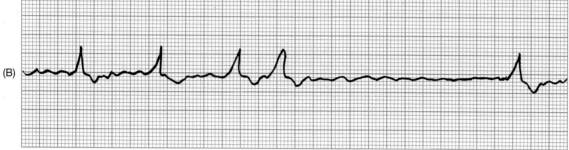

## FIGURE 5–1

**Two rhythms, both with mean rate of 50.**

information—the heart rate range does. The heart rate range is calculated using one of the other methods. Bottom line: *The mean heart rate, as determined using the 6-second strip method, should be used only along with the heart rate range—not by itself.*

**Quick Tip**

Do not use the 6-second strip method by itself to calculate heart rate! Use the memory method or the little-block method.

- **The memory method.**   Widely used in hospitals, this is the fastest method. See Table 5–1. There are 300 big blocks every minute, so count the number of big blocks between consecutive QRS complexes and divide that number into 300. You end up with the sequence below.

  Memorize the sequence 300–150–100–75–60–50–43–37–33–30. Using this method, what would the heart rate be if there were five big blocks between QRS complexes? Go to the fifth number in the sequence. The heart rate would be 60. What if there were 2 big blocks between QRS complexes? Go to the second number. The heart rate is 150. *Memorizing this sequence of numbers* will save lots of time.

- **The little block method.**   In this method, count the number of little blocks between QRS complexes and divide into 1,500, as there are 1,500 little blocks in one minute. It's helpful to remember that each big block is made up of five little blocks. Simply count each big block as five and the leftover little blocks as one. See Figure 5–2.

## TABLE 5–1   **Memory Method of Calculating Heart Rate**

| Number of Big Blocks Between QRS | Heart Rate | Number of Big Blocks Between QRS | Heart Rate |
| --- | --- | --- | --- |
| 1 | 300 | 6 | 50 |
| 2 | 150 | 7 | 43 |
| 3 | 100 | 8 | 37 |
| 4 | 75 | 9 | 33 |
| 5 | 60 | 10 | 30 |

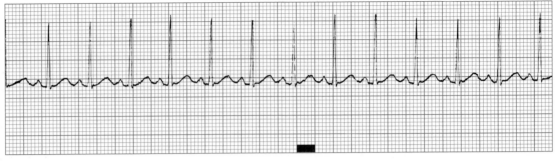

**FIGURE 5–2**

**Little block method of calculating heart rate.**

In Figure 5–2, there are 11 little blocks between QRS complexes, so the calculation is 1,500 ÷ 11 = 137. You can also use this method to calculate the heart rate range in irregular rhythms. Just find the two consecutive QRS complexes that are the farthest apart from each other and calculate that heart rate there—that's the slowest rate. Then find the two consecutive QRS complexes that are the closest together and calculate the heart rate there—that's the fastest rate.

**chapter** CHECKUP

We're about halfway through this chapter. To evaluate your understanding of the material thus far, answer the following questions. If you have trouble with them, review the material again before continuing.

1. Define *heart rate*, *ventricular rate*, and *atrial rate*.
2. Discuss the three methods of heart rate calculation.

## Regularity-Based Heart Rate Calculation

Heart rate calculation is regularity based. The kind of heart rate you calculate will depend on the rhythm's regularity. Rhythm regularity is concerned with the spacing of the QRS complexes. Although we can also determine atrial regularity by examining the spacing of P waves, regularity of the QRS complexes is more important. To determine the regularity of a rhythm, compare the R-R intervals (the distance between consecutive QRS complexes). To compare R-Rs, count the number of little blocks between QRS complexes. Go from spike to spike.

## Regularity Types

There are three basic types of regularity.

1. *Regular.*   Regular rhythms are those in which the R-R intervals vary by only one or two little blocks. In regular rhythms, the QRS complexes usually look alike. Imagine these regular R-Rs as the rhythmic ticking of a clock. In Figure 5–3, the R-R intervals are all 23 to 24 little blocks apart. The rhythm is regular.

2. *Regular but interrupted.*   This is a regular rhythm that is interrupted by either premature beats or pauses. At first glance, these rhythms may look irregular, but closer inspection reveals that only one or two beats, or a burst of several beats, make them look irregular, and that the rest of the R-R intervals are constant. The beats that interrupt this otherwise regular rhythm may look the same as the surrounding regular beats or may look quite different. Some texts would say that a rhythm that is interrupted by premature beats or pauses is indeed not regular and must therefore be called irregular. This text, however, makes the distinction between a rhythm that is regular except for an occasional "hiccup" and rhythms that are "all over the place" in their irregularity.

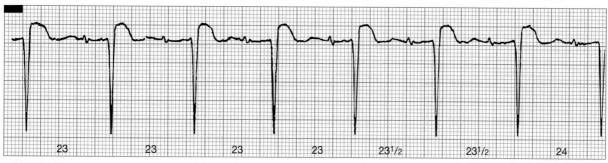

**FIGURE 5–3**

**Regular rhythm.**

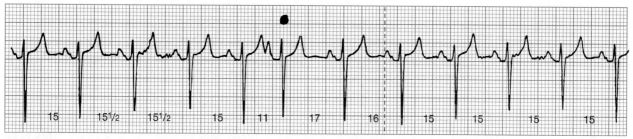

**FIGURE 5–4**

**Regular rhythm interrupted by a premature beat.**

In Figure 5–4, the rhythm is regular until the sixth QRS pops in prematurely. Premature beats are those that arrive early, before the next normal beat is due. Typically, after a premature beat, there is a short pause, and then the regular rhythm resumes. That's what happened on this strip. The R-R intervals are 15 to 16 little blocks apart except when beat number six popped in. Think of premature beats as hiccups. Imagine you're breathing normally and suddenly you hiccup. This hiccup pops in between your normal breaths and temporarily disturbs the regularity of your breathing pattern. Afterward, your breathing returns to normal. You wouldn't characterize your breathing pattern as irregular just because of one hiccup.

In Figure 5–5, the rhythm is regular until a sudden pause temporarily disturbs the regularity of the rhythm. Before and after the pause, the R-R intervals are constant—25 to 26 little blocks apart. During the pause, the R-R is 43 little blocks. Imagine these pauses are like a sudden power outage. Say you've got an electric clock ticking regularly. Suddenly, the power goes out for a few seconds and then comes back on. The outage temporarily disturbs the clock's otherwise normal, regular ticking pattern.

3. *Irregular.* . Irregular rhythms are those in which the R-R intervals vary, not just because of premature beats or pauses, but because the rhythm is intrinsically chaotic. R-R intervals will vary throughout the strip. Imagine these varying R-Rs as

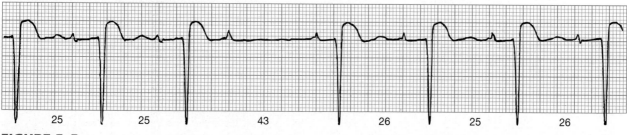

**FIGURE 5–5**

**Regular rhythm interrupted by a pause.**

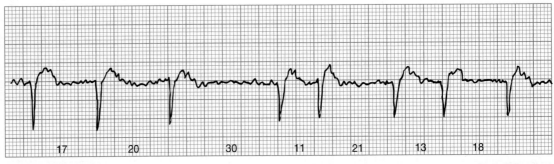

**FIGURE 5–6**

**Irregular rhythm.**

the interval of time between rain showers. Maybe it rains once a week for two weeks in a row; then it rains again in three weeks, then after a month passes, then after a week and a half, then two months. The pattern is one of unpredictability—it happens when it happens.

In Figure 5–6, the R-R intervals are all over the place. Some QRS complexes are close together; others are farther apart. There is no sudden change, no regular pattern interrupted by a premature beat or pause. From beat to beat, the R-Rs vary. This is an intrinsically irregular rhythm. Do you see the difference between this rhythm and the strips of the regular but interrupted rhythms? *Whenever you see a rhythm that looks irregular, look closely to make sure it's not a regular but interrupted rhythm.* Let's practice a few.

## Practice Strips: Regularity of Rhythms

For each of these strips, determine if it is regular, regular but interrupted, or irregular.

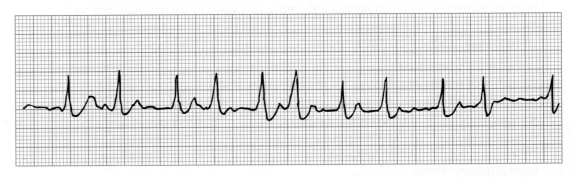

**1.** Answer _____

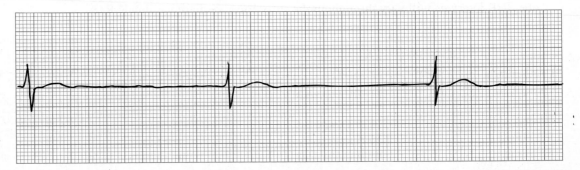

**2.** Answer _____

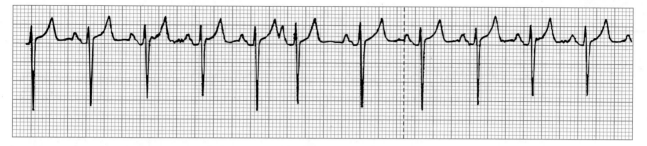

**3.** Answer _____

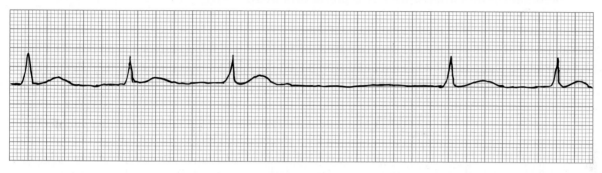

**4.** Answer _____

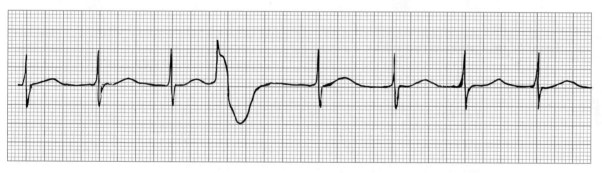

**5.** Answer _____

## Kind of Heart Rate to Calculate for Different Types of Regularity

- *For regular rhythms.*   Calculate the heart rate by choosing any two successive QRS complexes and using the little block or memory method.
- *For irregular rhythms.*   Calculate the mean rate by using the 6-second strip method, and then calculate the heart rate range using the little block or memory method. It is important to note that the mean rate is not a mathematical average of the heart rate range and can be a number above or below what might be expected mathematically.
- *For rhythms that are regular but interrupted by premature beats.*   Ignore the premature beats and calculate the heart rate, using the little block or memory method, on an uninterrupted part of the strip. Premature beats do not impact the heart rate much, as they are typically followed by a short pause that at least partially, if not completely, makes up for the prematurity of the beat. In Figure 5–7, the fifth QRS is a premature beat. Ignore this premature beat for purposes of heart rate calculation. The heart rate is 100.

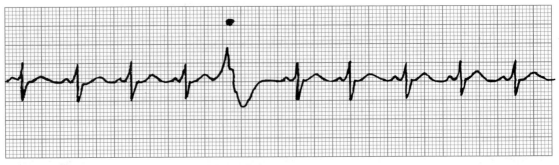

**FIGURE 5–7**

**Regular rhythm interrupted by a premature beat.**

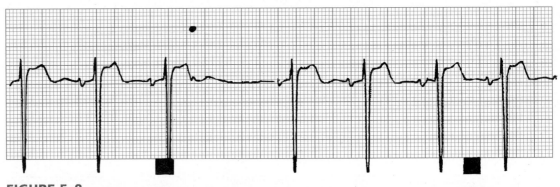

**FIGURE 5–8**

**Regular rhythm interrupted by a pause.**

■ *For rhythms that are regular but interrupted by pauses.*    Calculate the heart rate range slowest to fastest, along with the mean rate. Because pauses can be lengthy, they can greatly impact the heart rate; it's important to take them into account when calculating heart rate. See Figure 5–8.

In Figure 5–8, the regular rhythm is interrupted by a pause. Here the mean rate is 70, because there are 7 QRS complexes on this 6-second strip. There are 34 little blocks between the third and fourth QRS complexes, giving a rate of 44. There are 20 little blocks between the remainder of QRS complexes, for a heart rate of 75. The heart rate range is 44 to 75.

To sum up, see Table 5–2.

Calculating heart rate is a basic skill you will use throughout this book, and indeed throughout your work with EKGs. With practice, you will become expert at it. Let's get to the practice.

**TABLE 5–2    Kind of Heart Rate to Calculate for Different Types of Regularity**

| Rhythm Regularity | Kind of Heart Rate to Calculate |
| --- | --- |
| Regular | One heart rate |
| Irregular | Range slowest to fastest, plus mean rate |
| Regular but interrupted by premature beats | One heart rate (ignoring premature beats) |
| Regular but interrupted by pauses | Range slowest to fastest, plus mean rate |

## Practice Strips: Calculating Heart Rate

Calculate the heart rate on these strips.

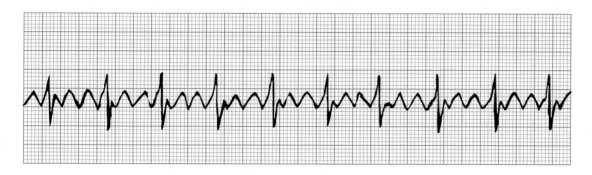

**1.** Heart rate _____

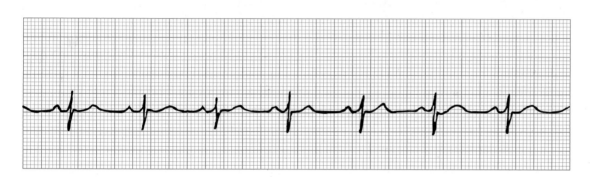

**2.** Heart rate _____

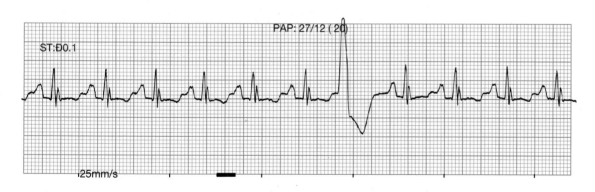

**3.** Heart rate _____

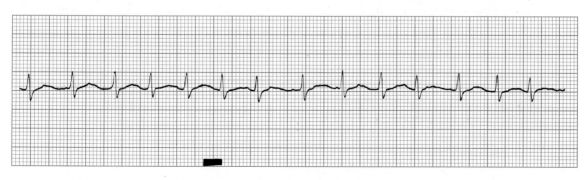

**4.** Heart rate _____

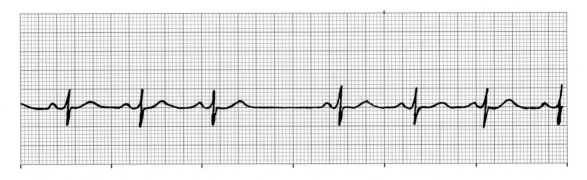

**5.** Heart rate _____

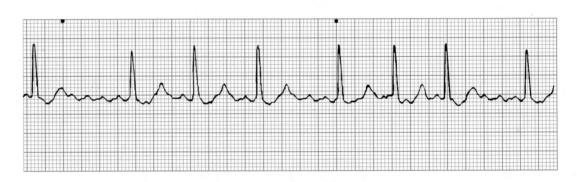

**6.** Heart rate _____

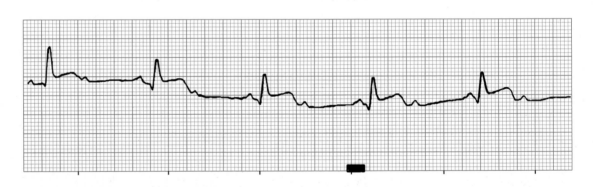

**7.** Heart rate _____

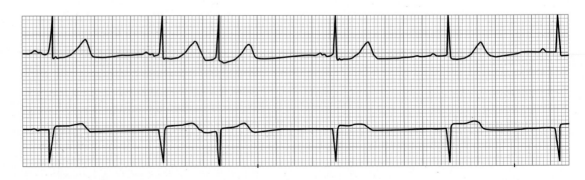

**8.** Heart rate _____

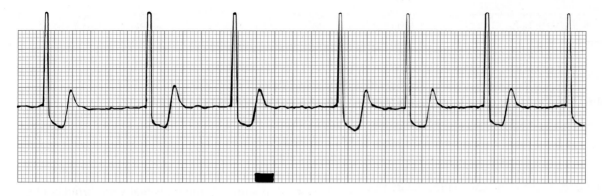

**9.** Heart rate _____

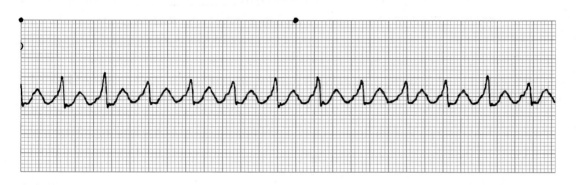

**10.** Heart rate _____

 **chapter five notes** TO SUM IT ALL UP . . .

- **Heart rate**—Number of QRS complexes in one minute.
- **Heart rate is same as ventricular rate.**
- **Atrial rate**—Number of P waves in one minute.
- **Three methods of calculating heart rate:**
  - *6-second strip method*—Least accurate. Count QRS complexes on a 6-second strip and multiply by 10—provides **mean heart rate**.
  - *Memory method*—Memorize the chart.
  - *Little block method*—Count number of little blocks between consecutive QRS complexes and divide into 1,500.
- **Heart rate calculations are regularity based.**
- **Regularity**—Refers to the constancy of QRS complexes and/ or P waves.
- **R-R interval**—Distance between consecutive QRS complexes. Count number of little blocks between QRS complexes and that's the R-R interval.

- **Three kinds of regularity:**
  - *Regular*—R-R intervals vary by only one or two little blocks.
  - *Regular but interrupted*—R-R intervals are regular until interrupted by a premature beat or a pause.
  - *Irregular*—R-R intervals are all over the place—completely unpredictable.
- **Regularity-based heart rate calculation:**
  - *Regular rhythm*—Choose method of choice and calculate one heart rate.
  - *Irregular rhythm*—Calculate heart rate range slowest to fastest, along with mean rate.
  - *Regular rhythm interrupted by premature beat*—Ignore premature beat and the short pause that usually follows it. Go to uninterrupted part of the strip—calculate heart rate there using method of choice.
  - *Regular rhythm interrupted by pause*—Calculate heart rate range slowest to fastest, along with mean rate.

## Practice Quiz

1. Name the three methods for calculating heart rate.

   _____

   _____

   _____

2. The least accurate method of calculating heart rate is the _____

3. When using the little block method, count the number of little blocks between QRS complexes and divide into _____

4. Write the sequence of the memory method. _____

   _____

5. With regular rhythms interrupted by premature beats, how is the heart rate calculated? _____

   _____

6. Name the three types of regularity. _____

   _____

   _____

   _____

7. A rhythm with R-R intervals that vary throughout the strip is a(n) _____ rhythm.

8. A rhythm that is regular except for premature beats or pauses is a(n) _____ rhythm.

9. A rhythm in which the R-R intervals vary by only one or two little blocks is a(n) _____ rhythm.

10. Define *R-R interval*. _____

   _____

## Putting It All Together—Critical Thinking Exercises

These exercises may consist of diagrams to label, scenarios to analyze, brain-stumping questions to ponder, or other challenging exercises to boost your understanding of the chapter material.

1. A rhythm whose R-R intervals are 23, 24, 23, 23, 12, 24, 23, 24, 23, 23 would be considered which kind of regularity? _____ What's the heart rate? _____

2. A rhythm with R-R intervals of 12, 17, 22, 45, 10, and 18 would be considered which type of regularity? _____ What's the heart rate? _____

3. A rhythm with R-R intervals of 22, 23, 22, 22, 23, 22, 22, 22 would be considered which kind of regularity? _____ What's the heart rate? _____

## CHAPTER 6 OBJECTIVE

> Upon completion of this chapter, the student will be able to
>
> - Use the five steps to interpret a variety of rhythms.

## What It's All About

"I'll never learn this stuff," Erica, a new ICU nurse, moaned to her coworker Kim while staring at a rhythm strip. "It just looks like squiggly lines to me." Erica studied her textbook and practiced the rhythms there. She asked her fellow nurses to explain things that she didn't understand. She collected rhythm strips to practice on. About a month later, Kim and Erica were discussing a patient and examining a rhythm strip. "So what do you think this is, Erica?" Kim asked. "Well," Erica answered, "it looks like third degree AV block to me." Erica was correct. Her practicing had helped her learn quickly.

## Introduction

When we analyze a rhythm strip, we are looking for pathology in the form of arrhythmias. Arrhythmias can originate in any of the heart's pacemakers. Some of these rhythms are benign, causing no problem, and others are lethal, killing almost instantly. It's important to know not just what rhythm the patient is in now, but what rhythm preceded it and what's normal for this particular patient. Even so-called normal rhythms or heart rates can be cause for concern. For example, if a patient has a heart rate of 110 (abnormally fast) for two consecutive days, and it suddenly drops to 66, which is normal, it may be a sign of trouble—the heart rate may be at 66 on its way to 0. *Always look at the trend.* Only so much information can be obtained from a single rhythm strip. Comparing the present rhythm strip to previous ones paints a better picture of the patient's condition.

## The Five Steps to Rhythm Interpretation

It's important to have a plan of attack in analyzing EKG rhythms. In the previous chapters, you learned how to identify the waves and complexes on rhythm strips, and how to calculate the heart rate and measure intervals. Let's put all that together now. Asking the following questions for each rhythm strip will help identify the rhythm.

1. Are there QRS complexes? The QRS is the most readily identifiable structure on the rhythm strip. There are a few rhythms that have no QRS complexes at all, so look for the QRS complexes first.
   - If yes, are they the same shape, or does the shape vary?
   - If no, skip to question four.

2. Is the rhythm regular, regular but interrupted, or irregular?
   - Compare the R-R intervals.

3. What is the heart rate?
   - If the heart rate is greater than 100, the patient is said to have a tachycardia.
   - If the heart rate is less than 60, the patient has a bradycardia.

4. Are there P waves?
   - If so, what is their relationship to the QRS? In other words, are the Ps always in the same place relative to the QRS, or are the Ps in different places with each beat?
   - Are any Ps not followed by a QRS?
   - Are the Ps all the same shape, or does the shape vary?
   - Is the **P-P interval** (the distance between consecutive P waves) regular?

5. What are the PR and QRS intervals?
   - Are the intervals within normal limits, or are they too short or too long?
   - Are the intervals constant on the strip, or do they vary from beat to beat?

Once you have answered all these questions you are ready to identify (interpret) the rhythm. But first we need to know what is normal and what is abnormal.

### What Is Normal?

You'll recall that the heart's normal pacemaker is the sinus node. The normal rhythm originating from the sinus node is called **sinus rhythm**. See Table 6–1 for criteria for sinus rhythms.

**TABLE 6–1  Criteria for Sinus Rhythms.**

| |
|---|
| Narrow QRS complexes of uniform shape. |
| Regularly spaced QRS complexes. |
| Heart rate between 60 and 100. |
| Upright, rounded, matching P waves "married to" the QRS complexes (in the same place preceding each QRS) in Lead II. |
| PR interval between 0.12 to 0.20 seconds, constant from beat to beat. |
| QRS interval less than 0.12 secs. |

Arrhythmias, on the other hand, will exhibit some combination of the following. See Table 6–2.

**TABLE 6–2  Criteria for Arrhythmias.**

| |
|---|
| QRS complexes that are absent or abnormally shaped *and/or* |
| P waves that are absent, multiple in number, or abnormally shaped *and/or* |
| Abnormally prolonged or abnormally short PR intervals *and/or* |
| Abnormally prolonged QRS interval *and/or*. |
| Heart rate that is abnormally slow or fast *and/or* |
| Irregular rhythm or a rhythm that has interruptions by premature beats or pauses. |

## The Five Steps Practice

Let's practice the five steps on the five rhythm strips that follow:

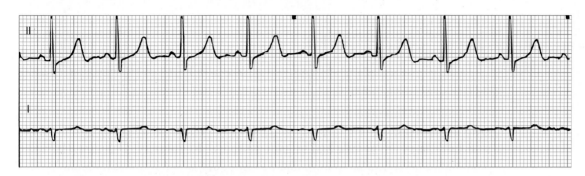

1. Note that this is a double-lead strip. The top strip is labeled Lead II, and the bottom is Lead I. Use either lead (whichever one is clearer to you) to gather your data about the strips. **QRS complexes:** There are QRS complexes on the strip. They are all shaped the same (in each lead). **Regularity:** The rhythm is regular, as evidenced by the R-R intervals all measuring about 18 small blocks. **Heart rate:** Because the rhythm is regular, we choose any two successive QRS complexes and calculate the heart rate there: 1,500 divided by 18 equals a heart rate of 83. **P waves:** There are upright matching P waves preceding each QRS. P waves are "married" to the QRS complexes—they are in the same place relative to the QRS. All P waves are followed by a QRS. P-P interval is regular, meaning the P waves are regularly spaced. **PR interval:** PR interval is about 0.12 secs (normal) and is constant from beat to beat. **QRS interval:** QRS interval is about 0.08 secs (normal, constant beat to beat).

2. **QRS complexes:**   There are QRS complexes, all but one of which is narrow and shaped the same. The fifth QRS is taller and wider than the others. **Regularity:** Regular but interrupted by a premature beat. The R-R intervals are 21, $21^1/_2$, 21, 13 (the premature beat), 30 (the normal pause following a premature beat), and 21. **Heart rate:** 1,500 divided by 21 equals 71. **P waves:** Upright and matching preceding all but the fifth QRS. That QRS has no P wave. The P waves are "married" to the QRS—they are in the same place relative to their QRS complexes. P-P interval is constant except for the wide QRS beat that has no P wave. **PR interval:** 0.12 secs (normal), constant from beat to beat. **QRS interval:** 0.06 (normal) on the narrow beats, 0.12 (abnormally wide) on the wide beat.

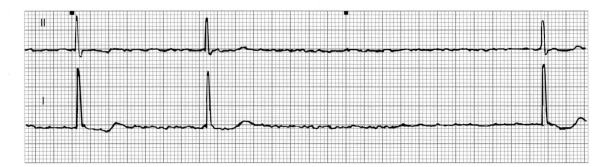

3. **QRS complexes:** There are only 3 QRS complexes in each lead of this double-lead strip. They are narrow and of uniform shape. **Regularity:** Irregular. (It would have been helpful to have had a longer strip to see if this is a regular rhythm interrupted by a pause, but since this is all we have, we must call it irregular). R-R intervals are 34 and 91. **Heart rate:** Mean rate of 30, range is 16 to 44. **P waves:** There are no P waves. There are undulations (waviness) of the baseline between QRS complexes. We cannot assess P-P interval because there are no P waves. Absence of P waves is abnormal. **PR interval:** Because there are no P waves, there can be no PR interval. **QRS interval:** 0.08 (normal), constant from beat to beat.

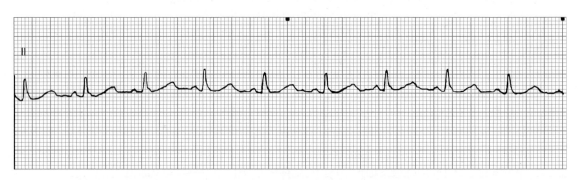

4. **QRS complexes:** All QRS complexes are narrow and of uniform shape. **Regularity:** Regular, as evidenced by the R-R intervals of about 16 small blocks. **Heart rate:** 1,500 divided by 16 equals 94. **P waves:** Upright and matching preceding each QRS. P waves are "married" to the QRS. P-P interval is regular. **PR interval:** 0.12 secs (normal), constant. **QRS interval:** 0.08 secs (normal), constant.

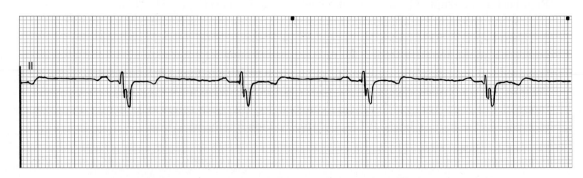

5. **QRS complexes:** All QRS complexes are wide and of uniform shape. **Regularity:** Regular, as evidenced by the R-R intervals of about 33 little blocks. **Heart rate:** 1,500 divided by 33 equals 45. **P waves:** P waves are

upright, matching, and "married" to the QRS complexes. P-P interval is regular.
**PR interval:** 0.20 secs (abnormally long). **QRS interval:** 0.16 secs (abnormally long).

You now should have a feel for what to look for on rhythm strips. In Chapters 7 to 11, you'll learn about the different rhythms themselves.

 **chapter six notes** TO SUM IT ALL UP . . .

- **Five steps to rhythm interpretation:**
  - Are there QRS complexes? Are they the same shape?
  - What's the regularity?
  - What's the heart rate?
  - Are there P waves? Are they the same shape? Are they in the same place relative to the QRS? Are any P waves not followed by a QRS?
  - What are the PR and QRS intervals?
- **The only normal rhythm is sinus rhythm. Characteristics:**
  - QRS narrow, uniform shape.
  - Regular.

- Heart rate 60–100.
- Upright uniform shape P waves "married" to the QRS.
- PR 0.12–0.20 secs, constant. QRS <0.12 secs.
- **Arrhythmia characteristics:**
  - QRS absent or abnormally shaped and/or
  - Irregular or regular-but-interrupted and/or
  - Heart rate varies from zero to tachycardias and/or
  - P waves may be absent, multiple in number, or abnormally shaped and/or
  - Intervals abnormal.

## Practice Quiz

**1.** A heart rate that is greater than 100 is said to be a
_____

**2.** A heart rate less than 60 is a _____

**3.** A drop in heart rate from a tachycardia to a normal heart rate (is/is not) cause for concern.

**4.** *Arrhythmia* means _____
_____

**5.** The five steps to rhythm interpretation are _____
_____
_____

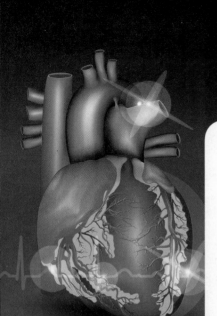

# Rhythms Originating in the Sinus Node

# 7

## CHAPTER 7 OBJECTIVES

Upon completion of this chapter, the student will be able to

- State the criteria for each of the sinus rhythms.
- Using the five steps, correctly interpret a variety of sinus rhythms on single- and double-lead strips.
- State the adverse effects for each of the sinus rhythms.
- State the possible treatment for the sinus rhythms.

## What It's All About

Paula, Donna, and Jackie were in their nursing fundamentals class learning how to check pulses. They were practicing on one another and were surprised to find that their heart rates were so different. Paula's was 106, Donna's was 88, and Jackie's was 54. Knowing that the normal sinus heart rate is between 60 and 100, the girls were concerned that Paula and Jackie had some exotic medical condition that was affecting their hearts. The girls approached their instructor, who checked the girls' pulses, then explained that they all had different heart rates because they are all different. Jackie is an athlete, so her pulse was slower because of her excellent conditioning. Donna's heart rate was normal, and Paula has been running a fever lately, so her heart rate was higher than normal.

## Introduction

Sinus rhythms originate in the sinus node, travel through the atria to depolarize them, and then head down the normal conduction pathway to depolarize the ventricles. You'll recall the sinus node is the normal pacemaker of the heart. See Figure 7–1.

In Figure 7–1, the sinus node fires its impulse, which travels throughout the atria, causing atrial depolarization and writing the P wave on the EKG. The impulse then heads down through the AV node to the ventricle. The QRS is written when ventricular depolarization occurs.

## The Word on Sinus Rhythms

The sinus node is the acknowledged king of the conduction system's pacemaker cells. There are only two ways for the sinus node king to relinquish its throne:

1. By illness or death of the sinus node, requiring a lower pacemaker to step in for it (escape)

2. By being overthrown by a lower pacemaker (usurpation/irritability)

Although they can be irregular at times, sinus rhythms are, for the most part, regular. They're like the ticking of a clock—predictable and expected. You'll recall the inherent rate of the sinus node is 60 to 100. But also remember that this rate can move higher or lower if the sinus node is acted on by the sympathetic or parasympathetic nervous system. The individual's tolerance of these rhythms will depend in large part on the heart rate. Heart rates that are too fast or too slow can cause symptoms of **decreased cardiac output** (inadequate blood flow to the body). Such symptoms can include

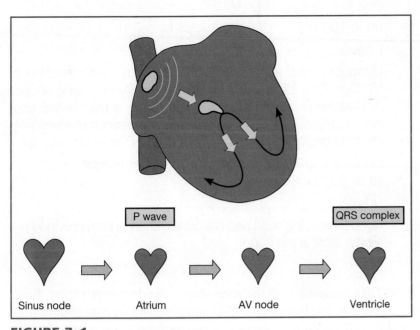

**FIGURE 7–1**

**Conduction in sinus rhythms.**

pallor, dizziness, chest pain, shortness of breath, confusion, decreased urine output, hypotension (low blood pressure), and diaphoresis (sweaty, clammy skin).

Treatment is not needed unless symptoms develop. At that time, the goal is to return the heart rate to normal levels.

Sinus rhythms are the standard against which all other rhythms are compared. Because most of the rhythms you'll see in real life will be sinus rhythms, you'll need a thorough understanding of them. Let's look at the criteria for sinus rhythms. See Table 7–1. *All these criteria must be met for the rhythm to be sinus in origin.*

*All matching upright P waves in Lead II are considered sinus P waves until proven otherwise.* The width and deflection of the QRS complex is irrelevant in determining whether a rhythm originates in the sinus node. Though the QRS is normally narrow (<0.12 seconds) in sinus rhythms, it can be wide (≥0.12 secs) if conduction through the bundle branches is impaired. *The deflection of the QRS will depend on the lead in which the patient is being monitored. For example, you'll recall from Chapter 3 that the QRS in Lead II should be upright but in V$_1$ should be inverted.*

Now let's look at the sinus rhythms.

## Sinus Rhythm

Sinus rhythm is *the* normal rhythm. The impulse is propagated in the sinus node and heads down the conduction pathway to the ventricle. Every P wave is married to a QRS complex, and the heart rate is the normal 60 to 100. The QRS complex can be positive, negative, or isoelectric depending on the lead being monitored.

**TABLE 7–1   Criteria for Sinus Rhythms**

| |
|---|
| Upright matching P waves in Lead II followed by a QRS *and* |
| PR intervals constant *and* |
| Heart rate less than or equal to 160 at rest |

| | |
|---|---|
| Rate | 60 to 100 |
| Regularity | Regular |
| P waves | Upright in most leads, although may be normally inverted in V₁. One P to each QRS. All P waves have the same shape. *All matching upright P waves in Lead II are sinus P waves until proven otherwise* (this is the most crucial criterion to identifying rhythms originating in the sinus node); P-P interval is regular. |
| Intervals | PR 0.12 to 0.20 secs, constant from beat to beat<br>QRS <0.12 secs |
| Cause | Normal |
| Adverse effects | None (unless the heart rate is a drastic change from previously—always look at the trend) |
| Treatment | None |

Figure 7–2 shows QRS complexes, all the same shape. The rhythm is regular. Heart rate is 88. P waves are present, one before each QRS complex, and they are all matching and upright. *Remember—all matching upright P waves in Lead II are sinus P waves until proven otherwise.* P-P interval is regular. PR interval is 0.20, QRS interval is 0.10, both normal. Interpretation: sinus rhythm.

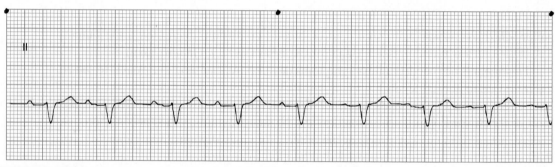

**FIGURE 7–2**

**Sinus rhythm.**

## Sinus Bradycardia

Sinus bradycardia is a slower-than-normal rhythm from the sinus node. The impulse originates in the sinus node and travels the conduction system normally. The QRS complex can be positive, negative, or isoelectric depending on the lead being monitored.

| | |
|---|---|
| Rate | Less than 60 |
| Regularity | Regular |
| P waves | Upright in most leads, although may be inverted in V₁. One P to each QRS. P waves shaped the same. P-P interval regular. |
| Intervals | PR 0.12 to 0.20 secs, constant from beat to beat<br>QRS <0.12 secs |
| Cause | Vagal stimulation such as vomiting or straining to have a bowel movement, **myocardial infarction** (MI), **hypoxia** (low blood oxygen level), **digitalis toxicity** (an overabundance of the medication digitalis in the bloodstream), and other medication side effects. Sinus bradycardia is common in athletes because their well-conditioned heart pumps more blood out with each beat and therefore doesn't need to beat as often. |

| | |
|---|---|
| Adverse effects | Too slow a heart rate can cause signs of decreased cardiac output. Many individuals, however, tolerate a slow heart rate and do not require treatment. |
| Treatment | None unless the patient is symptomatic. A medication called *atropine* can be used if needed to speed up the heart rate. Atropine increases the rate at which the sinus node propagates its impulses and speeds up impulse conduction through the AV node. Thus, it causes an increase in heart rate. If atropine is unsuccessful, an electronic pacemaker or medications such as epinephrine and dopamine can be utilized, although they are not usually necessary for sinus bradycardia unless the individual is in shock. Consider starting oxygen. If the heart does not receive adequate oxygen, conduction system cells become **ischemic** (oxygen starved) and may respond by firing at rates above or below their norm. Providing supplemental oxygen can help these stricken cells return to more normal functioning and a more normal heart rate. |

Figure 7–3 shows QRS complexes, all shaped the same. The rhythm is regular. Heart rate is 54. P waves are present, one before each QRS complex, and they are upright and matching. P-P interval is regular. PR interval is 0.16, and QRS interval is 0.09, both normal. Interpretation: sinus bradycardia. *The only difference between sinus rhythm and sinus bradycardia is the heart rate—the other interpretation criteria are the same.*

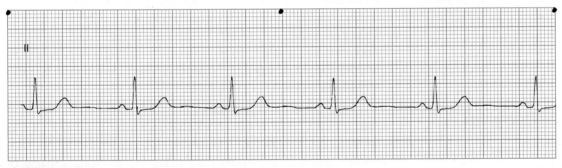

**FIGURE 7–3**

**Sinus bradycardia.**

---

**chapter CHECKUP**

We're about halfway through this chapter. To evaluate your understanding of the material thus far, answer the following questions. If you have trouble with them, review the material again before continuing.

Mrs. Spock calls you to her hospital room—she's having crushing chest pain, nausea, and shortness of breath. You check her vital signs—pulse, blood pressure, and respiratory rate—and find that her heart rate, which had been 78, is now 34. Her blood pressure is also lower, as is her respiratory rate. She is cold and clammy. You note her rhythm has a narrow (<0.12 secs) QRS and matching upright P waves in Lead II.

1. What is her rhythm?
2. What's the likely cause?
3. What treatment would be indicated?

## Sinus Tachycardia

Sinus tachycardia is a rhythm in which the sinus node fires at a heart rate faster than normal. The impulse originates in the sinus node and travels down the conduction pathway normally. The QRS complex can be positive, negative, or isoelectric depending on the lead being monitored.

| | |
|---|---|
| Rate | 101 to 160. According to most experts, the sinus node does not fire at a rate above 160 in *supine resting adults*. Although this is somewhat controversial, we will adopt 160 as the upper limit of the sinus node. *All strips in this text are from supine resting adults unless otherwise specified.* |
| Regularity | Regular |
| P waves | Upright in most leads, although may be inverted in V$_1$. One P to each QRS. P waves shaped the same. P-P interval regular. |
| Intervals | 0.12 to 0.20 secs, constant from beat to beat<br>QRS <0.12 secs |
| Cause | Medications such as atropine or bronchodilators (medications used to open up narrowed respiratory passages in patients with asthma or chronic obstructive pulmonary disease [COPD]); emotional upset, **pulmonary embolus** (blood clot in the lung), MI, **congestive heart failure** (CHF), fever, inhibition of the vagus nerve, hypoxia, and **thyrotoxicosis** (thyroid storm—an emergent medical condition in which the thyroid gland massively overproduces thyroid hormones so that the heart rate, blood pressure, and temperature all rise to dangerously high levels) |
| Adverse effects | Increased heart rate causes increased cardiac workload. The faster a muscle works, the more blood and oxygen it requires. This can stress an already weakened heart. Cardiac output can drop. This is especially true in the patient with an acute MI, as the increased blood and oxygen demand taxes the already damaged heart muscle. |
| Treatment | Treat the cause. For example, if the patient in sinus tachycardia has a fever, give medications to decrease the fever. If the tachycardia is caused by anxiety, consider sedation. For cardiac patients with persistent sinus tachycardia, a class of medications called *beta-blockers* may be used to slow the heart rate. Consider starting oxygen to decrease the heart's workload. |

**Quick Tip**

Every one degree increase in body temperature causes the heart rate to rise by about 10 beats per minute.

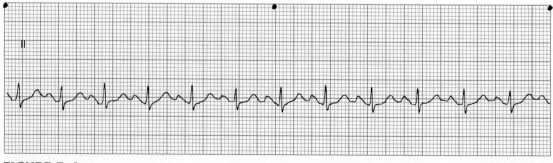

**FIGURE 7–4**

**Sinus tachycardia.**

Figure 7–4 shows QRS complexes, all shaped the same. The rhythm is regular. Heart rate is about 125. P waves are present, one before each QRS, and they are all upright and matching. P-P interval is regular. PR interval is 0.14, and QRS interval is 0.06, both within normal limits. Interpretation: sinus tachycardia. *Just as in sinus rhythm and sinus bradycardia, all the criteria for interpretation are the same for sinus tachycardia—the only difference is the heart rate.*

## Sinus Arrhythmia

Sinus arrhythmia is the only *irregular rhythm* from the sinus node, and it has a pattern that is cyclic and usually corresponds with the breathing pattern. The QRS complex can be positive, negative, or isoelectric depending on the lead being monitored.

| | |
|---|---|
| Rate | Varies with respiratory pattern—faster with inspiration, slower with expiration. The negative pressure in the chest during inspiration sucks up blood from the lower extremities, causing an increase in blood returning to the right atrium. The heart rate speeds up to circulate this extra blood. Sinus arrhythmia is especially common during sleep, especially among those with **sleep apnea** (a temporary, often repetitive cessation of breathing during sleep). |
| Regularity | Irregular in a repetitive pattern; longest R-R cycle exceeds the shortest by ≥0.16 secs (four or more little blocks) |
| P waves | Upright in most leads, although may be inverted in $V_1$. P waves shaped the same. One P to each QRS. P-P interval is irregular. |
| Intervals | PR 0.12 to 0.20 secs, constant from beat to beat<br>QRS <0.12 secs |
| Cause | Usually caused by the breathing pattern, but can be caused by heart disease |
| Adverse effects | Usually no ill effects |
| Treatment | Usually none required |

Figure 7–5 shows QRS complexes, all the same shape. The rhythm is irregular. Heart rate is 62 to 88, with a mean rate of 80. The longest R-R interval (24 little blocks) exceeds the shortest (17 blocks) by 7 little blocks. P waves are present, one before each QRS, and all are upright and shaped the same. P-P interval varies. PR interval is 0.24 secs (abnormally long), and QRS interval is 0.10 (normal). Interpretation: sinus arrhythmia with a prolonged PR interval.

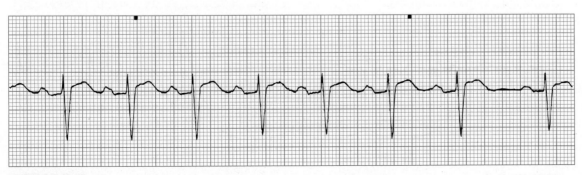

**FIGURE 7–5**

**Sinus arrhythmia.**

## Sinus Arrest

Sinus arrest is a pause that occurs when the regularly firing sinus node suddenly stops firing for a brief period. One or more P-QRS-T sequences will be missing. An escape beat from a lower pacemaker may then take over for one or more beats. The sinus node may resume functioning after missing one or more beats, or the lower pacemaker may continue as the pacemaker, creating a new escape rhythm. The QRS complex can be positive, negative, or isoelectric depending on the lead being monitored.

| | |
|---|---|
| Rate | Can occur at any heart rate |
| Regularity | Regular but interrupted (by a pause). In any rhythm with a pause, always measure the length of the pause in seconds. |
| P waves | Normal sinus P waves before the pause, normal or different-shaped Ps (if even present) on the beat ending the pause. P-P interval is usually regular before the pause and may vary after the pause, depending on whether the sinus node regains pacemaking control. |
| Intervals | PR 0.12 to 0.20 secs before the pause, may be shorter or absent after the pause. QRS on the sinus beats will be <0.12 secs.<br><br>On the escape beat(s), the QRS may be narrow (<0.12 secs) or wide (>0.12 secs) depending on which pacemaker of the heart resumes following the pause. |
| Cause | Sinus node ischemia, hypoxia, digitalis toxicity, excessive vagal tone, other medication side effects |
| Adverse effects | Frequent or very long sinus arrests can cause decreased cardiac output. |
| Treatment | Occasional sinus arrests may not cause a problem— the patient has no ill effects. Frequent sinus arrests may require that the medication causing it be stopped and can require atropine and/or a pacemaker to speed up the heart rate. Consider starting oxygen |

In Figure 7–6, the first three beats are sinus beats firing along regularly. Suddenly there is a long pause, at the end of which is a beat from a lower pacemaker. How do we know the beat that ends the pause (the escape beat) is not a sinus beat? Sinus beats all have matching upright P waves. This beat has no P wave at all, plus its QRS complex is huge, completely unlike the other QRS complexes. Going through our steps: There are QRS complexes, all but one having the same shape. Regularity is regular but interrupted.

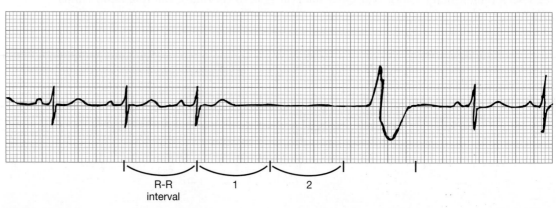

**FIGURE 7–6**

**Sinus arrest.**

Heart rate is 30 to 75, with a mean rate of 60. P waves are upright, matching, one before all QRS complexes except the escape beat. PR interval is 0.16, and QRS interval is 0.08 on the sinus beats and 0.14 on the escape beat. Interpretation: sinus rhythm interrupted by a 2-second sinus arrest (you'll recall every 5 big blocks equals 1 second; there are 10 big blocks between these QRS complexes) and a wide-QRS-complex escape beat. Note that the sinus node resumes functioning after one escape beat.

## Sinus Block (Also Called Sinus Exit Block)

Sinus block is a pause that occurs when the sinus node fires its impulse on time, but the impulse's exit from the sinus node to the atrial tissue is blocked. *In other words, the beat that the sinus node propagated is not conducted anywhere.* This results in one or more P-QRS-T sequences being missing, creating a pause, the length of which will depend on how many sinus beats are blocked. When conduction of the regularly firing sinus impulses resumes, the sinus beats return on time at the end of the pause. The pause will be a multiple of the previous R-R intervals—that is, exactly 2 or more R-R cycles will fit into the pause. The QRS complex can be positive, negative, or isoelectric depending on the lead being monitored.

| | |
|---|---|
| Rate | Can occur at any heart rate |
| Regularity | Regular but interrupted (by a pause) |
| P waves | Normal sinus Ps both before and after the pause; P waves shaped the same |
| Intervals | PR 0.12 to 0.20 secs |
| | QRS <0.12 secs |
| Cause | Medication side effects, hypoxia, or strong vagal stimulation |
| Adverse effects | Same as sinus arrest |
| Treatment | Same as sinus arrest |

Figure 7–7 shows a pause that lasts 8 big blocks. This is exactly twice the R-R interval of the sinus beats that precede and follow the pause. The pause is, therefore, a multiple of the R-R intervals. The pause ends with a sinus beat. Going through our steps: There are QRS complexes, all shaped the same. Regularity is regular but interrupted. Heart rate is 37 to 75, with a mean rate of 60. P waves are upright, matching, one before each QRS complex. PR interval is 0.16, and QRS interval is 0.08. Interpretation: sinus rhythm with a 1.6-second sinus block.

See Table 7–2 and Figure 7–8 for a review of the sinus rhythms. Then move on to the practice strips.

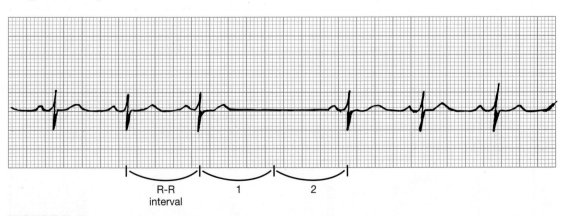

**FIGURE 7–7**

**Sinus block.**

**TABLE 7–2  Rhythm Summary: Sinus Rhythms**

| | Rate | Regularity | P Wave | PR Interval | QRS Interval | Cause | Adverse Effects | Treatment |
|---|---|---|---|---|---|---|---|---|
| Sinus rhythm | 60–100 | Regular | Upright in Lead II; one per QRS; uniform shape | 0.12–0.20; constant | <0.12 | Normal | None | None |
| Sinus bradycardia | <60 | Regular | Upright in Lead II; one per QRS; uniform shape | 0.12–0.20; constant | <0.12 | MI, vagal stimulation, hypoxia; common in athletes | None necessarily; maybe decreased cardiac output | Atropine if symptoms; consider $O_2$ |
| Sinus tachycardia | 101–160 | Regular | Upright in Lead II; one per QRS; uniform shape | 0.12–0.20; constant | <0.12 | SNS stimulation, MI, hypoxia, pulmonary embolus, CHF, thyroid storm, fever, vagal inhibition | Maybe none; maybe decreased cardiac output | Treat the cause; consider $O_2$ and beta blockers |
| Sinus arrhythmia | Varies↑ with inspiration, ↓ with expiration | Irregular; R-R varies by ≥0.16 s | Upright in Lead II; one per QRS; uniform shape | 0.12–0.20; constant | <0.12 | The breathing pattern | Usually none | Atropine if HR slow and symptoms |
| Sinus arrest | Can occur at any rate | Regular but interrupted | Normal before the pause; may be different or absent after | Normal before pause; may be different or absent after | <0.12 unless ventricular escape beat present | Sinus node ischemia, hypoxia, digitalis toxicity, excessive vagal tone, medication side effects | Maybe none; maybe decreased cardiac output; lower pacemaker may take over after pause | Consider $O_2$; atropine or pacemaker if symptoms |
| Sinus exit block | Can occur at any rate | Regular but interrupted | Normal before and after the pause; all shaped the same | 0.12–0.20 | <0.12 | Medication side effects, excessive vagal tone, hypoxia | Same as sinus arrest; pause is a multiple of R-R; sinus resumes after pause | Consider $O_2$; atropine or pacemaker if symptoms |

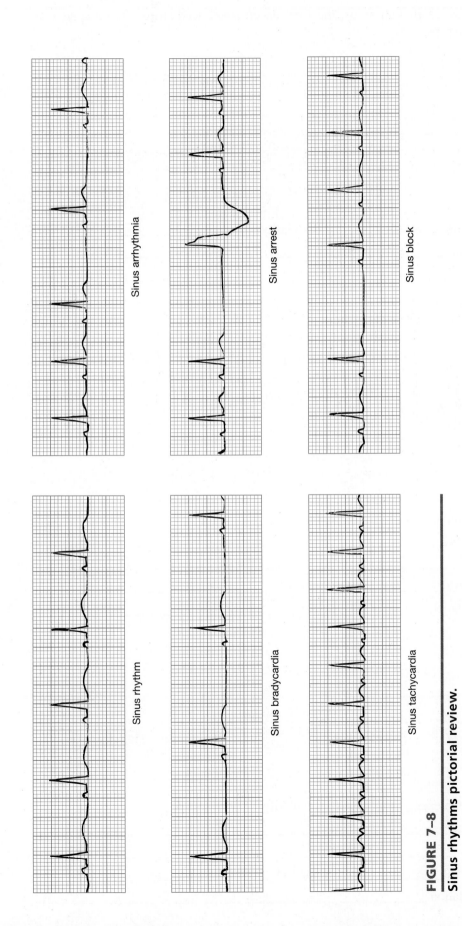

Sinus arrhythmia

Sinus arrest

Sinus block

Sinus rhythm

Sinus bradycardia

Sinus tachycardia

**FIGURE 7-8**

## Sinus rhythms pictorial review.

## Practice Strips: Sinus Rhythms

Following are 25 rhythm strips, the first ten on single-lead strips, the remainder on double-lead strips.

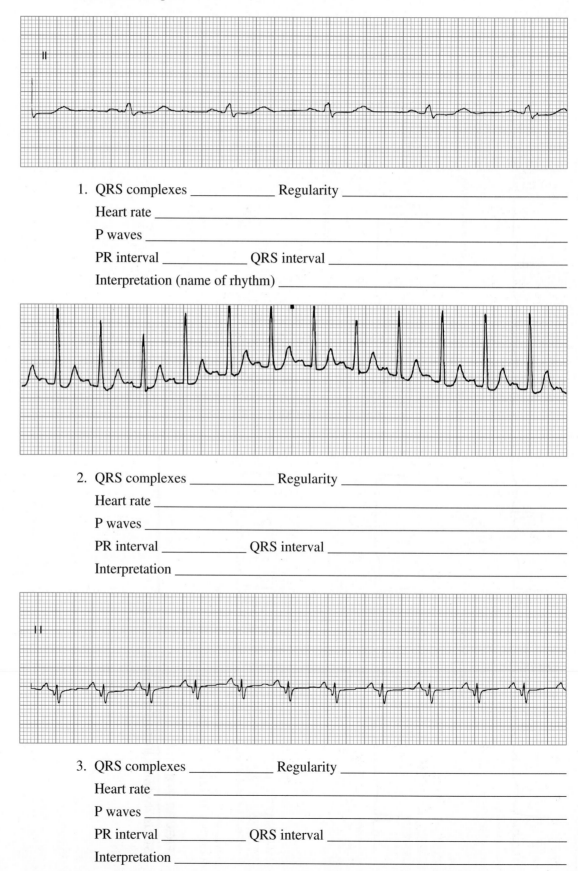

1. QRS complexes _____ Regularity _____

   Heart rate _____

   P waves _____

   PR interval _____ QRS interval _____

   Interpretation (name of rhythm) _____

2. QRS complexes _____ Regularity _____

   Heart rate _____

   P waves _____

   PR interval _____ QRS interval _____

   Interpretation _____

3. QRS complexes _____ Regularity _____

   Heart rate _____

   P waves _____

   PR interval _____ QRS interval _____

   Interpretation _____

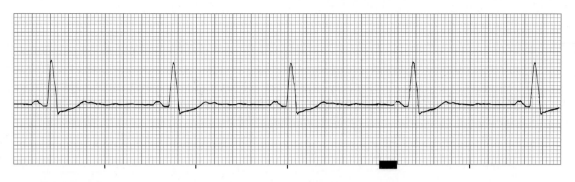

4. QRS complexes _____ Regularity _____

   Heart rate _____

   P waves _____

   PR interval _____ QRS interval _____

   Interpretation _____

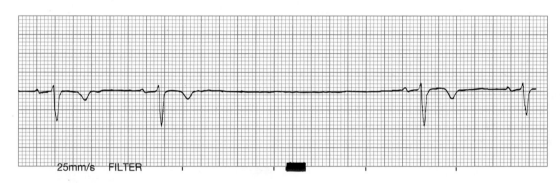

5. QRS complexes _____ Regularity _____

   Heart rate _____

   P waves _____

   PR interval _____ QRS interval _____

   Interpretation _____

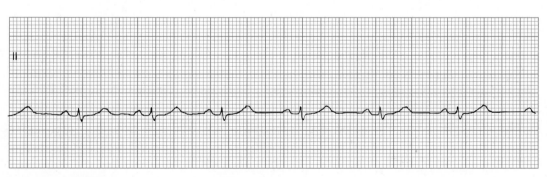

6. QRS complexes _____ Regularity _____

   Heart rate _____

   P waves _____

   PR interval _____ QRS interval _____

   Interpretation _____

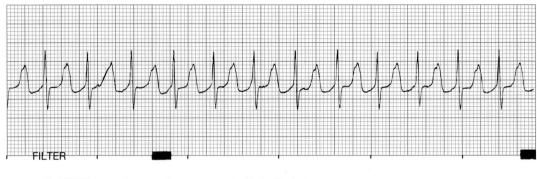

FILTER

7. QRS complexes _____ Regularity _____

   Heart rate _____

   P waves _____

   PR interval _____ QRS interval _____

   Interpretation _____

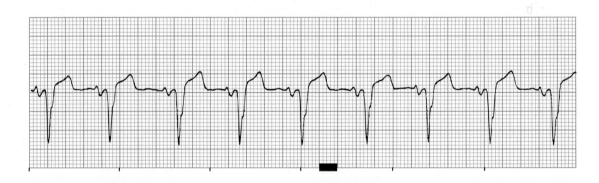

8. QRS complexes _____ Regularity _____

   Heart rate _____

   P waves _____

   PR interval _____ QRS interval _____

   Interpretation _____

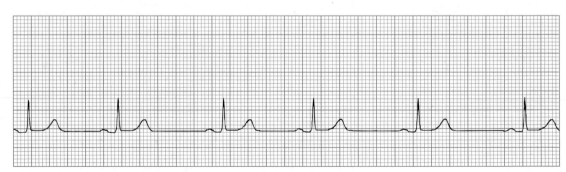

9. QRS complexes _____ Regularity _____

   Heart rate _____

   P waves _____

   PR interval _____ QRS interval _____

   Interpretation _____

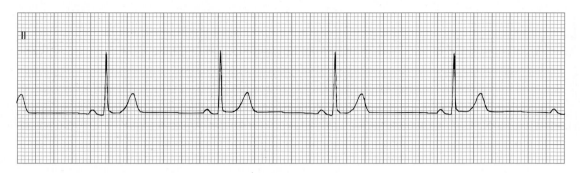

10. QRS complexes _____ Regularity _____

    Heart rate _____

    P waves _____

    PR interval _____ QRS interval _____

    Interpretation _____

Practice strips 11–20 are double-lead strips. On each strip, choose the lead that has the biggest and/or clearest waves and complexes and use that lead for interpretation. *Remember—both leads are the same patient at the same time, so both leads will have the same rhythm and intervals. This is a good chance to see how different these sinus rhythms can look in different leads.*

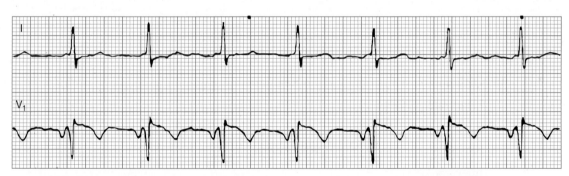

11. QRS complexes _____ Regularity _____

    Heart rate _____

    P waves _____

    PR interval _____ QRS interval _____

    Interpretation (name of rhythm) _____

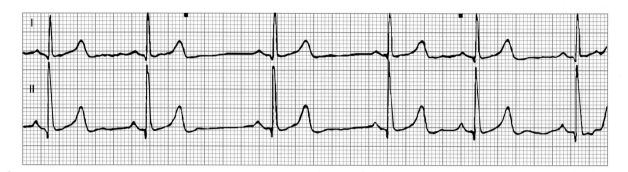

12. QRS complexes _____ Regularity _____

    Heart rate _____

    P waves _____

    PR interval _____ QRS interval _____

    Interpretation _____

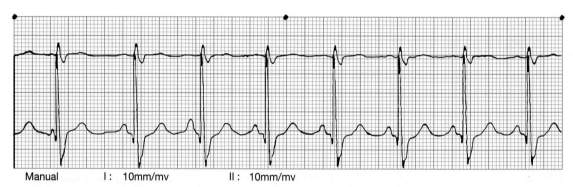

13. QRS complexes _____ Regularity _____

    Heart rate _____

    P waves _____

    PR interval _____ QRS interval _____

    Interpretation _____

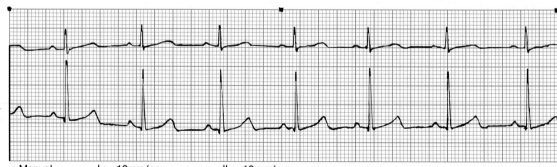

14. QRS complexes _____ Regularity _____

    Heart rate _____

    P waves _____

    PR interval _____ QRS interval _____

    Interpretation _____

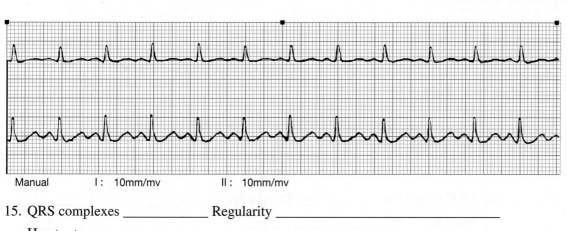

Manual        I :   10mm/mv              II :   10mm/mv

15. QRS complexes _____ Regularity _____

    Heart rate _____

    P waves _____

    PR interval _____ QRS interval _____

    Interpretation _____

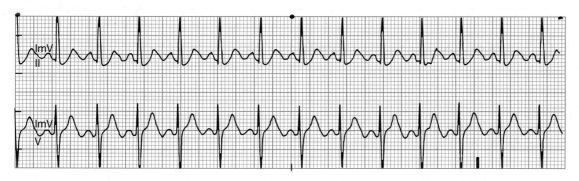

16. QRS complexes _____ Regularity _____

    Heart rate _____

    P waves _____

    PR interval _____ QRS interval _____

    Interpretation _____

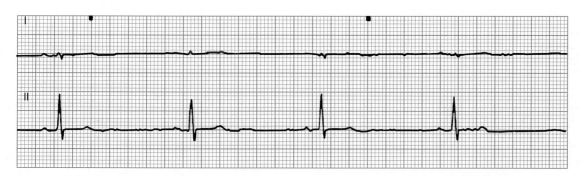

17. QRS complexes _____ Regularity _____

    Heart rate _____

    P waves _____

    PR interval _____ QRS interval _____

    Interpretation _____

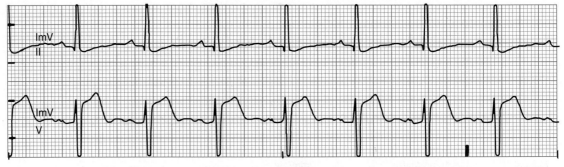

18. QRS complexes _____ Regularity _____

    Heart rate _____

    P waves _____

    PR interval _____ QRS interval _____

    Interpretation _____

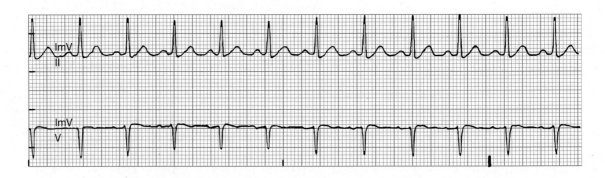

19. QRS complexes _____ Regularity _____

    Heart rate _____

    P waves _____

    PR interval _____ QRS interval _____

    Interpretation _____

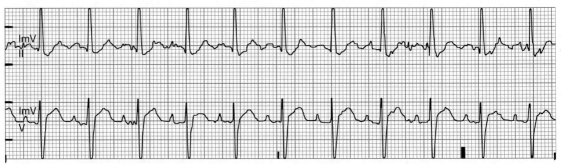

20. QRS complexes _____ Regularity _____

    Heart rate _____

    P waves _____

    PR interval _____ QRS interval _____

    Interpretation _____

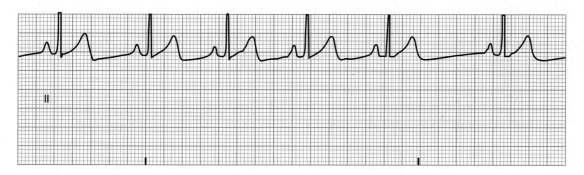

21. QRS complexes _____ Regularity _____

    Heart rate _____

    P waves _____

    PR interval _____ QRS interval _____

    Interpretation _____

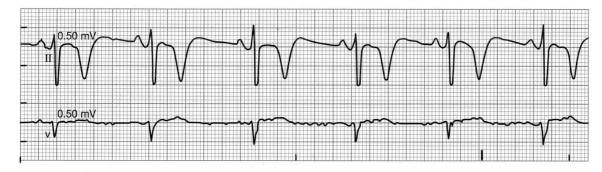

22. QRS complexes _____ Regularity _____

    Heart rate _____

    P waves _____

    PR interval _____ QRS interval _____

    Interpretation _____

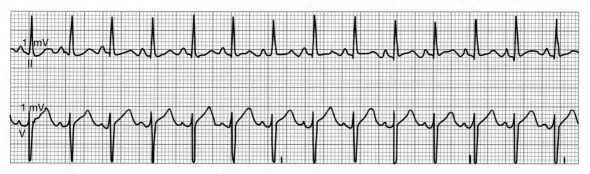

23. QRS complexes _____ Regularity _____

    Heart rate _____

    P waves _____

    PR interval _____ QRS interval _____

    Interpretation _____

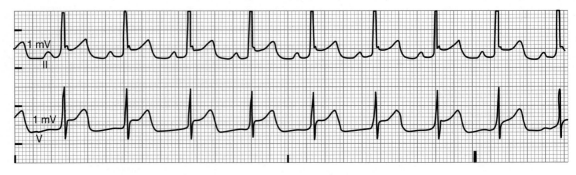

24. QRS complexes _____ Regularity _____

    Heart rate _____

    P waves _____

    PR interval _____ QRS interval _____

    Interpretation _____

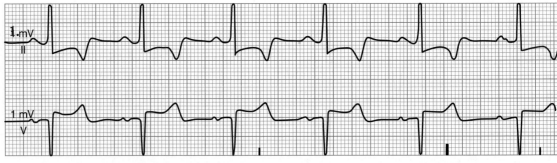

25. QRS complexes _____ Regularity _____

    Heart rate _____

    P waves _____

    PR interval _____ QRS interval _____

    Interpretation _____

## chapter seven notes TO SUM IT ALL UP . . .

- All matching upright P waves in Lead II are sinus P waves until proven otherwise.
- QRS interval should be <0.12 secs, but width and deflection of QRS is irrelevant in determining whether or not a rhythm is sinus in origin. QRS width is determined by the state of conduction through the bundle branches. QRS deflection depends on lead being monitored. Lead II's QRS should be positive; $V_1$'s should be negative.
- Sinus rhythm criteria:
  - *Heart rate*—60–100
  - *Regularity*—Regular
  - *P waves*—Matching upright P waves in Lead II; P-P interval regular
  - *Intervals*—PR interval 0.12–0.20 secs constant; QRS <0.12 secs

- *Causes*—Normal rhythm
- *Adverse effects*—none
- *Treatment*—none needed
- Sinus bradycardia criteria:
  - *Heart rate*—<60
  - *Regularity*—Regular
  - *P waves*—Matching upright P waves in Lead II; P-P interval regular
  - *Intervals*—PR interval 0.12–0.20 secs constant; QRS <0.12 secs
  - *Causes*—Vagal stimulation, hypoxia, medication side effects, MI; very common in athletes
  - *Adverse effects*—Can cause decreased cardiac output
  - *Treatment*—Atropine if symptoms; oxygen, pacemaker if necessary

- **Sinus tachycardia criteria:**
  - *Heart rate*—101–160
  - *Regularity*—Regular
  - *P waves*—Matching upright P waves in Lead II; P-P interval regular
  - *Intervals*—PR interval 0.12–0.20 secs; QRS <0.12 secs
  - *Causes*—Medications, anxiety, pain, MI, pulmonary embolus, fever, CHF, hypoxia
  - *Adverse effects*—Decreased cardiac output
  - *Treatment*—Oxygen, treat the cause, beta blockers if persistent in presence of acute MI
- **Sinus arrhythmia criteria:**
  - *Heart rate*—Varies with respirations
  - *Regularity*—Irregular
  - *P waves*—Matching upright P waves in Lead II; P-P interval varies
  - *Intervals*—PR interval 0.12–0.20 secs; QRS <0.12 secs
  - *Causes*—Normal during sleep; follows respiratory pattern
  - *Adverse effects*—Usually none
  - *Treatment*—None

- **Sinus arrest criteria:**
  - *Heart rate*—Can occur at any heart rate
  - *Regularity*—Regular but interrupted by a pause
  - *P waves*—Matching upright Ps before the pause; may have different or absent Ps after if lower pacemaker takes over
  - *Intervals*—PR interval 0.12–0.20 secs before pause, may change after; QRS <0.12 secs.
  - *Causes*—Sinus node ischemia, hypoxia, medication side effects, excessive vagal tone
  - *Adverse effects*—Decreased cardiac output
  - *Treatment*—Atropine if symptoms; oxygen, pacemaker if needed.
- **Sinus exit block criteria:**
  - *Heart rate*—Can occur at any heart rate
  - *Regularity*—Regular but interrupted by a pause
  - *P waves*—Matching upright P waves in Lead II; P-P interval varies
  - *Intervals*—PR interval 0.12–0.20 secs, QRS <0.12 secs
  - *Causes*—Same as sinus arrest
  - *Adverse effects*—Same as sinus arrest
  - *Treatment*—Same as sinus arrest

## Practice Quiz

1. True or false: All rhythms from the sinus node are irregular.

2. The only difference in interpretation between sinus rhythm, sinus bradycardia, and sinus tachycardia is

   _____

   _____

3. Sinus arrhythmia is typically caused by _____

4. In what way does a sinus exit block differ from a sinus arrest? _____

   _____

5. True or false: Atropine is a medication that is useful in treating sinus tachycardia.

6. What rhythm would be expected in an individual with a fever of 103°F? _____

   _____

7. A regular rhythm from the sinus node that has a heart rate of 155 is called _____

   _____

8. True or false: All rhythms originating in the sinus node have matching P waves that are upright in most leads.

9. What effect does atropine have on the heart rate?

   _____

10. True or false: Anyone with a heart rate of 45 should be given atropine, whether or not he/she is symptomatic.

## Putting It All Together—Critical Thinking Exercises

These exercises may consist of diagrams to label, scenarios to analyze, brain-stumping questions to ponder, or other challenging exercises to boost your understanding of the chapter material.

Let's play with sinus rhythms a bit. The following scenario will provide you with information about a fictional patient and ask you to analyze the situation, answer questions, and decide on appropriate actions.

Mr. Cavernum, age 62, is admitted to your telemetry floor with a diagnosis of pneumonia. He has a past medical history of sleep apnea and an "irregular heartbeat." On admission, his vital signs are as follows: blood pressure (BP) normal at 132/84, heart rate 94 (normal), temperature 98.9 degrees (normal), respirations normal at 20. His rhythm strip is shown in Figure 7–9.

1. What is this rhythm _____

At 3 A.M., Mr. Cavernum calls his nurse, saying he feels awful. The nurse notes his skin to be very hot and his face flushed. His vitals are as follows: BP 140/90 (slightly high), respirations 26 (rapid), temp 101.1 degrees (high). See his rhythm strip shown in Figure 7–10.

2. What is the rhythm and heart rate? _____

3. What do you suspect is causing this change in heart rate? _____

Your coworker brings three medications—atropine, a beta-blocker called diltiazem, and acetaminophen (Tylenol)—into Mr. Cavernum's room.

4. Which of the three medications is indicated in this situation? _____

After receiving his medication, Mr. Cavernum falls asleep and within two hours his rhythm is as shown in Figure 7–11.

5. What is this rhythm? _____

6. Does this rhythm require emergency treatment?

_____

7. What in Mr. Cavernum's past medical history is a possible cause of this rhythm? _____

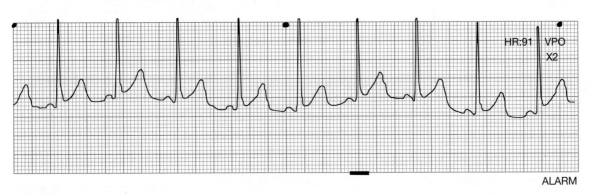

**FIGURE 7–9**

**Admission rhythm strip.**

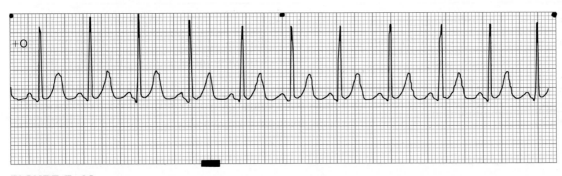

**FIGURE 7–10**

**Second rhythm strip.**

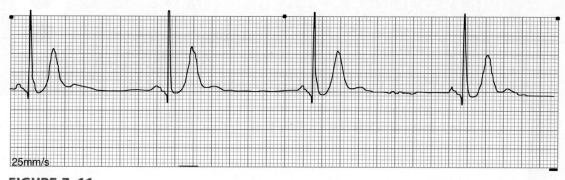

**FIGURE 7–11**

**Final rhythm.**

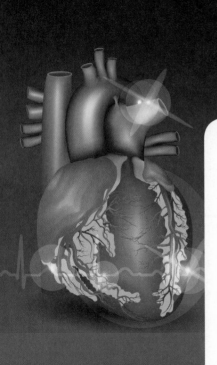

## CHAPTER 8 OBJECTIVES

Upon completion of this chapter, the student will be able to

- State the criteria for each of the atrial rhythms.
- Using the criteria and other rhythm analysis tools, interpret a variety of atrial rhythms.
- State the adverse effects for each rhythm.
- State the possible treatment for each rhythm.

## What It's All About

When 87-year-old Ms. Avis was rushed to the ICU, she was very pale, unresponsive to verbal commands, and drenched in a cold sweat, but breathing fine so far on oxygen. Her physician had ordered her transferred to the ICU and had arrived there with her. The ICU nurses attached the patient to the heart monitor, which showed supraventricular tachycardia (SVT) with a heart rate in the 190s. Blood pressure was 68/36 (extremely low, especially for this patient with a history of hypertension). One nurse ran to get the code cart. She removed Ms. Avis's shirt and wiped her chest dry with it. Another nurse attached defibrillation pads to Ms. Avis's chest and back. They double-checked that the IV line was working properly, then looked at the physician. "Now?" they asked him. "Yes—hit her with 100 joules." A nurse depressed the synchronize button, charged up the machine, and cardioverted the patient. Ms. Avis's chest lurched from the shock. Everyone looked at the monitor. No change in rhythm. "Does she still have a pulse?" somebody asked. By then all the ICU staff had come into the room to help. "Yes, she's still pulsating but it's weak and her blood pressure is really low. Let's shock her again" called the physician. The second cardioversion was successful—the rhythm converted to sinus rhythm with a heart rate of 88. Ms. Avis's blood pressure improved and she woke up. It was discovered later that Ms. Avis had a history of SVT and could not refill her medication for several days because she was waiting for her Social Security check to arrive.

## Introduction

Atrial rhythms originate in one or more irritable **foci** (locations) in the atria, then depolarize the atria and head down the conduction pathway to the ventricles. Atrial rhythms, and indeed all rhythms that originate in a pacemaker other than the sinus node, are called **ectopic rhythms**. See Figures 8–1 and 8–2. In Figure 8–1, a single atrial impulse depolarizes the atria and writes a P wave on the EKG. The impulse then heads down the pathway normally, and a QRS is written once the impulse depolarizes the ventricle. In Figure 8–2, there are multiple atrial impulses. They write a P wave (or an alternate form of atrial wave) and then head down the pathway normally and write a QRS once the ventricles have been depolarized.

## The Word on Atrial Rhythms

Although the atrium is not considered an inherent pacemaker like the sinus node, AV junction, and ventricle (it is highly unusual for the atrium to fire in an escape capacity), the atrium is indeed another pacemaker of the heart. It is best known for usurping the underlying sinus rhythm and producing rhythms with rapid heart rates. Because of these rapid heart rates, patients are often symptomatic. Every now and then the atrium will fire more slowly and produce rhythms with rates less than 100.

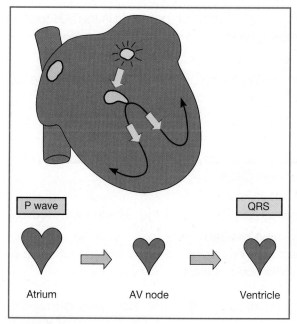

**FIGURE 8–1**

**Conduction of a single atrial focus.**

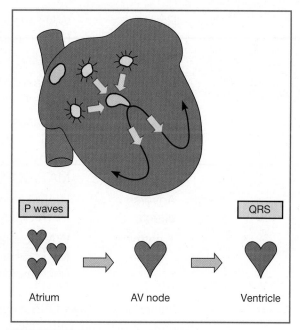

**FIGURE 8–2**

**Conduction of multiple atrial foci.**

Treatment is aimed at converting the rhythm back to sinus rhythm or, if that is not possible, returning the heart rate to more normal levels.

Atrial rhythms are extremely variable in their presentation. Some rhythms have obvious P waves. Others have no Ps at all—instead, they have a wavy or fluttery baseline between the QRS complexes. Some atrial rhythms are regular and others are completely irregular, even chaotic. Although most atrial rhythms are rapid, a few are slower.

Unlike sinus rhythms, which have a common set of criteria, atrial rhythms have multiple and variable possible criteria. If the rhythm or beat in question meets *any* of these criteria, it is atrial in origin. Let's look at these criteria now. See Table 8–1.

**TABLE 8–1   Criteria for Atrial Rhythms**

| |
|---|
| Matching upright Ps, atrial rate (the heart rate of the P waves) >160 at rest *or* |
| No Ps at all; wavy or sawtooth baseline between QRSs present instead *or* |
| P waves of ≥ 3 different shapes *or* |
| Premature abnormal P wave (with or without QRS) interrupting another rhythm, *or* |
| Heart rate ≥ 130, rhythm regular, P waves not discernible (may be present, but can't be sure) |

*It's important to note that atrial rhythms can have a positive QRS or a negative QRS depending on the lead in which the patient is being monitored. For example, in Lead II the QRS should be positive, but in $V_1$ it should be negative.* Reread Chapter 3 to review this if needed.

Now let's look at these rhythms in detail.

## Wandering Atrial Pacemaker/Multifocal Atrial Tachycardia

*Wandering atrial pacemaker* (WAP) and *multifocal atrial tachycardia* (MAT) are rhythms that occur when the pacemaking impulses originate from at least three different foci in the atria. Each focus produces its own unique P wave, resulting in a rhythm with at least three different shapes of P waves. WAP is an example of a slow atrial arrhythmia. MAT is rapid. *WAP and MAT are exactly the same rhythm, just with differing heart rates.*

| Rate | WAP: mean rate <100, usually a mean rate in the 50s to 60s; MAT: mean rate >100 |
|---|---|
| Regularity | Irregular |
| P waves | At least three different shapes. Some beats may have no visible P waves at all. |
| Intervals | PR varies<br>QRS <1.12 seconds |
| Cause | WAP: Medication side effects, hypoxia, vagal stimulation, or MI<br>MAT: COPD, heart disease |
| Adverse effects | WAP: Usually no ill effects<br>MAT: Signs of decreased cardiac output if heart rate is too fast |
| Treatment | WAP: Usually none needed<br>MAT: Beta blockers or calcium channel blockers if signs of decreased cardiac output exist |

Figure 8–3A shows QRS complexes, all shaped the same. Regularity is irregular. Heart rate is 50 to 60, with a mean rate of 50. At least three different shapes of P waves precede the QRS complexes. P-P interval varies. PR interval varies from 0.24 to 0.32. QRS interval is 0.08. Interpretation: wandering atrial pacemaker.

Figure 8–3B shows QRS complexes of uniform shape. Regularity is irregular. Heart rate is 107 to 187, with a mean rate of 120. P waves vary in shape. P-P interval varies. PR interval varies. QRS interval is 0.06. Interpretation: multifocal atrial tachycardia.

Remember: *To differentiate between WAP and MAT, check the heart rate!*

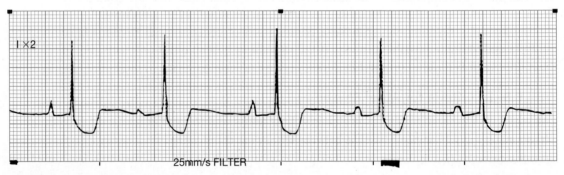

**FIGURE 8–3A**

**Wandering atrial pacemaker.**

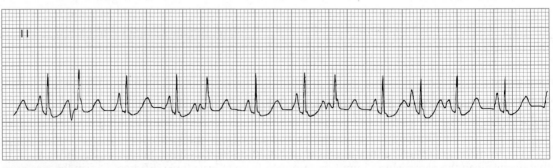

**FIGURE 8–3B**

**Multifocal atrial tachycardia.**

# Premature Atrial Complexes (PACs)

*Premature atrial complexes* (PACs) are premature beats that are fired out by irritable atrial tissue before the next sinus beat is due. The premature P wave may or may not be followed by a QRS, depending on how premature the PAC is. If the PAC is very premature, it will not be conducted to the ventricle because it will arrive during the ventricle's refractory period.

| | |
|---|---|
| Rate | Can occur at any rate |
| Regularity | Regular but interrupted (by the PACs) |
| P waves | Shaped differently from sinus P waves. The premature P waves of PACs may be hidden in the T wave of the preceding beat. If so, they will deform the shape of that T wave. Always be suspicious when a T wave suddenly changes shape. If the QRS complexes look the same, then the T waves that belong to them should also look the same. If one T wave is different, there's probably a P wave hiding in it. If the PAC's P wave is inverted, the PR interval should be the normal 0.12 to 0.20 secs. |
| Intervals | PR 0.12 to 0.20 secs<br><br>QRS <0.12 secs<br><br>QRS will be absent after a nonconducted PAC. *The most common cause of an unexplained pause is a nonconducted PAC.* If you see a pause and you're tempted to call it a sinus arrest or sinus block, make sure there's no P hiding in the T wave inside the pause. It might just be a nonconducted PAC. |
| Cause | The atria become "hyper" and fire early, before the next sinus beat is due. This can be caused by medications (stimulants, caffeine, bronchodilators), tobacco, hypoxia, or heart disease. Occasional PACs are normal. |
| Adverse effects | Frequent PACs can be an early sign of impending heart failure or impending atrial tachycardia or atrial fibrillation. Patients usually have no ill effects from occasional PACs. |
| Treatment | Usually none needed. Omit caffeine, tobacco, and other stimulants. Can give digitalis, calcium channel blockers, or beta blockers to treat PACs if needed. These medications all slow the heart rate and can decrease atrial irritability, decreasing PACs and other atrial arrhythmias. Treat heart failure if present. Consider starting oxygen. |

In Figure 8–4, the fourth beat is premature, as evidenced by the shorter R-R interval there. Recall that premature beats are followed by a short pause immediately afterward. The QRS complexes are all the same shape. Regularity is regular but interrupted (by a premature beat). Heart rate is 54. P waves precede each QRS complex, and all but the fourth P wave are the same shape. Thus the matching upright P waves are sinus Ps, and the premature P wave is *not* a sinus P as it has a different shape. P-P interval is irregular because of the premature P wave. PR interval is 0.16, and QRS interval is 0.08. Interpretation: sinus bradycardia with a PAC.

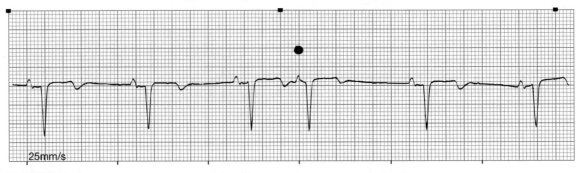

**FIGURE 8–4**

**PAC.**

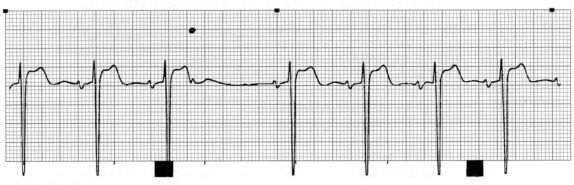

**FIGURE 8–5**

**Nonconducted PAC.**

Figure 8–5 shows QRS complexes, all the same shape. Regularity is regular but interrupted (by a pause). Heart rate is 43 to 75, with a mean rate of 70. P waves are biphasic (half up, half down) and matching, except for the P wave that's at the end of the third beat's T wave. See the little hump there under the dot? That's a P wave. That P wave is shaped differently from the sinus P waves, and it is premature. How do we know it's premature? Look at the P-P intervals, the distance between consecutive P waves. All the sinus P waves are about 4 big blocks apart. This abnormal P wave is only $2\frac{1}{2}$ blocks from the P wave that precedes it. Thus it is premature. A premature P wave that is not followed by a QRS complex is a **nonconducted PAC**. Note the long pause that this nonconducted PAC causes. *Nonconducted PACs are the most common cause of otherwise unexplained pauses.* It is important to note that many nonconducted PACs do not have such easily noticeable P waves. Much of the time the premature P wave is hidden inside the T wave of the preceding beat, deforming that T wave's shape. PR interval here is 0.16, and QRS interval is 0.10. Interpretation: sinus rhythm with a nonconducted PAC.

---

**chapter** CHECKUP

We're about halfway through this chapter. To evaluate your understanding of the material thus far, answer the following questions. If you have trouble with them, review the material again before continuing.

Mr. Sulu's rhythm is very irregular, with a heart rate in the 130s and multiple P wave shapes. His QRS is narrow (<0.12 secs).

Medication is given and the heart rate slows to the 50s but the multiple P wave shapes continue. His blood pressure with this new rhythm is good and he feels fine now.

1. What was his rhythm before the medication?
2. What is his rhythm after?
3. What treatment, if any, is indicated for this new rhythm?

# Paroxysmal Atrial Tachycardia

*Paroxysmal atrial tachycardia* (PAT) is a sudden burst of three or more PACs in a row that usurps the underlying rhythm and then becomes its *own* rhythm for a period of time. The term **paroxysmal** refers to a rhythm that starts and stops suddenly. PAT resembles sinus tach, but with a faster heart rate. *In order to diagnose PAT, the PAC that initiates it must be seen.*

| | |
|---|---|
| Rate | 160 to 250 on the atrial tachycardia itself. The rhythm it interrupts will have a different rate. |
| Regularity | The atrial tachycardia itself is regular; but because it interrupts another rhythm, the rhythm strip as a whole will be regular but interrupted. |
| P waves | The atrial tachycardia Ps will be shaped the same as each other, but differently from sinus P waves. |
| Intervals | PR 0.12 to 0.20 secs, constant<br>QRS <0.12 secs |
| Cause | Same as PACs or sinus tach |
| Adverse effects | Prolonged runs of PAT can cause decreased cardiac output. Healthy people can tolerate this rhythm for a while without symptoms, but those with heart disease may develop symptoms rapidly. |
| Treatment | Digitalis, calcium channel blockers, beta-blockers, sedation, amiodarone (a medication that helps abolish atrial and ventricular dysrhythmias), adenosine (another medication to slow the heart rate), and oxygen. Elective cardioversion (a small electrical shock to the heart to restore sinus rhythm) can be done if the patient is unstable because of the rhythm. |

Figure 8–6 shows four sinus beats and then a run of five PACs. This run of PACs is called PAT. There are QRS complexes, all the same shape. Regularity is regular but interrupted (by a run of premature beats). Heart rate is 75 for the sinus rhythm, and 187 for the atrial tachycardia. P waves precede each QRS complex but are not all the same shape. The sinus beats have one shape of P wave, and the atrial tachycardia has a different shape P that is deforming the T waves. Note the dots over the premature P waves. Wait a minute, you say! What P waves? We can't see them! Here's a rule to help you: *If the QRS complexes on the strip look alike, the T waves that follow them should also look alike. A T wave that changes shape when the QRSs don't is hiding a P wave inside it.* Look at the T waves of the first four beats. They have rather broad sloping T waves. The PAT's T waves are pointy—totally different in shape. They're hiding a P wave. Now to continue with our interpretation: P-P interval is regular during the sinus rhythm, and

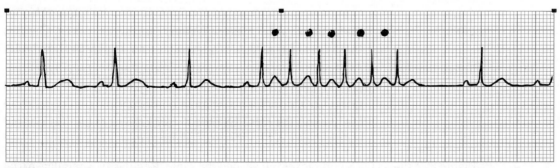

**FIGURE 8–6**

**Paroxysmal atrial tachycardia.**

regular, though different, during the atrial tachycardia. PR interval of the sinus beats is 0.16. We cannot measure the PR interval of the PAT beats, because the P wave is hidden. QRS 0.08. Interpretation: sinus rhythm with a five-beat run of PAT.

## Atrial Flutter

*Atrial flutter* is a rhythm that results when one irritable atrial focus fires out regular impulses at a rate so rapid that a fluttery pattern is produced instead of P waves. The atrium is firing out its impulses so fast that the AV node, bombarded with all these impulses, lets some through but blocks others. Imagine a tennis ball machine firing out tennis balls so fast that there's no way you can hit them all. You end up ducking to protect yourself. The AV node is the gatekeeper—the protector—of the ventricles. Impulses must pass through it to reach the ventricles. Impulses that are too fast would provide a dangerously fast heart rate, so the AV node selectively blocks out some of the impulses, letting only some through.

| | |
|---|---|
| Rate | Atrial rate 250 to 350. Ventricular rate depends on the conduction ratio. |
| Regularity | Regular if the conduction ratio (ratio of flutter waves to QRS complexes) is constant; irregular if the conduction ratio varies; can look regular but interrupted at times |
| P waves | No P waves present. Flutter waves are present instead. These are sawtooth-shaped waves between the QRS complexes. Flutter waves are also described as picket-fence-shaped, V-shaped, or upside-down-V shaped. There will be two or more flutter waves to each QRS. All flutter waves march out—they're all the same distance apart. Flutter waves are regular. They do not interrupt themselves to allow a QRS complex to pop in. Some flutter waves will, therefore, be hidden inside QRS complexes or T waves. The easiest way to find all the flutter waves is to find two flutter waves back-to-back and note the distance between them (go from top to top of the flutter waves or bottom to bottom). Then march out where the rest of the flutter waves should be using this interval. Although most flutter waves will be easily visible using this method, some will not be as obvious, as they are hidden inside the QRS or the T wave. Even though you can't see these flutter waves, they are there and they still count. |
| Intervals | PR not measured, because there are no real P waves<br>QRS <0.12 secs |
| Cause | Almost always implies heart disease; other causes include pulmonary embolus, valvular heart disease, thyrotoxicosis, or lung disease |
| Adverse effects | Can be very well tolerated at normal ventricular rates; at higher rates, signs of decreased cardiac output can occur. Cardiac output is influenced not by the atrial rate, but by the heart rate. |
| Treatment | Digitalis, calcium channel blockers, beta-blockers, adenosine, **carotid sinus massage** (rubbing the carotid artery in the neck to stimulate the vagus nerve) to slow the ventricular rate. Electrical cardioversion can be done if medications are ineffective or the patient is unstable. |

Figure 8–7 shows QRS complexes, all shaped the same. Regularity is regular. Atrial rate is 250; heart rate is 65. P waves are not present; flutter waves are present instead, as evidenced by the V-shaped waves between the QRS complexes. Flutter waves are

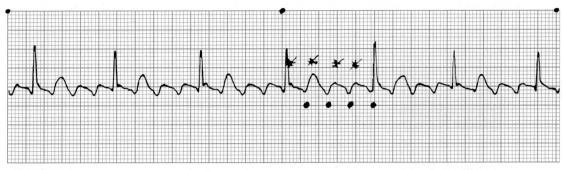

**FIGURE 8–7**

**Atrial flutter.**

all regular. PR interval is not measured in atrial flutter. QRS interval is approximately 0.08, although it's difficult to measure as the flutter waves distort the QRS complex. Interpretation: atrial flutter with 4:1 conduction (four flutter waves to each QRS). See the dots under the flutter waves? There are four dots for each QRS. What if we measured from the top of the flutter waves instead of the bottom? Same thing. See the asterisks above the flutter waves? There are four of them (the fourth flutter wave is *inside* the QRS, but it still counts) to each QRS complex.

## Atrial Fibrillation

During *atrial fibrillation,* hundreds of atrial impulses from different locations all fire at the same time. As a result, the atria depolarize not as a unit as they usually do, but rather in small sections. This causes the atria to wiggle instead of contract. The AV node is bombarded with all these impulses and simply cannot depolarize fast enough to let them all through. Every now and then one of these impulses does get through to the ventricle and provides a QRS.

| | |
|---|---|
| Rate | Atrial rate is 350 to 700; ventricular rate varies. Atrial fibrillation with a mean ventricular rate >100 is said to have RVR (rapid ventricular response). Remember ventricular rate is the same as heart rate. |
| Regularity | Irregularly irregular, completely unpredictable |
| P waves | No P waves are present. Fibrillatory waves are present instead. These are undulations or waviness of the baseline between QRSs. *If there are P waves, the rhythm is not atrial fibrillation.* |
| Intervals | Because there are no P waves, there is no PR interval. QRS <0.12 secs |
| Cause | MI, lung disease, valvular heart disease, hyperthyroidism |
| Adverse effects | Atrial fibrillation can cause a drop in cardiac output because of the loss of the atrial kick, which accounts for 15% to 30% of the cardiac output. One possible complication of atrial fibrillation is blood clots, which can collect in the sluggish atria. This can result in MI, strokes, or blood clots in the lung. See Figure 8–8. |
| Treatment | Depends on the duration of atrial fibrillation. Because the atria are wiggling, not contracting, blood flow is stagnant and clots can develop. If there are atrial clots and the rhythm is converted back to sinus, the restored atrial contraction (atrial kick) can dislodge these clots, propelling them out of the atrium into the circulation. |

## Atrial Fibrillation and Stroke

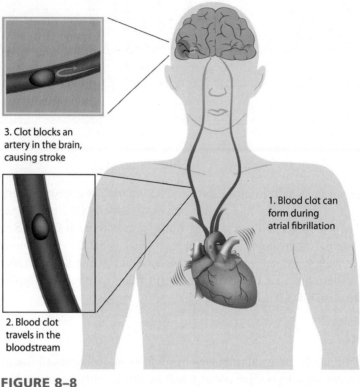

3. Clot blocks an
artery in the brain,
causing stroke

1. Blood clot can
form during
atrial fibrillation

2. Blood clot
travels in the
bloodstream

**FIGURE 8–8**

**Atrial fibrillation and stroke** (Alila Medical Media/Shutterstock).

*If atrial fibrillation duration is less than 48 hours, the goal is to convert the rhythm back to sinus.* Digitalis, calcium channel blockers, beta-blockers, amiodarone, or electrical cardioversion can be utilized. In atrial fibrillation less than 48 hours old, the likelihood that there are blood clots in the atria is low, so there is minimal chance of showering clots to the brain, heart, lungs, and other organs once the atrial kick is reestablished in sinus rhythm.

*In stable patients who have been in atrial fibrillation for longer than 48 hours, the risk of blood clots is greater, so initial treatment is aimed at controlling the heart rate rather than converting the rhythm back to sinus.* Anticoagulants (blood thinners) are given to prevent any more blood clots from forming, and cardioversion is delayed 2 to 3 weeks to allow any clots that are there to dissolve on their own. Meanwhile, medications can be given to regulate the heart rate to a more normal level. In emergencies, patients in atrial fibrillation longer than 48 hours will be started on heparin (an anticoagulant) intravenously, given a transesophageal echocardiogram (TEE—a sonarlike test using a probe inserted into the esophagus) to rule out blood clots in the atria, then electrically cardioverted. Consider starting oxygen.

Figure 8–9 shows QRS complexes, all the same shape. Regularity is irregular. Heart rate is 65 to 100, with a mean rate of 90. P waves are absent; fibrillatory waves are present instead. PR interval is not applicable, and QRS interval is 0.10. Interpretation: atrial fibrillation.

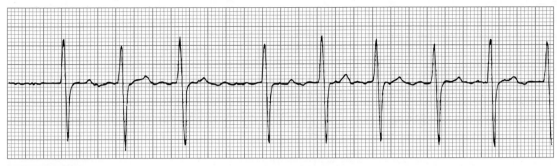

**FIGURE 8–9**

**Atrial fibrillation.**

# Supraventricular Tachycardia

Supraventricular tachycardia (SVT) is a catchall term given to tachycardias that are **supraventricular**; that is, they originate above the ventricles (the prefix *supra-* means "above") in either the sinus node, the atrium, or the AV junction, but whose exact origin cannot be identified because P waves are not discernible.

| | |
|---|---|
| Rate | About 130 or higher (usually >150) |
| Regularity | Regular |
| P waves | Not discernible |
| Intervals | PR cannot be measured because P waves cannot be positively identified.<br>QRS <0.12 secs |
| Cause | Same as PAT |
| Adverse effects | Decreased cardiac output secondary to the rapid heart rate |
| Treatment | Adenosine, digitalis, ibutilide (a medication to control atrial arrhythmias), calcium channel blockers, beta-blockers. Consider starting oxygen. Elective cardioversion can also be done if the patient is unstable. |

Figure 8–10 shows QRS complexes, all shaped the same. Rhythm is regular. Heart rate is 150. P waves are not identifiable. PR interval is not measurable. QRS interval is 0.08. Interpretation: SVT. The origin of this rhythm is not clear, but we know that it originated in a pacemaker above the ventricle, because the QRS complex is narrow, less than 0.12 secs. (Rhythms that originate in the ventricle have a wide QRS complex, greater than 0.12 secs.) Bottom line: *If the QRS is <0.12 secs, the heart rate is around 130 or higher, the rhythm is regular, and you can't pick out the P waves, call the rhythm SVT.*

See Table 8–2 and Figure 8–11 to review the atrial rhythms. Then move on to the practice strips.

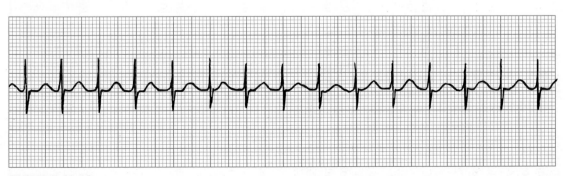

**FIGURE 8–10**

**SVT (supraventricular tachycardia).**

**TABLE 8-2    Rhythm Summary: Atrial Rhythms**

| | Rate | Regularity | P Wave | QRS Interval | Cause | Adverse Effects | Treatment |
|---|---|---|---|---|---|---|---|
| Wandering atrial pacemaker (WAP) | Mean rate <100 | Irregular | At least 3 different shapes; sometimes no P at all on some beats | <0.12 | MI, medication side effects, hypoxia, vagal stimulation | Usually no ill effects | Usually none; atropine or pacemaker if HR slow and symptoms |
| Multifocal atrial tachycardia | Mean rate >100 | Irregular | Same as WAP | <0.12 | COPD | Decreased cardiac output at higher heart rates | Beta blockers or calcium channel blockers |
| PACs | Can occur at any rate | Regular but interrupted | Shaped differently from sinus Ps; often hidden in preceding T wave | <0.12; QRS absent after non-conducted PAC | Stimulants, caffeine, hypoxia, heart disease, or normal | None if occasional; can be a sign of early heart failure | Remove the causes; consider O$_2$, digitalis, calcium channel blockers |
| Paroxysmal atrial tachycardia (PAT) | 161–250 once in atrial tach | Regular but interrupted | Shaped differently from sinus Ps but same as each other | <0.12 | Stimulants, caffeine, hypoxia, heart disease, or normal | Decreased cardiac output; some people tolerate OK for a while | Digitalis, amiodarone, calcium channel blockers, beta blockers, sedation, O$_2$, adenosine, electrical cardioversion |
| Atrial flutter | Atria: 251–350; ventricle: varies | Regular or irregular | None; flutter waves present (zigzag or sawtooth waves) | <0.12 | Heart disease, hypoxia, pulmonary embolus, lung disease, valve disease, thyroid storm | Tolerated OK at normal rate; decreased cardiac output at faster rates | Digitalis, amiodarone, calcium channel blockers, beta blockers; consider O$_2$, carotid massage, electrical cardioversion |
| Atrial fib | Atria: 350–700; ventricle: varies | Irregularly irregular | None; fibrillatory waves present (waviness of the baseline) | <0.12 | MI, lung disease, valve disease, thyrotoxicosis | Decreased cardiac output; can cause blood clots in atria | Digitalis, amiodarone, calcium channel blockers, beta blockers; consider O$_2$; electrical cardioversion; consider anticoagulation to prevent clots |
| SVT | ≥130 | Regular | May be present but hard to see | <0.12 | Stimulants, caffeine, hypoxia, heart disease, or normal | Decreased cardiac output; some people tolerate OK for a while | Digitalis, amiodarone, calcium channel blockers, beta blockers, sedation, O$_2$, adenosine, electrical cardioversion |

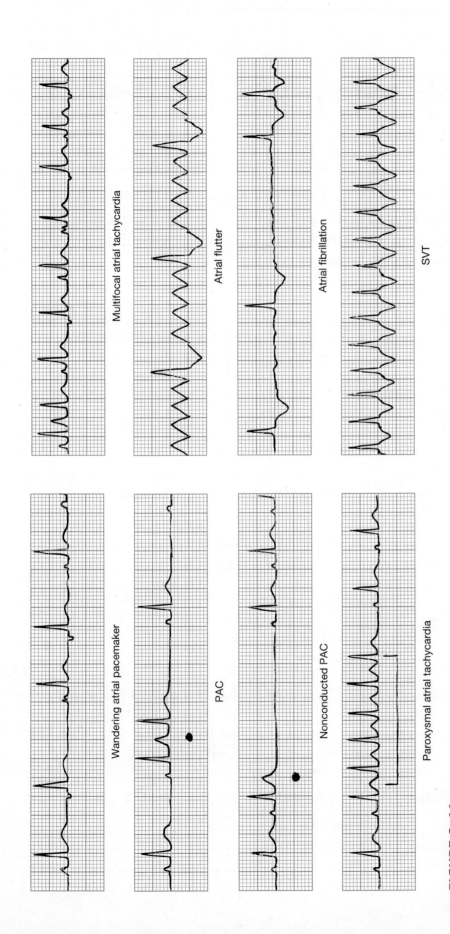

Wandering atrial pacemaker

Multifocal atrial tachycardia

PAC

Atrial flutter

Nonconducted PAC

Atrial fibrillation

Paroxysmal atrial tachycardia

SVT

**FIGURE 8–11**

**Atrial Rhythms Pictorial Review.**

## Practice Strips: Atrial Rhythms

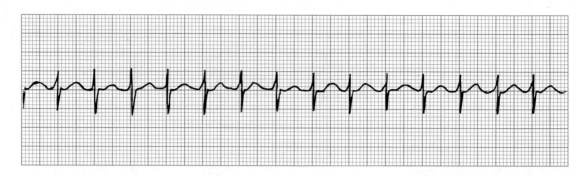

1. QRS complexes _____ Regularity _____ Heart rate _____

   P waves _____

   PR interval _____ QRS interval _____

   Interpretation (name of rhythm) _____

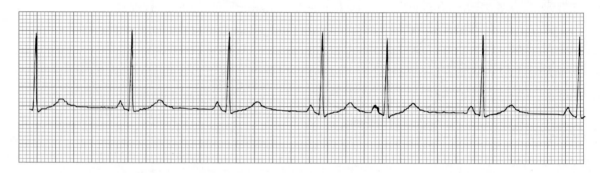

2. QRS complexes _____ Regularity _____ Heart rate _____

   P waves _____

   PR interval _____ QRS interval _____

   Interpretation _____

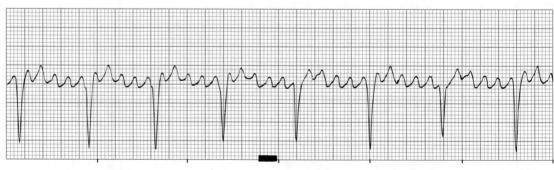

3. QRS complexes _____ Regularity _____ Heart rate _____

   P waves _____

   PR interval _____ QRS interval _____

   Interpretation _____

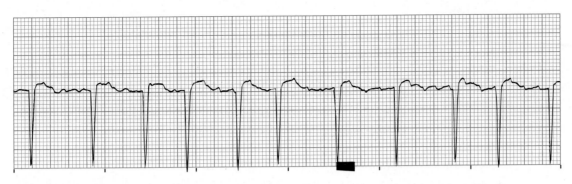

4. QRS complexes _____ Regularity _____ Heart rate _____

   P waves _____

   PR interval _____ QRS interval _____

   Interpretation _____

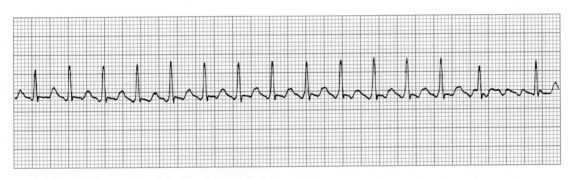

5. QRS complexes _____ Regularity _____ Heart rate _____

   P waves _____

   PR interval _____ QRS interval _____

   Interpretation _____

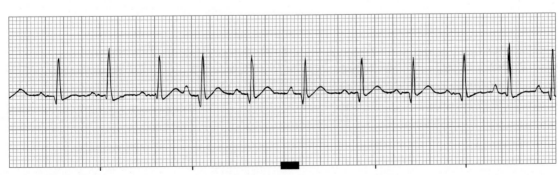

6. QRS complexes _____ Regularity _____ Heart rate _____

   P waves _____

   PR interval _____ QRS interval _____

   Interpretation _____

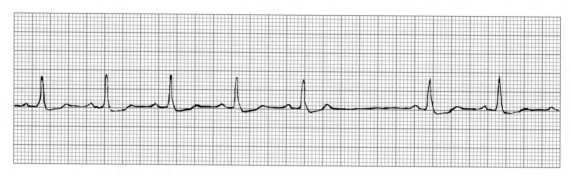

7. QRS complexes _____ Regularity _____ Heart rate _____

   P waves _____

   PR interval _____ QRS interval _____

   Interpretation _____

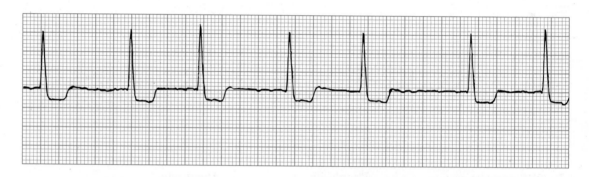

8. QRS complexes _____ Regularity _____ Heart rate _____

   P waves _____

   PR interval _____ QRS interval _____

   Interpretation _____

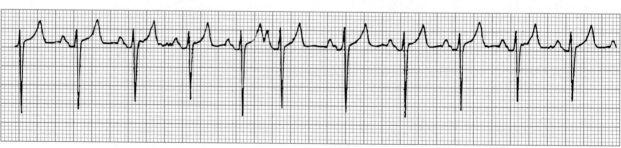

9. QRS complexes _____ Regularity _____ Heart rate _____

   P waves _____

   PR interval _____ QRS interval _____

   Interpretation _____

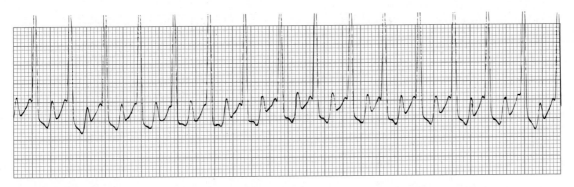

**10.** QRS complexes _____ Regularity _____ Heart rate _____

P waves _____

PR interval _____ QRS interval _____

Interpretation _____

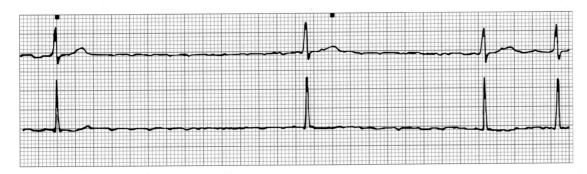

**11.** QRS complexes _____ Regularity _____ Heart rate _____

P waves _____

PR interval _____ QRS interval _____

Interpretation (name of rhythm) _____

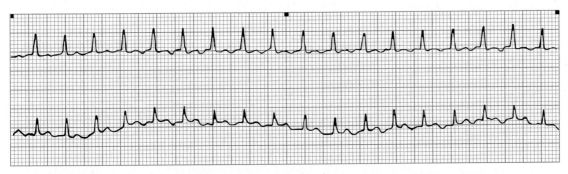

**12.** QRS complexes _____ Regularity _____ Heart rate _____

P waves _____

PR interval _____ QRS interval _____

Interpretation _____

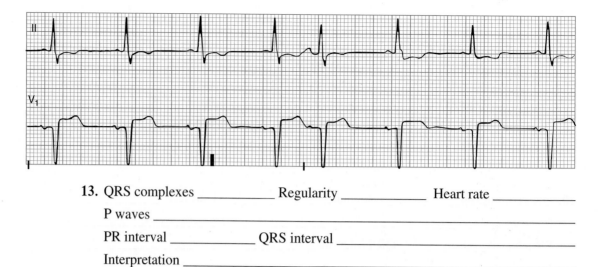

**13.** QRS complexes _____ Regularity _____ Heart rate _____

P waves _____

PR interval _____ QRS interval _____

Interpretation _____

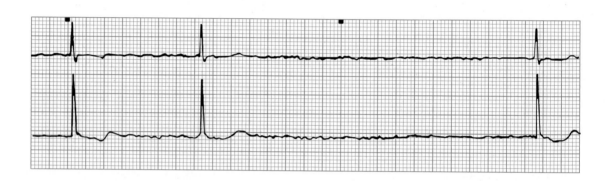

**14.** QRS complexes _____ Regularity _____ Heart rate _____

P waves _____

PR interval _____ QRS interval _____

Interpretation _____

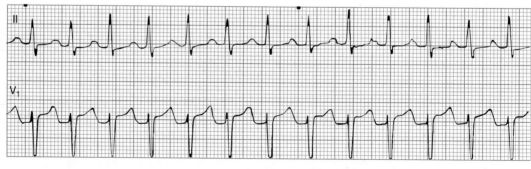

**15.** QRS complexes _____ Regularity _____ Heart rate _____

P waves _____

PR interval _____ QRS interval _____

Interpretation _____

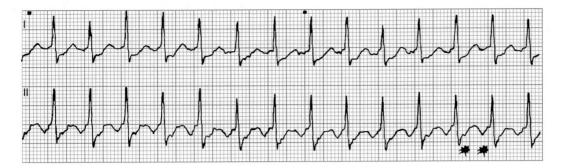

**16.** QRS complexes _____ Regularity _____ Heart rate _____

P waves _____

PR interval _____ QRS interval _____

Interpretation _____

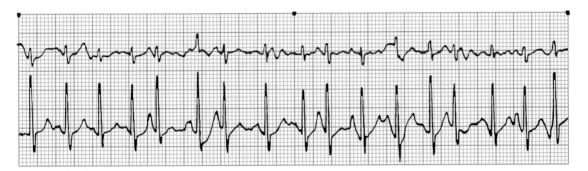

**17.** QRS complexes _____ Regularity _____ Heart rate _____

P waves _____

PR interval _____ QRS interval _____

Interpretation _____

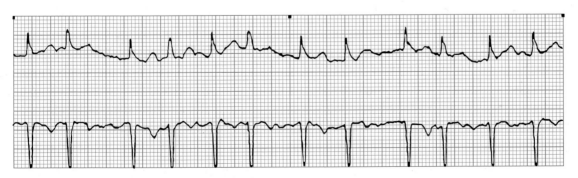

**18.** QRS complexes _____ Regularity _____ Heart rate _____

P waves _____

PR interval _____ QRS interval _____

Interpretation _____

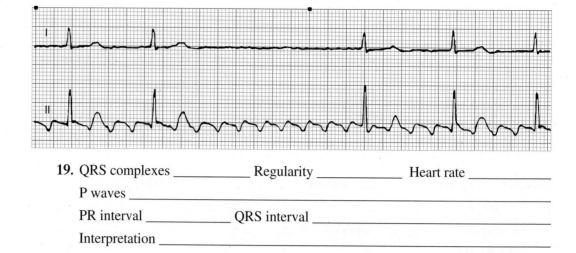

**19.** QRS complexes _____ Regularity _____ Heart rate _____

P waves _____

PR interval _____ QRS interval _____

Interpretation _____

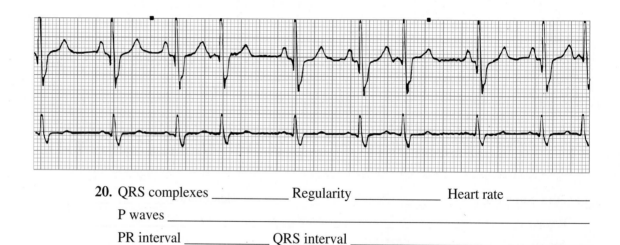

**20.** QRS complexes _____ Regularity _____ Heart rate _____

P waves _____

PR interval _____ QRS interval _____

Interpretation _____

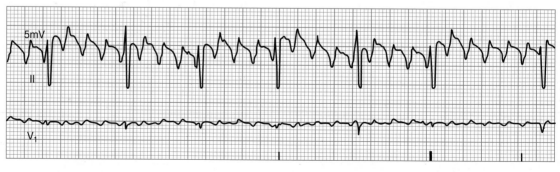

**21.** QRS complexes _____ Regularity _____ Heart rate _____

P waves _____

PR interval _____ QRS interval _____

Interpretation _____

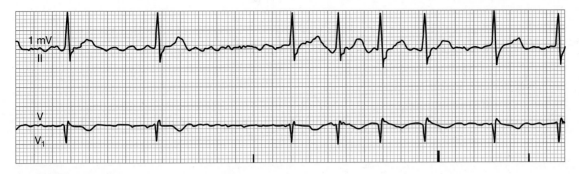

**22.** QRS complexes _____ Regularity _____ Heart rate _____

P waves _____

PR interval _____ QRS interval _____

Interpretation _____

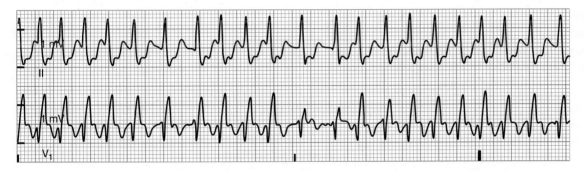

**23.** QRS complexes _____ Regularity _____ Heart rate _____

P waves _____

PR interval _____ QRS interval _____

Interpretation _____

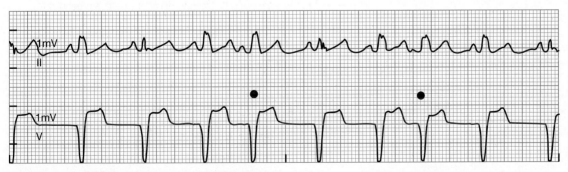

**24.** QRS complexes _____ Regularity _____ Heart rate _____

P waves _____

PR interval _____ QRS interval _____

Interpretation _____

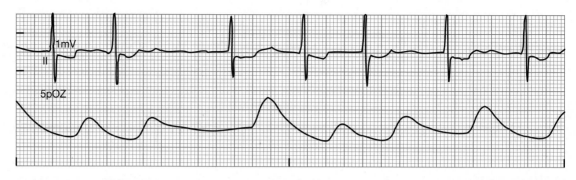

25. QRS complexes _____ Regularity _____ Heart rate _____

    P waves _____

    PR interval _____ QRS interval _____

    Interpretation _____

## chapter eight notes TO SUM IT ALL UP . . .

- **Atrial rhythms can have positive or negative QRS complexes depending on the lead being monitored. In** Lead II, the QRS should be positive; in V₁ they'll be negative.
- **Wandering atrial pacemaker (WAP)/Multifocal atrial tachycardia (MAT):**
  - *Heart rate*—WAP—mean rate <100
    MAT—mean rate >100
  - *Regularity*—Irregular
  - *P waves*—At least three different shapes
  - *Intervals*—PR varies; QRS <0.12 secs
  - *Causes*—WAP—medication side effects, MI, vagal stimulation
    MAT—typically COPD
  - *Adverse effects*—WAP—usually none
    MAT—signs of decreased cardiac output if heart rate too fast
  - *Treatment*—WAP—usually none needed
    MAT—beta blockers, calcium channel blockers
- **PACs:**
  - *Heart rate*—Can occur at any rate
  - *Regularity*—Cause the rhythm to be regular but interrupted by a premature beat
  - *P waves*—Different shape than sinus P waves. Ps may be hidden inside T waves.
  - *Intervals*—PR 0.12–0.20 secs; QRS <0.12 secs
  - *Causes*—Stimulants, medications, hypoxia, heart disease
  - *Adverse effects*—Usually none
  - *Treatment*—Oxygen, calcium channel blockers, beta blockers, omit stimulants, treat CHF if present
- **PAT:**
  - *Heart rate*—160–250. Rhythm it interrupts will have a different heart rate.
  - *Regularity*—The atrial tach itself is regular, but it will cause the whole strip to look regular but interrupted because it interrupts another rhythm.

- *P waves*—Different from sinus Ps; uniform shape
- *Intervals*—PR 0.12–0.20 secs; QRS <0.12 secs
- *Causes*—Same as PACs
- *Adverse effects*—Decreased heart rate
- *Treatment*—Digitalis, calcium channel blockers, beta blockers, adenosine, oxygen, electrical cardioversion
- **Atrial flutter:**
  - *Heart rate*—Atrial rate 250–350; ventricular rate varies depending on conduction ratio
  - *Regularity*—Regular, irregular, or regular but interrupted—depends on conduction ratio
  - *P waves*—No P waves. Flutter waves are present (zigzag waves of uniform shape).
  - *Intervals*—No PR interval because no P waves; QRS <0.12 secs
  - *Causes*—Heart disease, pulmonary embolus, lung disease, heart valve disease
  - *Adverse effects*—Decreased cardiac output if heart rate too fast or too slow
  - *Treatment*—Oxygen, calcium channel blockers, beta blockers, adenosine, digitalis
- **Atrial fibrillation:**
  - *Heart rate*—Atrial rate 350–700; ventricular rate varies
  - *Regularity*—Irregularly irregular
  - *P waves*—No P waves. Fibrillatory waves present (undulating baseline).
  - *Intervals*—No PR interval because no P waves; QRS <0.12 secs
  - *Causes*—MI, lung disease, heart valve disease, hyperthyroidism
  - *Adverse effects*—Decreased cardiac output, blood clots that can cause strokes, pulmonary emboli, or MI
  - *Treatment*—If duration <48 hours—digitalis, calcium channel blockers, beta blockers, amiodarone, or electrical

cardioversion; if duration >48 hours—anticoagulants for 2–3 weeks, then cardioversion. In emergencies—start on heparin, do a TEE to check for blood clots in the atria, then cardiovert.

- **SVT:**
  - *Heart rate*—130 or higher
  - *Regularity*—Regular
  - *P waves*—None seen

- *Intervals*—No PR interval because can't see P waves; QRS <0.12 secs
- *Causes*—Same as PAT
- *Adverse effects*—Decreased cardiac output
- *Treatment*—Adenosine, digitalis, ibutilide, calcium channel blockers, beta blockers, oxygen, electrical cardioversion

## Practice Quiz

1. What common complication of atrial fibrillation can be prevented by the use of anticoagulant medications?

_____

2. The rhythm that is the same as wandering atrial pacemaker except for the heart rate is _____

_____

3. The rhythm that produces V-shaped waves between QRS complexes is

_____

4. Atrial rhythms take which path to the ventricles?

_____

5. All rhythms that originate in a pacemaker other than the sinus node are called _____

6. Treatment for atrial fibrillation is dependent on which factor? _____

_____

7. True or false: All PACs conduct through to the ventricles.

8. The classic cause of multifocal atrial tachycardia is

_____

9. Which test can be used in emergencies to determine if atrial blood clots are present? _____

_____

10. If the rhythm is regular, heart rate is 130 or greater, and P waves cannot be identified, the rhythm is called

_____

## Putting It All Together—Critical Thinking Exercises

These exercises may consist of diagrams to label, scenarios to analyze, brain-stumping questions to ponder, or other challenging exercises to boost your knowledge of the chapter material.

Let's play with atrial rhythms a bit. The following scenario will provide you with information about a fictional patient and ask you to analyze the situation, answer questions, and decide on appropriate actions.

Mr. Baldo, a 20-year-old college student, awoke feeling palpitations in his chest. He arrives at your emergency department an hour later with the following vital signs: BP normal at 130/78, respirations 22, temp 98.0 degrees. Skin is warm and dry. No pain, shortness of breath, or other distress aside from feeling the palpitations off and on. He denies ever having felt anything like this before. His rhythm strip is shown in Figure 8–12.

1. What is Mr. Baldo's rhythm and heart rate?

_____

2. Is his situation an emergency? Why or why not?

_____

3. Because Mr. Baldo's rhythm started this morning, what medication do we *not* need to consider as a part of his treatment? _____

4. What treatment would be appropriate for Mr. Baldo's rhythm? _____

_____

Mr. Baldo is given medication and, within the hour, the nurse records the following rhythm strip. See Figure 8–13.

5. What's happening on this strip?_____

_____

Mr. Baldo is watched in your emergency department for 2 more hours and then discharged with the rhythm shown in Figure 8–14. He is sent home with medication and told to follow up with a cardiologist for more studies.

**6.** What is Mr. Baldo's rhythm on discharge?

_____

_____

_____

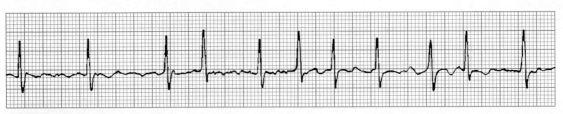

**FIGURE 8–12**

Mr. Baldo's initial strip.

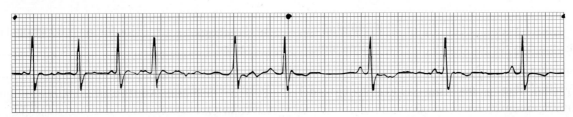

**FIGURE 8–13**

Rhythm after medication.

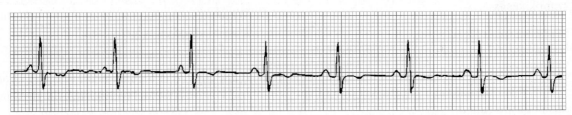

**FIGURE 8–14**

Discharge rhythm.

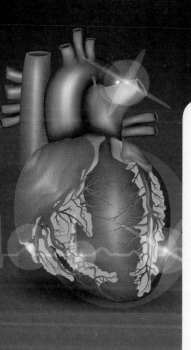

# Rhythms Originating in the AV Junction

# 9

## CHAPTER 9 OBJECTIVES

Upon completion of this chapter, the student will be able to

- State the criteria for each junctional rhythm.
- Differentiate among *high, low,* and *midjunctional impulses.*
- Correctly identify the junctional rhythms on a variety of strips.
- State the adverse effects of each junctional rhythm.

- State the possible treatment for the junctional rhythms.
- State which junctional rhythms occur mostly because of escape and which imply usurpation.

## What It's All About

Mr. Alvin thought he was getting the flu, so he took a sick day from work and stayed in bed. He took some cold medicine but didn't feel any better. So he took another dose. When his wife came home from work, she found Mr. Alvin still in bed. He complained that he had thought at first he had the flu but now he wasn't so sure because now he was getting chest pain. His wife scooped up all of his medications, put them in a paper bag, and drove Alvin to the hospital. In the emergency department, Mr. Alvin had labs drawn and had an EKG, which showed *junctional tachycardia* with a heart rate of 160. He was not having a heart attack, the physician told him—he had a toxic amount of digitalis in his system. "How did that happen? I take only one digitalis a day," Mr. Alvin said. "Show me which medicine you took this morning," his nurse said on a hunch. Alvin reached into the paper bag and showed the nurse his bottle of cold pills. The "cold medicine" was actually his digitalis. Because of Mr. Alvin's poor vision, he'd grabbed the wrong medication and had taken several doses of digitalis over and above his normal daily dose. The chest pain he experienced was caused by the fast heart rate and went away once Mr. Alvin's heart rate returned to normal.

## Introduction

Junctional rhythms arise from the **AV junction**, the tissue located between the right atrium and ventricle and surrounding the AV node.

The impulse originates around the AV node and travels **antegrade**, or forward, toward the ventricle, and **retrograde**, or backward, toward the atria. Thus, the impulse travels in two directions. The AV junctional area can be divided into regions—high, mid, and low—and whichever of these regions initiates the impulse will determine the location of the P wave. If the impulse originates high in the AV junction, close to the atria, it will arrive at the atria first and write an **inverted** (upside down) P wave. The P wave is inverted because the impulse is going in a backward direction to reach the atria. Then the forward impulses reach the ventricle and write the QRS complex. The PR interval is short, less than 0.12 second. Because the impulse starts out in the AV junction, halfway to the ventricle, it simply doesn't have as far to go as sinus impulses would. Bottom line: *If the impulse originates high in the AV junction, the resultant rhythm or beat will have an inverted P wave preceding the QRS, and the PR interval should be less than 0.12 secs.*

If the impulses originate midway in the AV junction, the impulses will reach the atria and ventricles simultaneously because both are the same distance from the AV junction.

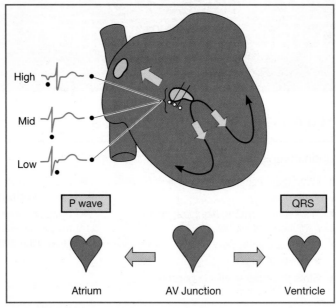

**FIGURE 9–1**

**Conduction and P wave location in junctional rhythms.**

Therefore, the P wave will be swallowed up by the QRS complex. Bottom line: *Midjunctional impulses have no visible P waves.*

If the impulses originate low in the AV junction, the impulses will reach the ventricle first, writing a QRS complex, and then reaching the atria and writing the P wave. Thus, the P wave will follow the QRS and, because the impulses must travel backward to reach the atria, the P wave will be inverted. Bottom line: *Impulses originating from low in the AV junction have inverted P waves following the QRS complex.* See Figure 9–1.

## The Word on Junctional Rhythms

Junctional rhythms are seen less often than sinus or atrial rhythms. Although the inherent rate of the AV junction is 40 to 60, the heart rate could actually be much faster or slower, which can result in symptoms. More normal heart rates are less likely to cause symptoms.

Treatment is aimed at alleviating the cause of the junctional rhythm. More active treatment is not usually necessary unless symptoms develop, at which time the goal is to return the sinus node to control or to return the heart rate to more normal levels.

Junctional rhythms are easy to identify. Let's look at the criteria. See Table 9–1.

**TABLE 9–1   Criteria for Junctional Rhythms**

Regular rhythm or premature beat with a narrow QRS along with one of the following:

Absent P waves

Inverted P waves following the QRS

Inverted P waves with short PR interval preceding the QRS

*It's important to note that the QRS in junctional rhythms can be positive (upright) or negative (downward) depending on the lead the patient is being monitored in.* For example, the QRS in Lead II should be positive, but in $V_1$ should be negative. Look back to Chapter 3 for a refresher on this if needed. Now let's look at the junctional rhythms in detail.

## Premature Junctional Complexes (PJCs)

*Premature junctional complexes* (PJCs) are premature beats that originate in the AV junction before the next sinus beat is due. This is caused by irritable tissue in the AV junction firing and usurping the sinus node for that beat.

| | |
|---|---|
| Rate | Can occur at any rate |
| Regularity | Regular but interrupted |
| P waves | Inverted before or after the QRS, or hidden inside the QRS |
| Intervals | PR <0.12 secs if the P wave precedes the QRS<br>QRS <0.12 secs |
| Cause | Stimulants (such as caffeine or drugs), nicotine, hypoxia, heart disease |
| Adverse effects | Usually no ill effects |
| Treatment | Usually none required aside from removal of the cause |

Figure 9–2 shows QRS complexes, all shaped the same. Regularity is regular but interrupted (by 2 premature beats). Heart rate is 71. P waves are matching and biphasic except for the fourth and eighth beats, which are premature and have no P waves. PR interval is 0.16, and QRS is 0.10. Interpretation: sinus rhythm with 2 PJCs.

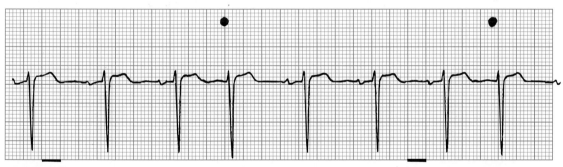

**FIGURE 9–2**

**PJC.**

## Junctional Bradycardia

*Junctional bradycardia* is a junctional rhythm with a heart rate slower than usual. A higher pacemaker has failed, and the AV junction has to escape to save the patient's life.

| | |
|---|---|
| Rate | <40 |
| Regularity | Regular |
| P waves | Inverted before or after the QRS, or hidden inside the QRS |
| Intervals | PR <0.12 secs if the P precedes the QRS<br>QRS <0.12 secs |
| Cause | Vagal stimulation, hypoxia, ischemia of the sinus node, heart disease |
| Adverse effects | Slow heart rate can cause decreased cardiac output. |
| Treatment | Prepare for immediate transcutaneous pacing (attaching a pacemaker to the patient's skin) if the patient is symptomatic. If the pacemaker is not immediately available and the patient is symptomatic, give atropine or consider starting an epinephrine or dopamine infusion to increase the heart rate. Start oxygen. Stop any heart rate–slowing medications. |

Figure 9–3 shows QRS complexes, all shaped the same. Regularity is regular. Heart rate is 23. P waves are absent, or at least not visible. There is some somatic tremor artifact causing the baseline to look a bit jittery. PR interval is not applicable. QRS interval is 0.12, wider than normal. Whenever the QRS interval is longer than normal, document this in your interpretation. Interpretation: junctional bradycardia with a wide QRS.

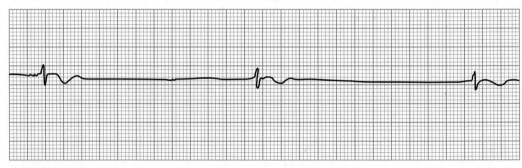

**FIGURE 9–3**

**Junctional bradycardia.**

# Junctional Rhythm

*Junctional rhythm* is a rhythm that originates in the AV junction at its inherent rate of 40 to 60. It is usually an escape rhythm.

| | |
|---|---|
| Rate | 40 to 60 |
| Regularity | Regular |
| P waves | Inverted before or after the QRS, or hidden inside the QRS |
| Intervals | PR <0.12 secs if the P precedes the QRS |
| | QRS <0.12 secs. |
| Cause | Vagal stimulation, hypoxia, sinus node ischemia, heart disease |
| Adverse effects | Usually none if the heart rate is closer to the 50s to 60s range. Signs of decreased cardiac output are possible at slower heart rates. |
| Treatment | Transcutaneous pacing, atropine, dopamine or epinephrine infusion if symptomatic from the slow heart rate. Withdraw or decrease any medications that can slow the heart rate. Consider starting oxygen. |

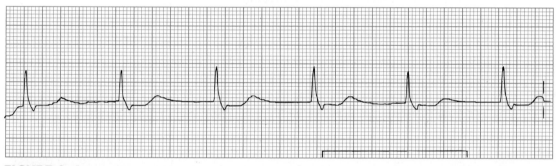

**FIGURE 9–4**

**Junctional rhythm.**

Figure 9–4 shows QRS complexes, all the same shape. Regularity is regular. Heart rate is 58. P waves are absent. (Those are not P waves after the QRS; those are S waves, a part of the QRS.) PR interval is not applicable. QRS interval is 0.12. Interpretation: junctional rhythm with a wide QRS. Although this example of junctional rhythm has no visible P waves, it could just as easily have had an inverted P wave with a short PR interval preceding the QRS, or an inverted P wave following the QRS. Remember, *the location of the P wave is dependent on the region of the AV junction in which the impulse originates.*

## Accelerated Junctional Rhythm

*Accelerated junctional rhythm* can occur because of escape or usurpation. If the sinus node slows down, the AV junction can escape and take over as the pacemaker. Or an irritable spot in the AV junction can usurp control from the slower sinus node and become the heart's pacemaker at a faster-than-normal rate.

| | |
|---|---|
| Rate | 60 to 100 |
| Regularity | Regular |
| P waves | Inverted before or after the QRS, or hidden inside the QRS |
| Intervals | PR <0.12 secs if the P precedes the QRS <br> QRS <0.12 secs |
| Cause | Heart disease, stimulant drugs, and caffeine |
| Adverse effects | Usually none because the heart rate is within normal limits |
| Treatment | Usually none required aside from removal of the cause |

Figure 9–5 shows QRS complexes, all the same shape. Regularity is regular. Heart rate is 75. P waves are absent. PR interval is not applicable. QRS interval is 0.08. Interpretation: accelerated junctional rhythm.

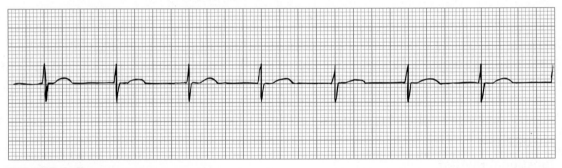

**FIGURE 9–5**

**Accelerated junctional rhythm.**

## Junctional Tachycardia

An irritable spot in the AV junction has taken over as the pacemaker, and the heart rate is very rapid. This is usually a result of usurpation. Junctional tachycardia is best called SVT (supraventricular tachycardia) if there are no visible P waves, as the origin of the rhythm is not identifiable.

| | |
|---|---|
| Rate | >100 |
| Regularity | Regular |
| P waves | Inverted before or after the QRS, or hidden inside the QRS |
| Intervals | PR <0.12 secs if the P precedes the QRS<br>QRS <0.12 secs |
| Cause | Most often caused by digitalis toxicity, but can be caused by heart disease, stimulants, or sympathetic nervous system stimulation |
| Adverse effects | Decreased cardiac output possible if the heart rate is fast enough |
| Treatment | Beta-blockers, calcium channel blockers, adenosine. Consider starting oxygen. Electrical cardioversion can be done if the patient is unstable. |

Figure 9–6 shows QRS complexes, all the same shape. Regularity is regular. Heart rate is 125. P waves are present, inverted, following the QRS complex. PR interval is not applicable. QRS interval is 0.08. Interpretation: junctional tachycardia.

See Table 9–2 and Figure 9–7 to review junctional rhythms. Then move on to the practice strips.

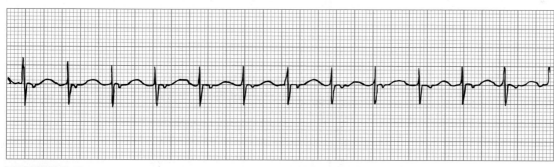

**FIGURE 9–6**

**Junctional tachycardia**

**TABLE 9–2    Rhythm Summary: Junctional Rhythms**

| | Rate | Regularity | P Wave | QRS | Cause | Adverse Effects | Treatment |
|---|---|---|---|---|---|---|---|
| PJCs | Can occur at any rate | Regular but interrupted | Inverted before or after QRS or hidden inside QRS | <0.12 | Stimulants, caffeine, hypoxia, heart disease, or normal | Usually no ill effects | Usually none required |
| Junctional bradycardia | <40 | Regular | Inverted before or after QRS or hidden inside QRS | <0.12 | Vagal stimulation, hypoxia, sinus node ischemia, MI | Decreased cardiac output | Pacemaker or atropine if symptoms; hold medications that can slow the HR; start $O_2$ |
| Junctional rhythm | 40–60 | Regular | Inverted before or after QRS or hidden inside QRS | <0.12 | Vagal stimulation, hypoxia, sinus node ischemia, MI | Well tolerated if HR closer to 50–60; decreased cardiac output possible | Pacemaker or atropine if symptoms; hold medications that can slow the HR; start $O_2$ |
| Accelerated junctional | 60–100 | Regular | Inverted before or after QRS or hidden inside QRS | <0.12 | Heart disease, stimulant drugs, caffeine | Usually no ill effects | Usually none needed |
| Junctional tach | >100 | Regular | Inverted before or after QRS or hidden inside QRS | <0.12 | Digitalis toxicity, heart disease, stimulants, sympathetic nervous system stimulation | Decreased cardiac output at faster heart rates | Beta-blockers, calcium channel blockers, adenosine; consider $O_2$ and electrical cardioversion |

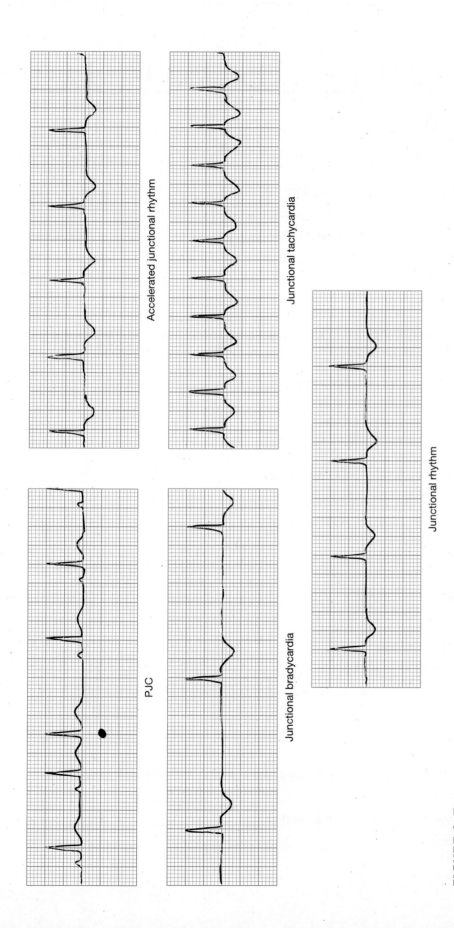

Accelerated junctional rhythm

Junctional tachycardia

PJC

Junctional bradycardia

Junctional rhythm

**FIGURE 9–7**

## Junctional Rhythms Pictorial Review.

## Practice Strips: Junctional Rhythms

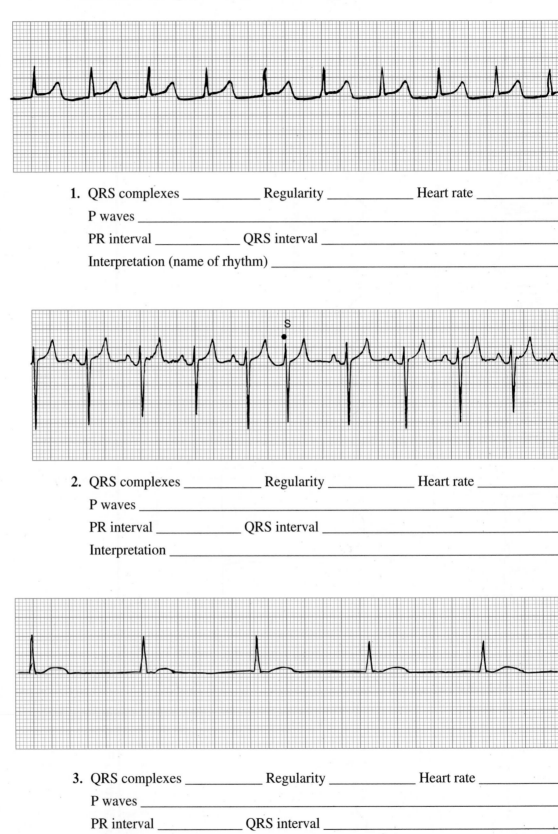

1. QRS complexes _____ Regularity _____ Heart rate _____

   P waves _____

   PR interval _____ QRS interval _____

   Interpretation (name of rhythm) _____

2. QRS complexes _____ Regularity _____ Heart rate _____

   P waves _____

   PR interval _____ QRS interval _____

   Interpretation _____

3. QRS complexes _____ Regularity _____ Heart rate _____

   P waves _____

   PR interval _____ QRS interval _____

   Interpretation _____

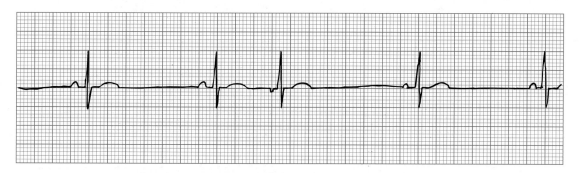

4. QRS complexes _____ Regularity _____ Heart rate _____

   P waves _____

   PR interval _____ QRS interval _____

   Interpretation _____

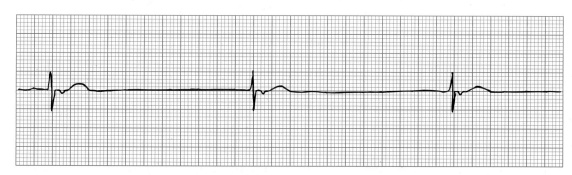

5. QRS complexes _____ Regularity _____ Heart rate _____

   P waves _____

   PR interval _____ QRS interval _____

   Interpretation _____

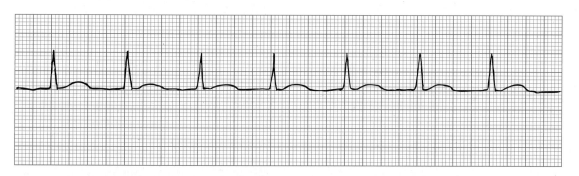

6. QRS complexes _____ Regularity _____ Heart rate _____

   P waves _____

   PR interval _____ QRS interval _____

   Interpretation _____

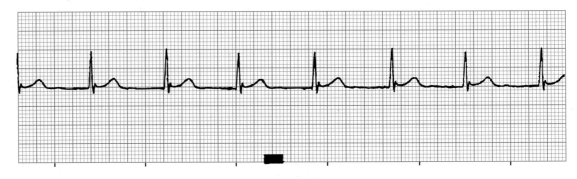

7. QRS complexes _____ Regularity _____ Heart rate _____

   P waves _____

   PR interval _____ QRS interval _____

   Interpretation _____

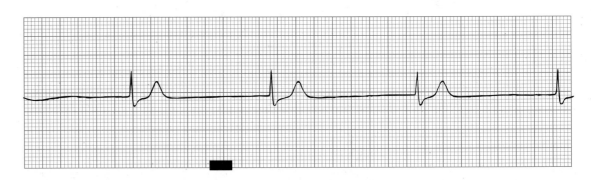

8. QRS complexes _____ Regularity _____ Heart rate _____

   P waves _____

   PR interval _____ QRS interval _____

   Interpretation _____

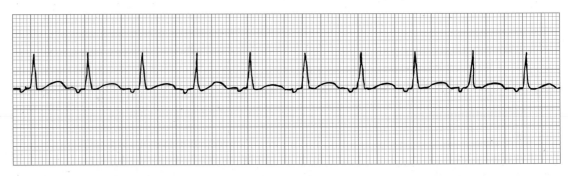

9. QRS complexes _____ Regularity _____ Heart rate _____

   P waves _____

   PR interval _____ QRS interval _____

   Interpretation _____

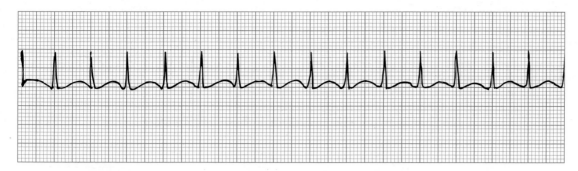

**10.** QRS complexes _____ Regularity _____ Heart rate _____

P waves _____

PR interval _____ QRS interval _____

Interpretation _____

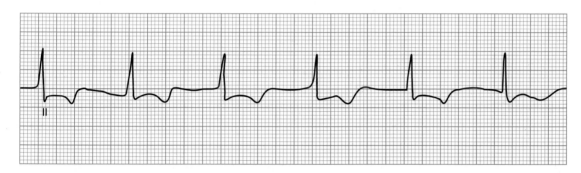

**11.** QRS complexes _____ Regularity _____ Heart rate _____

P waves _____

PR interval _____ QRS interval _____

Interpretation _____

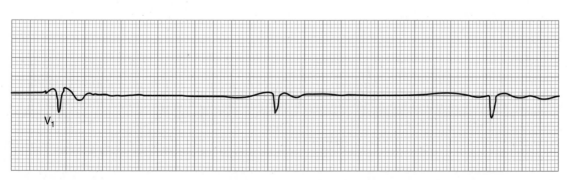

**12.** QRS complexes _____ Regularity _____ Heart rate _____

P waves _____

PR interval _____ QRS interval _____

Interpretation _____

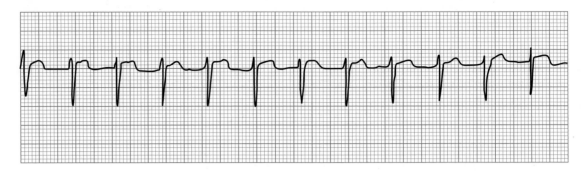

**13.** QRS complexes _____ Regularity _____ Heart rate _____

P waves _____

PR interval _____ QRS interval _____

Interpretation _____

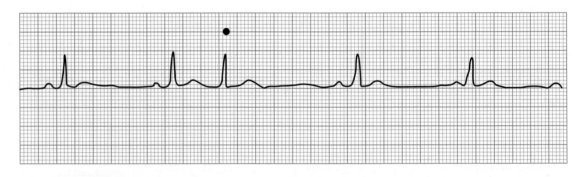

**14.** QRS complexes _____ Regularity _____ Heart rate _____

P waves _____

PR interval _____ QRS interval _____

Interpretation _____

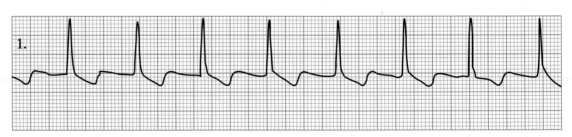

**15.** QRS complexes _____ Regularity _____ Heart rate _____

P waves _____

PR interval _____ QRS interval _____

Interpretation _____

**chapter nine notes** TO SUM IT ALL UP . . .

- **Junctional rhythms**—Arise from tissue located between the right atrium and right ventricle, an area known as the AV junction.
- **In junctional rhythms, the impulse travels antegrade toward the ventricles and retrograde toward the atria.**
- **P waves in junctional rhythms can be inverted preceding the QRS, inverted following the QRS, or hidden inside the QRS (invisible).**
- **The QRS in junctional rhythms will be positive or negative depending on the lead being monitored.** In Lead II, for example, the QRS should be positive; in V₁ it should be negative.
- **PJCs:**
  - *Heart rate*—Can occur at any heart rate
  - *Regularity*—Regular but interrupted by a premature beat
  - *P waves*—Inverted preceding or following the QRS, or hidden inside the QRS
  - *Intervals*—PR <0.12 secs if P wave precedes QRS; QRS <0.12 secs
  - *Causes*—Stimulants such as caffeine or drugs, nicotine, hypoxia, heart disease
  - *Adverse effects*—Usually none
  - *Treatment*—None except treat the cause
- **Junctional bradycardia:**
  - *Heart rate*—<40
  - *Regularity*—Regular
  - *P waves*—Inverted preceding or following the QRS, or hidden inside QRS
  - *Intervals*—PR <0.12 secs if P wave precedes QRS; QRS <0.12 secs
  - *Causes*—Vagal stimulation, hypoxia, sinus node ischemia, heart disease
  - *Adverse effects*—Decreased cardiac output
  - *Treatment*—Atropine, pacemaker, epinephrine or dopamine infusions, oxygen, stop any heart rate–slowing medications
- **Junctional rhythm:**
  - *Heart rate*—40–60
  - *Regularity*—Regular

  - *P waves*—Inverted preceding or following the QRS, or hidden inside QRS
  - *Intervals*—PR <0.12 secs if P wave precedes QRS; QRS <0.12 secs
  - *Causes*—Vagal stimulation, hypoxia, sinus node ischemia, heart disease
  - *Adverse effects*—Usually none if heart rate closer to 50–60; decreased cardiac output possible at slower rates
  - *Treatment*—Atropine, pacemaker, epinephrine or dopamine infusion, oxygen, stop heart rate–slowing medications
- **Accelerated junctional rhythm:**
  - *Heart rate*—60–100
  - *Regularity*—Regular
  - *P waves*—Inverted preceding or following the QRS, or hidden inside QRS
  - *Intervals*—PR <0.12 secs if P wave precedes QRS; QRS <0.12 secs
  - *Causes*—Heart disease, stimulant drugs, caffeine
  - *Adverse effects*—Usually none
  - *Treatment*—None except to treat the cause
- **Junctional tachycardia:**
  - *Heart rate*—>100
  - *Regularity*—Regular
  - *P waves*—Inverted preceding or following the QRS, or hidden inside QRS
  - *Intervals*—PR <0.12 secs if P wave precedes QRS; QRS <0.12 secs
  - *Causes*—Digitalis toxicity is main cause; heart disease, stimulants
  - *Adverse effects*—Decreased cardiac output if heart rate too fast
  - *Treatment*—Stop digitalis; start beta blockers, calcium channel blockers, or adenosine; consider cardioversion
- **Junctional tachycardia with no visible P waves is best called SVT, because there is no proof there even *are* P waves there.** There is no way to know the rhythm's origin for sure.

## Practice Quiz

1. What are the three possible locations for the P waves in junctional rhythms? _____
_____
_____

2. Why is the P wave inverted in junctional rhythms?
_____
_____

3. A junctional rhythm with a heart rate greater than 100 is _____
_____

4. True or false: PJCs are a sign that the heart is going to develop a lethal arrhythmia.

5. A junctional rhythm with a heart rate less than 40 is _____
_____

6. Treatment for junctional bradycardia could consist of
_____
_____
_____

7. PJCs cause the regularity to be _____

8. Is junctional bradycardia usually a result of escape or usurpation? _____
_____

9. Junctional tachycardia is best called SVT if the P waves are located where? _____
_____

10. Is junctional tachycardia a result of escape or usurpation? _____
_____
_____

## Putting It All Together—Critical Thinking Exercises

These exercises may consist of diagrams to label, scenarios to analyze, brain-stumping questions to ponder, or other challenging exercises to boost your understanding of the chapter material.

Let's play with junctional rhythms a bit. The following scenario will provide you with information about a fictional patient and ask you to analyze the situation, answer questions, and decide on appropriate actions.

Mrs. Dubos, age 86, is to be admitted to your intensive care unit. The ER nurse reports the following: Mrs. Dubos came to the ER complaining of shortness of breath and chest pain. Examination in the ER found her to be in sinus bradycardia with a heart rate of 47. BP at that time was 76/43 (very low), respirations 34 (fast), and temperature was normal. She was cool and clammy and appeared a bit dazed and confused. After appropriate medication, the heart rate came up to 86, her BP came up to 132/74 (normal), and her respirations slowed to a normal 20. Chest pain and shortness of breath subsided.

1. What medication do you believe was given in the ER to speed up Mrs. Dubos's heart rate? _____

   When Mrs. Dubos arrives on your floor, you look at the ER rhythm strip. See Figure 9–8.

2. What is the rhythm and rate? _____

   _____

3. Was the ER nurse correct in her interpretation of this rhythm and rate? Explain. _____

   _____

   _____

   _____

4. Do you agree that the treatment rendered in the ER was appropriate for this patient? Why or why not?

   _____

   _____

   _____

5. Did Mrs. Dubos have signs of decreased cardiac output in the ER? If yes, what were they?

   _____

   _____

   _____

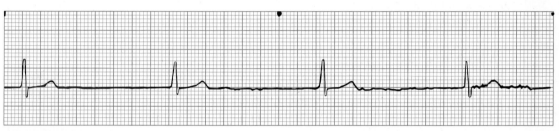

**FIGURE 9–8**

**Mrs. Dubos's ER rhythm strip.**

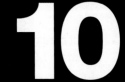

# Rhythms Originating in the Ventricles

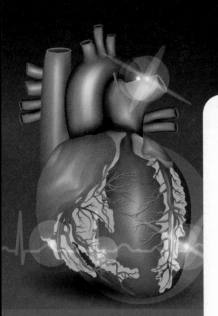

## CHAPTER 10 OBJECTIVES

Upon completion of this chapter, the student will be able to

- State the criteria for each of the ventricular rhythms.
- Correctly identify ventricular rhythms on a variety of strips.
- State the adverse effects for each ventricular rhythm.
- State the possible treatment for the ventricular rhythms.
- Explain fusion beats.

## What It's All About

Chris was at the gas station when he saw an elderly man clutch his chest and collapse. An experienced ICU nurse, Chris quickly determined the man was in cardiac arrest. He yelled for bystanders to call 911 and began doing CPR. The paramedics soon arrived and were briefed by Chris, who told them he suspected the patient had had a heart attack and was in ventricular fibrillation. Seeing that Chris was doing effective CPR, the paramedics attached the patient to the heart monitor and evaluated the man's heart rhythm. He was indeed in ventricular fibrillation—Chris recognized the telltale pattern on the monitor immediately. He knew what was coming next. The paramedics ordered Chris out of the way and immediately defibrillated the heart. The rhythm converted to sinus rhythm for a few beats, then slowed dramatically and the QRS widened. There was no pulse. Paramedics quickly resumed CPR, inserted an IV line, and gave medications. Soon the pulse returned and the man was loaded into the ambulance and taken to a nearby hospital, where it was discovered that he'd had a heart attack that had caused his ventricular fibrillation.

## Introduction

Ventricular rhythms originate in one or more irritable foci in the ventricular tissue below the conduction system pathway. Without the benefit of this conduction pathway to speed the impulses through the tissue, the impulses trudge very slowly, cell by cell, through the ventricle, producing a wide QRS complex that measures >0.12 seconds. The impulse does sometimes travel backward to depolarize the atria, but the resultant P wave is usually lost in the mammoth QRS complex. Slow ventricular rhythms are the heart's last gasp as a pacemaker, kicking in when the higher pacemakers can't. Rapid ventricular arrhythmias can result in drastically decreased cardiac output, cardiovascular collapse, and death. See Figures 10–1 and 10–2.

In Figure 10–1, a single ventricular focus sends its impulse out, depolarizing the ventricles and providing the QRS complex. The impulse then heads backwards toward the atria to depolarize them, resulting in a P wave that may or may not be seen.

In Figure 10–2, multiple ventricular foci are firing off, each depolarizing its own little piece of ventricular territory. Rather than a QRS, which implies coordinated ventricular depolarization, this scenario results in a waveform that resembles static—no QRS in sight. This is a lethal rhythm unless properly treated.

# The Word on Ventricular Rhythms

Ventricular rhythms, the most lethal of all the rhythms, command great respect from health care personnel. They can result from escape or usurpation and can have a heart rate varying from 0 to more than 250 beats per minute. Although some ventricular rhythms can be well tolerated, many will cause symptoms of decreased cardiac output or—even worse—cardiac standstill.

Most ventricular rhythms respond well to medications. Unfortunately, some of the very medications used to treat ventricular rhythms can *cause* them in some circumstances. Some ventricular rhythms can be treated only by electric shock to the heart. And others, despite aggressive treatment, are usually fatal.

Some ventricular rhythms have no QRS at all; others have wide, bizarre QRS complexes. If the rhythm or beat in question meets *any* of the following criteria, it is ventricular in origin. See Table 10–1.

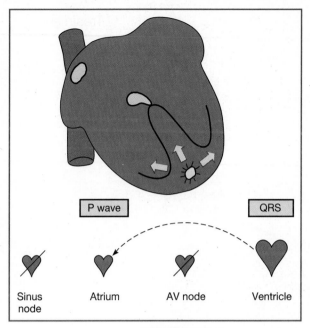

**FIGURE 10–1**

**Conduction of a single ventricular focus.**

**TABLE 10–1    Criteria for Ventricular Beats/Rhythms.**

| |
|---|
| Premature, wide QRS beat without preceding P wave, interrupting another rhythm *or* |
| No QRS at all (*or* can't be sure if there are QRS complexes) *or* |
| Rhythms that have wide QRS (>0.12 secs) without preceding P wave |

Let's look at these rhythms in detail now.

# Premature Ventricular Complexes (PVCs)

*Premature ventricular complexes* (PVCs) are premature beats that originate in irritable ventricular tissue before the next sinus beat is due.

| | |
|---|---|
| Rate | Can occur at any rate |
| Regularity | Regular but interrupted |
| P waves | Usually not seen on PVCs |
| Intervals | PR not applicable (because no P wave)<br>QRS interval >0.12 secs; QRS wide and bizarre in shape |
| T wave | Slopes off in the opposite direction to the QRS. If the QRS points upward, for example, the T wave will point downward. |
| Cause | The most frequent causes are heart disease, hypokalemia (low blood potassium level), and hypoxia. Other causes include medications, low blood magnesium level, stimulants, caffeine, stress, or anxiety. All these factors can cause the ventricle to become irritable and fire early beats. |
| Adverse effects | Occasional PVCs are of no concern. Frequent PVCs (6 or more per minute) or PVCs that are close to or land on the downstroke of the previous beat's T wave (a condition called R-on-T phenomenon) can progress to lethal ventricular arrhythmias. Multifocal PVCs (those with differing shapes) are also cause for concern, as they indicate multiple irritable areas. |

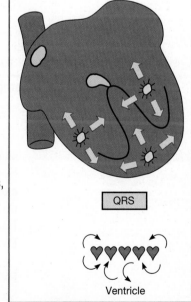

**FIGURE 10–2**

**Conduction of multiple ventricular foci.**

Treatment

Occasional PVCs can occur in normal healthy hearts and don't require treatment. For frequent PVCs, especially in the presence of myocardial ischemia or infarction, treat the cause. For example, if the potassium level is low, give supplemental potassium. If hypoxic, start oxygen. Antiarrhythmic medications such as amiodarone and lidocaine may be used to treat frequent PVCs, but the benefits of using these or any medications must be weighed against the medication's potential side effects. For many patients with frequent PVCs, the preferred treatment is cautious observation and follow-up by a cardiologist (physician specializing in cardiac disease). For frequent PVCs during a slow bradycardia, do not treat with antiarrhythmics; treat with atropine instead. Bradycardic rhythm PVCs are the heart's attempt to increase the heart rate by providing another beat from *somewhere*. Giving antiarrhythmics could knock out the PVCs, leaving a slower heart rate. Atropine would speed up the underlying rhythm and the PVCs should go away on their own. For patients with frequent *symptomatic* PVCs despite treatment, catheter ablation, a method of destroying the irritable focus causing the arrhythmia, may be advised. See Figure 10–3.

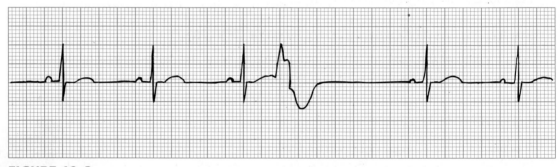

**FIGURE 10–3**

**PVC (example of R-on-T PVC).**

Figure 10–3 shows QRS complexes, all except the fourth beat having the same shape. The fourth beat has a wide QRS complex. Regularity is regular but interrupted by the premature beat. Heart rate is 60. There are matching upright P waves on all beats except the fourth beat, which has no P wave at all. PR interval is 0.16 on the sinus beats, no PR interval on the PVC. QRS interval is 0.08 on the sinus beats, 0.14 on the PVC. Interpretation: sinus rhythm with one PVC. This is an example of an R-on-T PVC, as the PVC lands on the downstroke of the previous beat's T wave.

PVCs that come from a single focus all look alike. They're called unifocal PVCs. PVCs from different foci look different. They're called multifocal PVCs. See Figure 10–4. Strip A's PVCs are shaped the same—they're unifocal. Strip B's PVCs are shaped differently—they're multifocal.

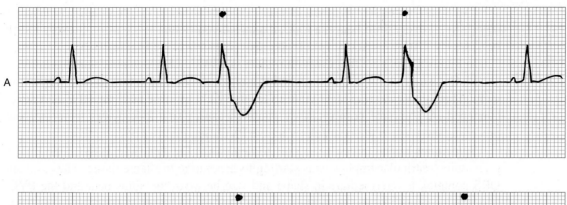

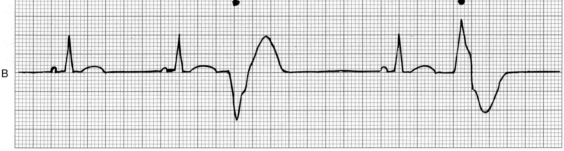

**FIGURE 10–4**

**(A) Unifocal PVCs; (B) Multifocal PVCs.**

*An important word about the shape of the QRS complex in ventricular beats/rhythms; depending on the lead being monitored and the ventricle propagating the ventricular beats, the QRS may be positive or negative.* The best lead(s) to use for identification of ventricular beats or rhythms is $V_1$ or $MCL_1$. With these leads, it's possible to tell from which ventricle the rhythm/beats originated. This can be very important. *Left-ventricular PVCs have an upward deflection in $V_1/MCL_1$. Right-ventricular PVCs have a downward deflection in $V_1/MCL_1$* In Figure 10–4, if the lead were $V_1$, strip A's PVCs would be from the left ventricle, as they're both positive. Strip B's first PVC would be right ventricular, because it is negative, and the second PVC would be left ventricular, because it is positive. Left ventricular PVCs are considered more significant than right ventricular PVCs. Because the left ventricle is the major pumping chamber of the heart, anything that adversely affects it can have profound implications on cardiac output.

Two consecutive PVCs are called a couplet. Couplets can be either unifocal or multifocal. See Figure 10–5.

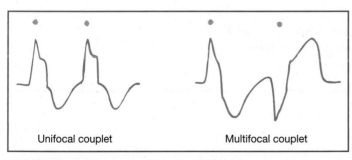

Unifocal couplet          Multifocal couplet

**FIGURE 10–5**

**Unifocal and multifocal couplets.**

PVCs can be regular at times. If every other beat is a PVC, it's called ventricular bigeminy. If every third beat is a PVC, it's called ventricular trigeminy. If every fourth beat is a PVC, it's ventricular quadrigeminy, and so on. See Figure 10–6.

In Figure 10–6, note that every third beat is a PVC. This is ventricular trigeminy.

PVCs usually have a pause, called a complete compensatory pause, following them. This allows the regular rhythm to resume right on time as if the PVC had never happened. A complete compensatory pause measures two R-R cycles from the beat preceding the PVC to the beat following the PVC. See Figure 10–7.

Sometimes a sinus impulse arrives to depolarize the ventricle at the same time a premature ventricular impulse was starting to depolarize the same tissue. The resultant QRS complex is intermediate in shape and size between the sinus beat and the PVC. Imagine the sinus beat as the mother and the PVC as the father. Fusion beats, as these beats are called, are their offspring. Just as in humans, where some children look more like their mother and others resemble their father, some fusion beats will look more like the sinus beat (just a little wider and/or taller or deeper), and others will look more like

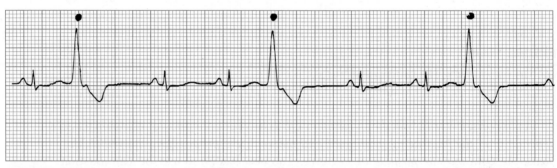

**FIGURE 10–6**

**Ventricular trigeminy.**

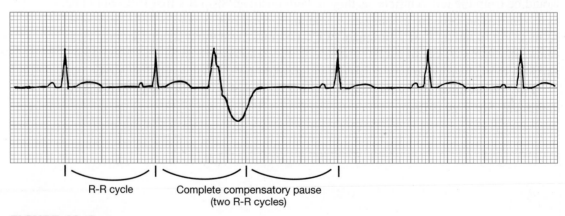

R-R cycle   Complete compensatory pause
(two R-R cycles)

**FIGURE 10–7**

**Complete compensatory pause.**

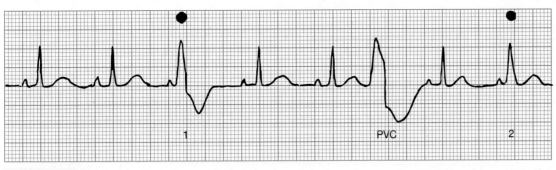

**FIGURE 10–8**

**Fusion beats.**

the PVC (but narrower). See Figure 10–8. Here the dotted QRS complexes represent fusion beats. Note the shape of the sinus beats and the PVC. Look at fusion beat 1. It looks more like a narrowed PVC, doesn't it? The ventricle obviously contributed more to its shape than the sinus node did. Now look at fusion beat 2. It looks more like the sinus beats, but with a thicker R wave. Its shape was contributed mostly by the sinus beat with a little contribution from the ventricle. Note on both fusion beats that a P wave precedes the QRS. This is not always the case. If there is a P wave, the PR interval will be shorter than on the surrounding sinus beats. Fusion beats are caused by the same factors that cause PVCs and are treated the same way.

## Agonal Rhythm (Dying Heart)

Agonal rhythm is an irregular rhythm in which the severely impaired heart is only able to "cough out" an occasional beat from its only remaining pacemaker, the ventricle. The higher pacemakers have all failed.

| | |
|---|---|
| Rate | <20, although an occasional beat might come in at a slightly higher rate |
| Regularity | Irregular |
| P waves | None |
| Intervals | PR not applicable |
| | QRS interval >0.12 secs; QRS wide and bizarre |
| T wave | Slopes off in the opposite direction to the QRS |
| Cause | The patient is dying, usually from profound cardiac or other damage or from hypoxia. |
| Adverse effects | Profound shock, unconsciousness; death if untreated. |
| | An agonal rhythm usually does not provide a pulse—and even if it does, the cardiac output it produces will be incompatible with life. |
| Treatment | CPR, epinephrine, atropine, oxygen |

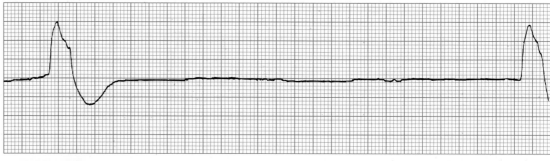

**FIGURE 10–9**

**Agonal rhythm.**

Figure 10–9 shows two QRS complexes, both the same shape, wide and bizarre. Regularity is indeterminate on this strip because there are only 2 QRS complexes. (Three are needed to determine regularity.) Heart rate is about 12. There are no P waves, therefore no PR interval. QRS interval is 0.28, extremely wide. Interpretation: agonal rhythm.

## Idioventricular Rhythm (IVR)

*Idioventricular rhythm* (IVR) is a rhythm originating in the ventricle at its inherent rate. Higher pacemakers have failed, so the ventricle escapes to save the patient's life.

| | |
|---|---|
| Rate | 20 to 40 |
| Regularity | Regular |
| P waves | None |
| Intervals | PR not applicable |
| | QRS interval >0.12 secs; QRS wide and bizarre |
| T wave | Slopes off in the opposite direction to the QRS |
| Cause | Usually implies massive cardiac or other damage, hypoxia |
| Adverse effects | Decreased cardiac output, cardiovascular collapse. IVR may or may not result in a pulse. |
| Treatment | Atropine, epinephrine, pacemaker, oxygen, dopamine. If the patient is pulseless, do CPR |

Figure 10–10 shows QRS complexes, all wide and bizarre. Regularity is regular. Heart rate is 37. There are no P waves, therefore no PR interval. QRS interval is 0.20, extremely wide. Interpretation: idioventricular rhythm.

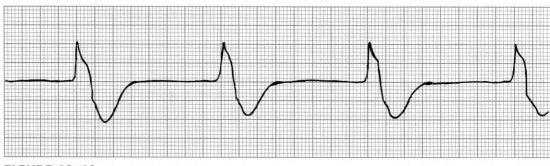

**FIGURE 10–10**

**Idioventricular rhythm.**

We're about halfway through this chapter. To evaluate your understanding of the material thus far, answer the following questions. If you have trouble with them, review the material again before continuing.

Mr. Kirk has a slow regular rhythm with a narrow QRS complex, matching upright P waves in Lead II, and a heart rate of 40. He's now having very frequent PVCs. He complains of feeling faint and you note his blood pressure has dropped alarmingly. You call for help. A coworker, having seen the rhythm, brings in amiodarone in case the physician orders it.

1. Is amiodarone the right medication for this situation? Why or why not?
2. If not, what medication would be indicated?

## Accelerated Idioventricular Rhythm (AIVR)

*Accelerated idioventricular rhythm* (AIVR) is a rhythm originating in the ventricle, with a heart rate faster than the ventricle's normal rate. It can result from escape or usurpation.

| | |
|---|---|
| Rate | 40 to 100 |
| Regularity | Usually regular, but can be a little irregular at times |
| P waves | Usually not seen |
| Intervals | No PR interval because no P waves<br>QRS interval >0.12 secs; QRS wide and bizarre |
| T wave | Slopes off in the opposite direction to the QRS |
| Cause | Very common after an MI. Can be caused by the same factors that cause PVCs. AIVR is also common after administration of thrombolytic (clot-dissolving) medications, and in that context it was once considered a **reperfusion arrhythmia**, implying the heart muscle was once again receiving blood flow after the clot was dissolved. Current studies, however, have shown that AIVR occurs just as often without reperfusion as with it, so it's no longer considered a sign of reperfusion. |
| Adverse effects | Usually no ill effects because the heart rate is close to normal |
| Treatment | Could be treated with atropine if the patient is symptomatic. Consider starting oxygen. Usually no treatment is necessary as AIVR tends to be a self-limiting rhythm |

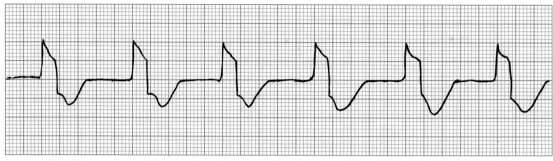

**FIGURE 10–11**

**Accelerated idioventricular rhythm (AIVR).**

Figure 10–11 shows QRS complexes, all wide and bizarre. Regularity is regular. Heart rate is 60. There are no P waves and thus no PR interval. QRS interval is about 0.18, very wide. Interpretation: accelerated idioventricular rhythm.

## Ventricular Tachycardia (V-tach)

In *ventricular tachycardia* (V-tach), an irritable ventricular focus has usurped the sinus node to become the pacemaker and is firing very rapidly.

| | |
|---|---|
| Rate | >100 |
| Regularity | Usually regular, but can be a little irregular at times |
| P waves | Usually none seen, but dissociated from the QRS if present |
| Intervals | Variable PR if even present<br>QRS >0.12 secs; QRS wide and bizarre |
| T wave | Slopes off in the opposite direction to the QRS |
| Cause | Same as PVCs |
| Adverse effects | This rhythm may be tolerated for short bursts, but prolonged runs of V-tach can cause profound shock, unconsciousness, and death if untreated. |
| Treatment | Amiodarone or lidocaine intravenously *if the patient is stable*. Electric shock to the heart (cardioversion or defibrillation) is indicated if the patient is unstable or pulseless. Also treat the cause (low potassium, magnesium, or oxygen levels, etc.). CPR is indicated if the patient is pulseless. For individuals with frequent runs of V-Tach unresponsive to other treatments, an **automated implantable cardioverter-defibrillator (AICD)** or catheter ablation may be advised. The defibrillator fires a small electrical shock from its location inside the body and aborts the rhythm. Catheter ablation destroys the tissue responsible for causing the V-Tach. |

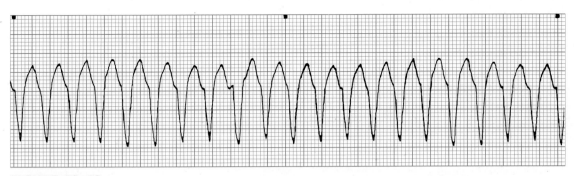

**FIGURE 10–12**

**Ventricular tachycardia.**

Figure 10–12 shows QRS complexes, all wide and bizarre. Regularity is regular. Heart rate is 214. P waves are absent. PR interval is not applicable. QRS interval is 0.13. Interpretation: ventricular tachycardia.

## Torsades de Pointes

*Torsades de pointes* (pronounced *tor-sahd de point*) is a French term meaning "twisting of the points." It's a form of polymorphic (multiple-shaped) ventricular tachycardia that is recognized primarily by its classic shape—it oscillates around an axis, with the QRS complexes pointing up, then becoming smaller, then rotating around until they point down. Torsades is not usually well tolerated in longer bursts and often deteriorates into ventricular fibrillation.

| | |
|---|---|
| Rate | >200 |
| Regularity | May be regular or irregular |
| P waves | None seen |
| Intervals | PR not applicable<br>QRS >0.12 secs, often hard to measure; QRS wide and bizarre<br>*QT interval on a pre-torsades strip will be prolonged.* |
| T wave | Opposite the QRS, but may not be seen due to the rapidity of the rhythm |
| Cause | Can be caused by antiarrhythmic medications such as quinidine, amiodarone, sotalol, flecainide, and others that cause increased QT interval. Also caused by hypokalemia or hypomagnesemia (low blood magnesium level). Even some antihistamines and antibiotics have been implicated in the development of Torsades. |
| Adverse effects | May be tolerated for short runs, but usually results in cardiac arrest if sustained |
| Treatment | Intravenous magnesium is the usual treatment, though electrical cardioversion or defibrillation may also be required to abort longer runs of the rhythm. Oxygen administration is needed. AICD or catheter ablation may be necessary if repeat symptomatic runs of Torsades occur despite treatment. |

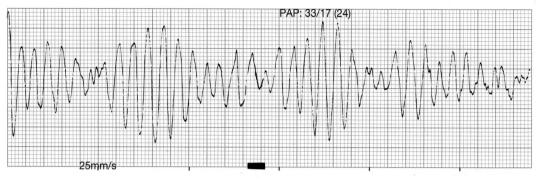

PAP: 33/17 (24)

25mm/s

**FIGURE 10–13**

**Torsades de pointes.**

Figure 10–13 shows QRS complexes, not all the same shape. Some point downward, some point upward, and others are very small. Regularity is regular. Heart rate is about 375. P waves are absent, therefore no PR interval. QRS interval is 0.16. Interpretation: torsades de pointes. The big clue here is the oscillating character of the QRS complexes—bigger, then smaller, then bigger again, and so on. That's classic for torsades.

## Ventricular Fibrillation (V-FIB)

In *ventricular fibrillation* (V-fib), hundreds of impulses in the ventricle are firing, each depolarizing its own little piece of territory. As a result, the ventricles wiggle instead of contract. The heart's electrical system is in chaos, and the resultant rhythm looks like static.

| | |
|---|---|
| Rate | Cannot be counted |
| Regularity | None detectable |
| P waves | None |
| Intervals | No PR interval because no P waves<br>No QRS interval because no QRS complexes—just a wavy or spiked baseline |
| T wave | None |
| Cause | Same as V-tach; also can be caused by drowning, drug overdoses, accidental electric shock. V-fib is the most common arrhythmia occurring in the first hours after an MI, and is responsible for most of the pre-hospital MI-related deaths. |
| Adverse effects | Profound cardiovascular collapse. There is no cardiac output whatsoever. There is no pulse and no breathing. The patient is functionally dead. New onset V-fib has coarse fibrillatory waves. These waves get progressively finer the longer it lasts. |

| Treatment | Immediate defibrillation (electric shock to the heart), epinephrine, CPR, amiodarone, lidocaine, oxygen. The rhythm will not be converted with just medications—defibrillation must be done. The medications make the defibrillation more successful and can prevent recurrences of V-fib. For individuals with recurrent V-fib, an AICD or catheter ablation may be advised. |
|---|---|

Figure 10–14 shows no identifiable QRS complexes—just a wavy, spiked baseline resembling static. Regularity is not determinable. Heart rate is not measurable because there are no QRS complexes. P waves are not present. PR and QRS intervals cannot be measured. Interpretation: ventricular fibrillation.

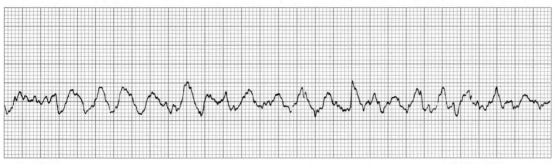

**FIGURE 10–14**

**Ventricular fibrillation.**

## Asystole

Asystole is flat-line EKG. Every one of the heart's pacemakers has failed.

| Rate | Zero |
|---|---|
| Regularity | None |
| P waves | None |
| Intervals | No PR interval because no P waves; no QRS interval because no QRS |
| T wave | None |
| Cause | Profound cardiac or other body system damage; profound hypoxia. Even with vigorous resuscitative efforts, this is usually a terminal rhythm. |
| Adverse effects | Death if untreated |
| Treatment | Epinephrine, CPR, oxygen. There is rarely a need to utilize a pacemaker. Depending on the situation, it may be appropriate to forgo resuscitative efforts. |

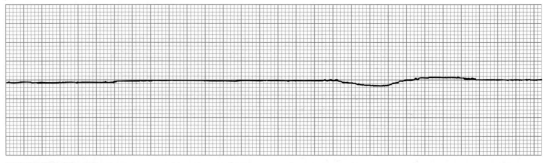

**FIGURE 10–15**

**Asystole.**

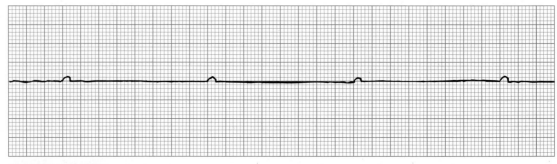

**FIGURE 10–16**

**P wave asystole.**

Figure 10–15 shows no QRS complexes, only a flat line. There is no regularity. Heart rate is zero. There are no P waves, no PR interval, and no QRS interval. Interpretation: asystole.

There is another kind of asystole in which there are no QRS complexes but there are still P waves. This is called **P wave asystole.** The still-functioning sinus node fires its impulses, but they do not cause ventricular depolarization either because the ventricle is too damaged to respond to the stimulus or because there is a complete block in conduction of the impulse to the ventricle. Because the atria depolarize but the ventricles do not, there will be P waves not followed by a QRS. Eventually the sinus impulses will slow and stop, as there is no cardiac output to feed blood to the sinus node. Remember—*if there is no QRS complex, there is no pulse—no cardiac output.* Treatment is the same as for asystole.

Figure 10–16 shows no QRS complexes. Regularity is not applicable. Heart rate is zero. P waves are present, regular, with an atrial rate of 37. There is no PR interval or QRS interval. Interpretation: P wave asystole.

## Pacemaker Rhythm

Pacemakers are electronic devices that can be implanted into or attached to the patient to send out an electrical impulse to cause the heart to depolarize. Pacemakers are used when the heart is temporarily or permanently unable to generate or transmit its own impulses, or when it does so too slowly to provide a reasonable cardiac output. They can be used to pace the atria, the ventricles, or both.

When the pacemaker sends out its signal, a vertical spike is recorded on the EKG paper. Ventricular pacing provides a spike followed by a wide QRS. Atrial pacing has a spike followed by a P wave. Dual-chamber pacing (both atrium and ventricle) has a spike before both the P and the QRS. See Figure 10–17.

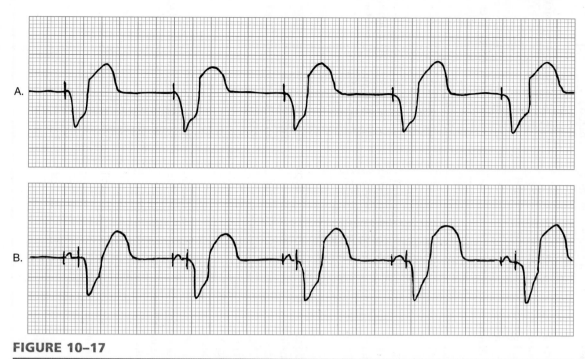

**FIGURE 10–17**

**(A) Ventricular pacing; (B) Dual-chamber pacing.**

In Figure 10–17A, there are QRS complexes, all wide, all shaped the same. Each QRS is preceded by a pacemaker spike. Regularity is regular. Heart rate is 50. There are no P waves, therefore no PR interval. QRS interval is 0.24 secs. Interpretation: ventricular pacing.

In Figure 10–17B, there are QRS complexes, all wide, all shaped the same. Regularity is regular. Heart rate is 50. There are matching P waves, each preceded by a pacemaker spike. A pacemaker-generated PR interval called the AV interval (the interval between atrial and ventricular pacing spikes) is 0.16 secs and should be constant as this interval is preset when the pacemaker is implanted. QRS interval is 0.24 secs. Interpretation: dual-chamber pacing (also called AV pacing).

Pacemakers will be covered in depth in Chapter 16. See Table 10-2 and Figure 10–18 for a review of the ventricular rhythms. Then move on to the practice strips.

**TABLE 10–2  Rhythm Summary: Ventricular Rhythms**

| | Rate | Regularity | P Wave | QRS | Cause | Adverse Effects | Treatment |
|---|---|---|---|---|---|---|---|
| PVCs | Can occur at any rate | Regular but interrupted | Usually none | >0.12; wide and bizarre in shape | Hypoxia, MI, hypokalemia, low magnesium, caffeine, stimulants, stress | Occasional are no problem; can lead to lethal arrhythmias if frequent or after an MI | Amiodarone, $O_2$, lidocaine; atropine for bradycardic PVCs. Consider catheter ablation. |
| Agonal rhythm | <20 | Irregular | None | >0.12; wide and bizarre in shape | Profound cardiac or other damage, profound hypoxia | Shock, unconsciousness, death if untreated | CPR, atropine, epinephrine, dopamine, $O_2$ |
| Idioventricular rhythm | 20–40 | Regular | None | >0.12; wide and bizarre in shape | Massive cardiac or other damage hypoxia | ↓CO | Atropine, epinephrine, dopamine, $O_2$, pacemaker |
| AIVR | 40–100 | Usually regular—can be irregular at times | Dissociated if even present | >0.12; wide and bizarre in shape | Most often seen during MI | Usually well tolerated | Atropine, epinephrine, dopamine if HR low and symptoms |
| V-tach | 100–250 | Usually regular—can be irregular at times | Dissociated if even present | >0.12; wide and bizarre in shape | Hypoxia, MI, hypokalemia, low magnesium, caffeine, stimulants, stress | May be tolerated OK for short bursts; can cause shock, unconsciousness, and death if untreated | Amiodarone, lidocaine, $O_2$, cardioversion or defib; CPR if no pulse. Consider catheter ablation. |
| Torsades de pointes | >200 | Regular or irregular | None seen | >0.12; QRS oscillates around an axis | Medications such as quinidine or amiodarone; hypoxia, MI, hypokalemia, low magnesium, caffeine, stimulants, stress | Circulatory collapse if sustained; tolerated OK for short bursts | IV magnesium, overdrive pacing, cardioversion or defib, $O_2$. Consider catheter ablation. |
| V-fib | Cannot be counted | None detectable | None | None; just a wavy baseline that looks like static | Hypoxia, MI, hypokalemia, low magnesium, caffeine, stimulants, stress | Cardiovascular collapse; no pulse, breathing, zero cardiac output | Defibrillation, amiodarone, lidocaine, epinephrine, $O_2$, CPR. Consider catheter ablation. |
| Asystole | Zero | None | None | None | Profound cardiac or other damage, hypoxia | Death if untreated | Epinephrine, CPR, $O_2$ |
| P wave asystole | Zero | Ps regular | Sinus Ps | None | Profound cardiac or other damage, hypoxia | Death if untreated | Same as asystole |

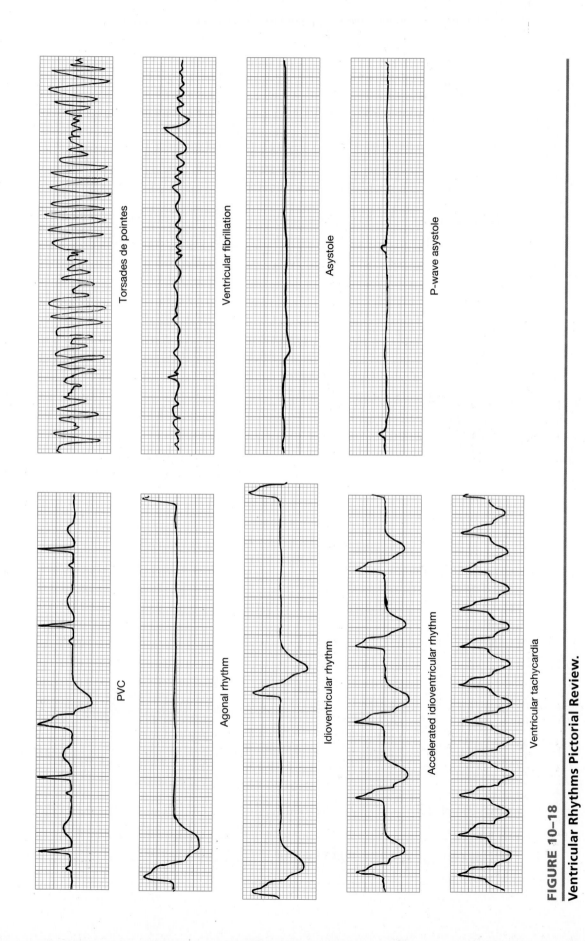

**FIGURE 10–18**

**Ventricular Rhythms Pictorial Review.**

Torsades de pointes

Ventricular fibrillation

Asystole

P-wave asystole

PVC

Agonal rhythm

Idioventricular rhythm

Accelerated idioventricular rhythm

Ventricular tachycardia

## Practice Strips: Ventricular Rhythms

The first 10 strips are single-lead strips; the last 15 are double-lead strips.

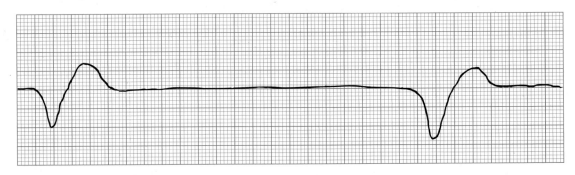

1.  QRS complexes _____ Regularity _____ Heart rate _____

    P waves _____

    PR interval _____ QRS interval _____

    Interpretation (name of rhythm)

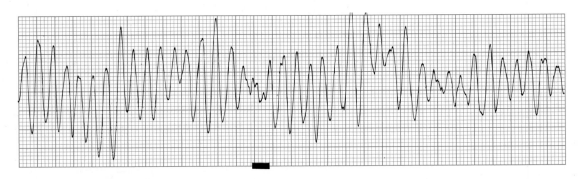

2.  QRS complexes _____ Regularity _____ Heart rate _____

    P waves _____

    PR interval _____ QRS interval _____

    Interpretation _____

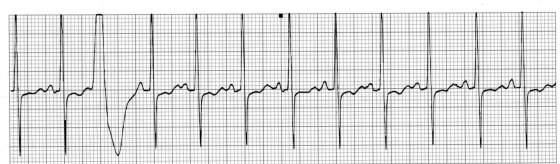

3.  QRS complexes _____ Regularity _____ Heart rate _____

    P waves _____

    PR interval _____ QRS interval _____

    Interpretation _____

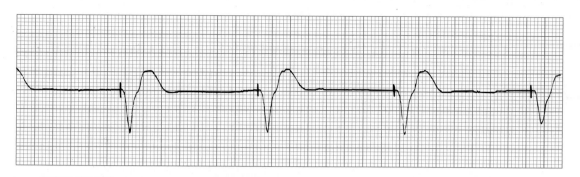

4. QRS complexes _____ Regularity _____ Heart rate _____

   P waves _____

   PR interval _____ QRS interval _____

   Interpretation _____

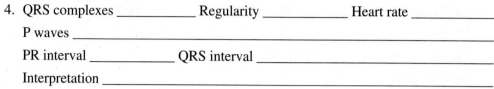

5. QRS complexes _____ Regularity _____ Heart rate _____

   P waves _____

   PR interval _____ QRS interval _____

   Interpretation _____

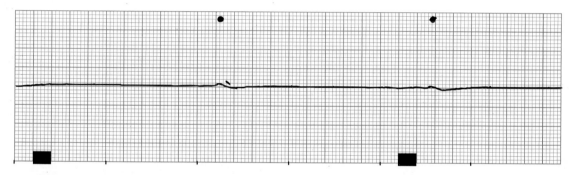

6. QRS complexes _____ Regularity _____ Heart rate _____

   P waves _____

   PR interval _____ QRS interval _____

   Interpretation _____

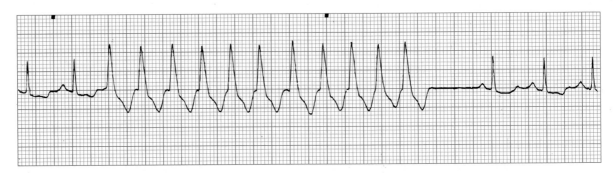

7. QRS complexes _____ Regularity _____ Heart rate _____

   P waves _____

   PR interval _____ QRS interval _____

   Interpretation _____

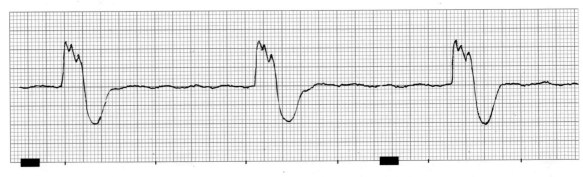

8. QRS complexes _____ Regularity _____ Heart rate _____

   P waves _____

   PR interval _____ QRS interval _____

   Interpretation _____

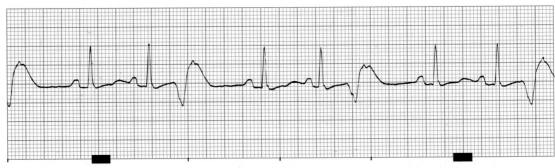

9. QRS complexes _____ Regularity _____ Heart rate _____

   P waves _____

   PR interval _____ QRS interval _____

   Interpretation _____

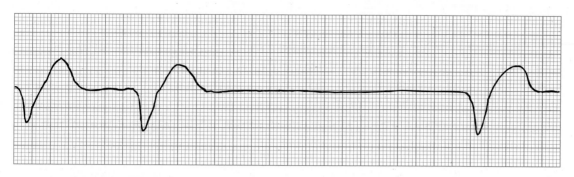

10. QRS complexes _____ Regularity _____ Heart rate _____

P waves _____

PR interval _____ QRS interval _____

Interpretation _____

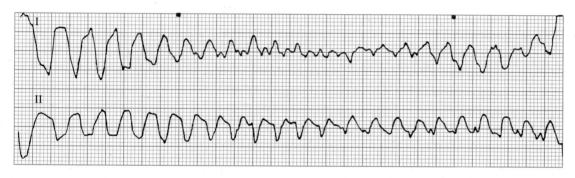

11. QRS complexes _____ Regularity _____ Heart rate _____

P waves _____

PR interval _____ QRS interval _____

Interpretation _____

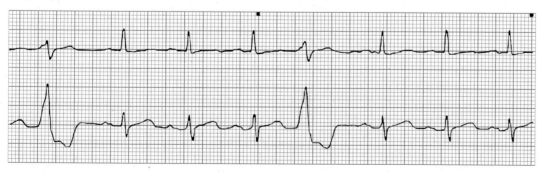

12. QRS complexes _____ Regularity _____ Heart rate _____

P waves _____

PR interval _____ QRS interval _____

Interpretation _____

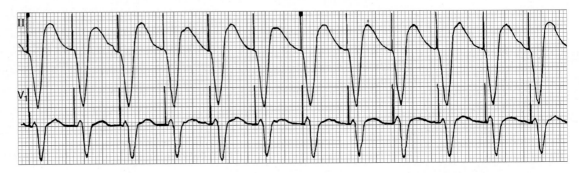

13. QRS complexes _____ Regularity _____ Heart rate _____

    P waves _____

    PR interval _____ QRS interval _____

    Interpretation _____

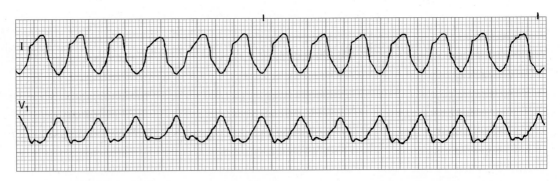

14. QRS complexes _____ Regularity _____ Heart rate _____

    P waves _____

    PR interval _____ QRS interval _____

    Interpretation _____

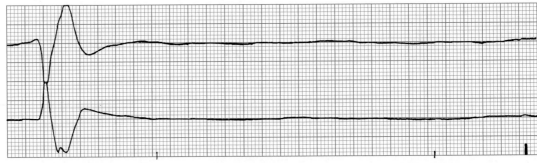

15. QRS complexes _____ Regularity _____ Heart rate _____

    P waves _____

    PR interval _____ QRS interval _____

    Interpretation _____

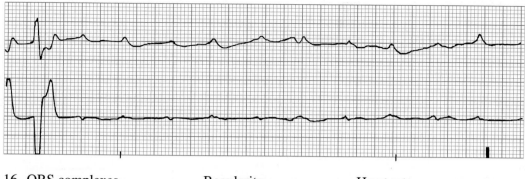

16. QRS complexes _____ Regularity _____ Heart rate _____

    P waves _____

    PR interval _____ QRS interval _____

    Interpretation _____

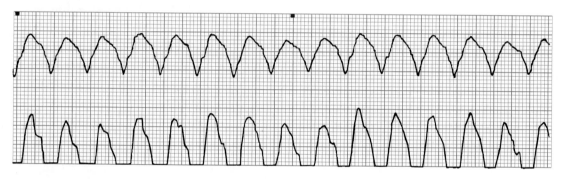

17. QRS complexes _____ Regularity _____ Heart rate _____

    P waves _____

    PR interval _____ QRS interval _____

    Interpretation _____

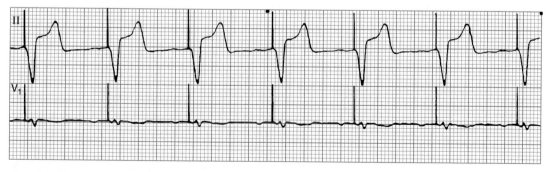

18. QRS complexes _____ Regularity _____ Heart rate _____

    P waves _____

    PR interval _____ QRS interval _____

    Interpretation _____

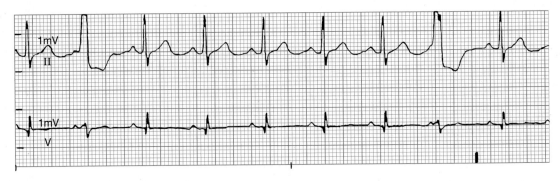

19. QRS complexes _____ Regularity _____ Heart rate _____

    P waves _____

    PR interval _____ QRS interval _____

    Interpretation _____

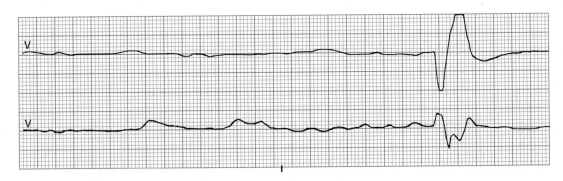

20. QRS complexes _____ Regularity _____ Heart rate _____

    P waves _____

    PR interval _____ QRS interval _____

    Interpretation _____

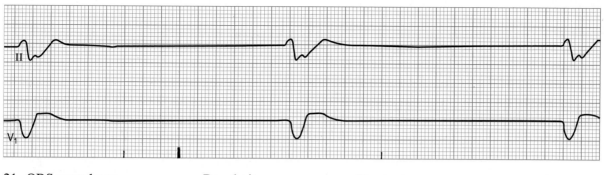

21. QRS complexes _____ Regularity _____ Heart rate _____

   P waves _____

   PR interval _____ QRS interval _____

   Interpretation _____

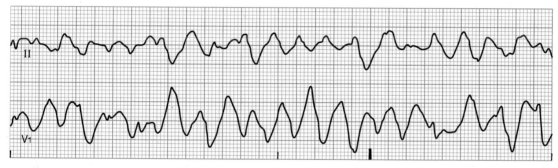

22. QRS complexes _____ Regularity _____ Heart rate _____

   P waves _____

   PR interval _____ QRS interval _____

   Interpretation _____

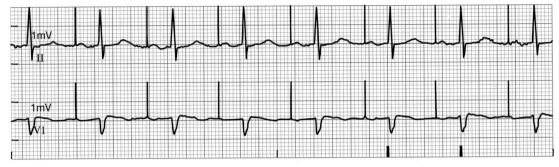

23. QRS complexes _____ Regularity _____ Heart rate _____

    P waves _____

    PR interval _____ QRS interval _____

    Interpretation _____

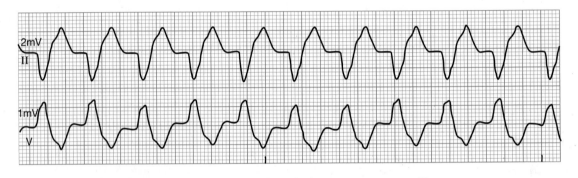

24. QRS complexes _____ Regularity _____ Heart rate _____

    P waves _____

    PR interval _____ QRS interval _____

    Interpretation _____

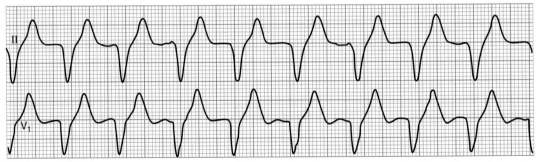

25. QRS complexes _____ Regularity _____ Heart rate _____

    P waves _____

    PR interval _____ QRS interval _____

    Interpretation _____

**chapter ten notes** TO SUM IT ALL UP . . .

- **Ventricular rhythms**—Originate in an irritable focus in the ventricle—travel cell by cell through the tissue. Ventricular rhythm impulses do not travel through the bundle branches. QRS complex is wide and bizarre in appearance.
- **In ventricular rhythms, QRS may be positive or negative depending on the lead being monitored and the ventricle originating the rhythm.** In $V_1$ or $MCL_1$, PVCs from left ventricle will have a positive QRS. PVCs from right ventricle will have negative QRS.
- **PVCs:**
  - *Heart rate*—Can occur at any rate
  - *Regularity*—Regular but interrupted by a premature beat
  - *P waves*—None
  - *Intervals*—PR—not applicable; QRS >0.12 secs.
  - *T wave*—Opposite the QRS
  - *Causes*—Heart disease, hypokalemia, hypoxia, low magnesium level, stress, caffeine, anxiety
  - *Adverse effects*—Can lead to worsening arrhythmias such as V-tach or V-fib
  - *Treatment*—Treat the cause; oxygen, amiodarone. Treat bradycardia PVCs with atropine. AICD or catheter ablation if frequent symptomatic PVCs.
- **Unifocal PVCs**—Have same shape
- **Multifocal PVCs**—have differing shapes
- **R-on-T PVCs**—Land on the T wave of the preceding beat— are more dangerous than PVCs that land after the T wave— can cause V-tach or V-fib
- **Couplets**—Paired PVCs; can be unifocal or multifocal
- **Fusion beats**—Combination of sinus beat and PVC
- **Agonal rhythm:**
  - *Heart rate*—<20
  - *Regularity*—Irregular
  - *P waves*—None
  - *Intervals*—PR—not applicable; QRS >0.12 secs
  - *T wave*—Opposite the QRS
  - *Causes*—Dying patient
  - *Adverse effects*—Shock, unconsciousness, death if untreated
  - *Treatment*—CPR, epinephrine, atropine, oxygen
- **Idioventricular rhythm:**
  - *Heart rate*—20–40
  - *Regularity*—Regular
  - *P waves*—None
  - *Intervals*—PR—not applicable; QRS >0.12 secs
  - *T wave*—Opposite the QRS
  - *Causes*—Hypoxia, massive heart or other organ damage
  - *Adverse effects*—Decreased cardiac output, cardiovascular collapse
  - *Treatment*—Oxygen, atropine, epinephrine, pacemaker if indicated, dopamine infusion, CPR if pulseless or cardiac output ineffective
- **Accelerated idioventricular rhythm:**
  - *Heart rate*—40–100
  - *Regularity*—Usually regular
  - *P waves*—Usually none
  - *Intervals*—PR—not applicable; QRS >0.12 secs
  - *T wave*—Opposite the QRS
  - *Causes*—MI

  - *Adverse effects*—Usually none—could have decreased cardiac output at slower heart rates
  - *Treatment*—Oxygen, atropine if symptoms from slow heart rate
- **Ventricular tachycardia:**
  - *Heart rate*—>100
  - *Regularity*—Usually regular
  - *P waves*—Usually none; if present will be dissociated from QRS
  - *Intervals*—PR—not applicable; QRS >0.12 secs
  - *T waves*—Opposite the QRS
  - *Causes*—Same as PVCs
  - *Adverse effects*—Decreased cardiac output, shock, unconsciousness, death
  - *Treatment*—Amiodarone or lidocaine if stable; electrical cardioversion if unstable; defibrillation if pulseless. **AICD or catheter ablation if recurrent symptomatic episodes.**
- **Torsades de pointes:**
  - *Heart rate*—<200
  - *Regularity*—Regular or irregular
  - *P waves*—None
  - *Intervals*—PR—none; QRS >0.12 secs
  - *T wave*—Opposite the QRS; T waves hard to see because of fast rate
  - *Causes*—Antiarrhythmic medications such as amiodarone or quinidine; hypokalemia or hypomagnesemia.
  - *Adverse effects*—Cardiac arrest if sustained
  - *Treatment*—Oxygen, IV magnesium, cardioversion or defibrillation. AICD or catheter ablation if recurrent symptomatic runs.
- **Ventricular fibrillation:**
  - *Heart rate*—Cannot count
  - *Regularity*—Cannot determine
  - *P waves*—None
  - *Intervals*—Not applicable
  - *T waves*—None
  - *Causes*—Same as V-tach plus drowning, accidental electric shock, drug overdoses
  - *Adverse effects*—Cardiac arrest; death if untreated
  - *Treatment*—Defibrillation, CPR, oxygen, amiodarone or lidocaine, epinephrine. AICD or catheter ablation if recurrent.
- **Asystole:**
  - *Heart rate*—Zero
  - *Regularity*—Not applicable
  - *P waves*—None unless it's P wave asystole
  - *Intervals*—Not applicable
  - *T wave*—None
  - *Causes*—Profound hypoxia or heart or other damage
  - *Adverse effects*—Death if untreated
  - *Treatment*—CPR, epinephrine, oxygen. Find and treat the cause. Consider termination of resuscitative efforts.
- **Pacemakers**—Devices that are attached to or implanted into a patient—stimulate the atria, ventricles, or both to depolarize when the patient's own conduction system is too slow or unable to do it.
  - *Atrial pacing*—Pacer spike, then P wave.
  - *Ventricular pacing*—Pacer spike, then QRS complex.

## Practice Quiz

1. The main causes of PVCs are _____ _____ _____

2. The rhythm that has no QRS complexes but instead has a wavy, static-looking baseline is _____ _____

3. Appropriate treatment for PVCs interrupting a sinus bradycardia with a heart rate of 32 would be _____

4. *Torsades de pointes* is a French term that means _____

5. How does asystole differ from P wave asystole? _____ _____

6. Your patient has a ventricular rhythm with a heart rate of 39, but no pulse. What treatment would be appropriate? _____ _____

7. True or false: Asystole is treated with electric shock to the heart.

8. The treatment of choice for ventricular fibrillation is _____ _____

9. True or false: Pacemakers can pace the atrium, the ventricle, or both.

10. True or false: Antiarrhythmics should be given to treat agonal rhythm.

## Putting It All Together—Critical Thinking Exercises

These exercises may consist of diagrams to label, scenarios to analyze, brain-stumping questions to ponder, or other challenging exercises to boost your understanding of the chapter material.

Let's play with ventricular rhythms a bit. The following scenario will provide you with information about a fictional patient and ask you to analyze the situation, answer questions, and decide on appropriate actions.

Mr. Winston, age 45, arrives in your ER complaining of intermittent dizziness. He feels he has come close to passing out a few times in the past 24 hours. Other than a past medical history of diet-controlled diabetes, he's been healthy. See his initial rhythm strip in the ER, Figure 10–19. Vital signs are stable. Mr. Winston denies feeling dizzy at this time.

1. What is this rhythm _____

2. Does this rhythm require emergency treatment? _____ _____ _____

3. Name three factors that can cause this rhythm. _____ _____

Lab tests reveal Mr. Winston's potassium level to be 1.9, extremely low. The physician orders potassium to be given intravenously. Half an hour later, an alarm sounds and the following rhythm strip prints out. See Figure 10–20.

4. What is this rhythm? _____

5. Does this rhythm require emergency treatment? _____

6. Mr. Winston has no breathing and no pulse. What intervention must be employed to terminate this rhythm? _____

After successful intervention, Mr. Winston returns to sinus rhythm and has no more problems. After an uneventful course in the intensive care unit, Mr. Winston goes home taking amiodarone.

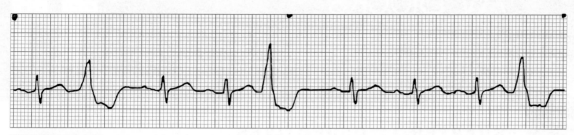

**FIGURE 10–19**

**Mr. Winston's initial strip.**

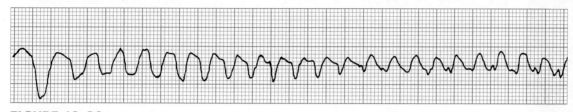

**FIGURE 10–20**

**Rhythm causing alarm.**

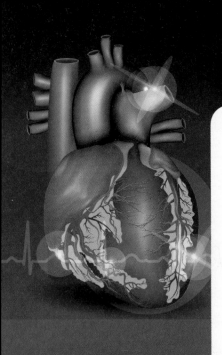

# AV Blocks

## CHAPTER 11 OBJECTIVES

Upon completion of this chapter, the student will be able to

- State the criteria for each type of AV block.
- State whether the block is at the AV node or the bundle branches.
- Identify each type of AV block on a variety of strips.
- State the criteria, causes, adverse effects, and treatment for AV blocks.

## What It's All About

Mr. Pomeroux, age 54, was watching TV when he began to feel light-headed. His wife brought him to the emergency room (ER) where his heart rate was discovered to be 42. The doctor diagnosed his rhythm as third-degree AV block and advised Mr. Pomeroux that he needed a pacemaker. Mr. Pomeroux signed himself out of the ER against medical advice. A few hours later, he was rushed back to the ER—this time by ambulance—having suffered a syncopal episode. He was in third-degree AV block with a heart rate of 27 and a wide QRS. Two ER nurses started oxygen and attached transcutaneous pacemaker patches to Mr. Pomeroux's chest while another nurse started an IV line and administered atropine. The atropine was ineffective, but the heart rate did improve with the pacemaker. Mr. Pomeroux was taken immediately for pacemaker insertion and recovered uneventfully.

## Introduction

With **AV blocks** (atrioventricular blocks), the sinus node fires its impulses as usual, but there is a problem down the line—a partial or complete interruption in the transmission of these impulses to the ventricles. The site of the block is the AV node or the bundle branches. See Figures 11–1 and 11–2.

In Figure 11–1, the sinus node sends its impulse through the atria and a P wave is written on the EKG. The impulse travels to the AV node where there is a block in conduction. The impulse dies out here. In Figure 11–2, the impulse travels as far as the bundle branches, where it is stopped by a block. In either case, the impulse can just end there, with a P wave and no QRS (because it never made it to the ventricle), or a lower pacemaker can escape to provide stimulus to the ventricle, thus providing a QRS.

## Degrees of AV Block

There are three degrees of block, varying in severity from benign to life threatening. See Table 11–1.

## The Word on AV Blocks

In AV blocks, the underlying rhythm is sinus. The impulse is propagated in the sinus node and starts down the conduction pathway as usual. The P waves are normal sinus P waves. Farther down the conduction pathway, however, there is a roadblock. This can result in any of three things: a simple delay in impulse transmission (all sinus impulses make it to the ventricles—just more slowly than normal), a partial interruption in the

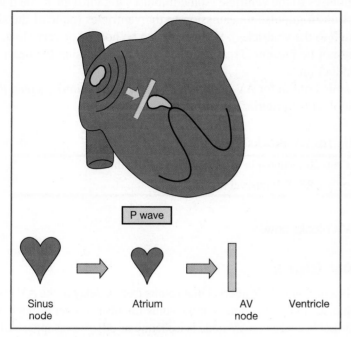

**FIGURE 11–1**

**Block at the AV node.**

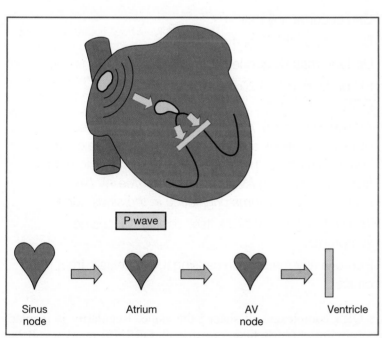

**FIGURE 11–2**

**Block at the bundle branches.**

**TABLE 11–1  Degrees of AV Block**

| Kind of AV Block | Site of Block | Feature | Clinical Importance |
|---|---|---|---|
| First degree | AV node | Delay in impulse transmission from sinus node to ventricles | No clinical danger—no symptoms |
| Second degree | AV node or bundle branches | Some impulses from sinus node get through; some don't | Can progress to higher degree of block—can cause decreased cardiac output |
| Third degree | AV node or bundle branches | None of the impulses get through to the ventricles. A lower pacemaker assumes control | Can be life-threatening, causing severe symptoms |

conduction of sinus impulses to the ventricle (some impulses get through, some don't), or a complete interruption in impulse transmission to the ventricles (none of the sinus impulses make it through to the ventricles). Heart rates can be normal or very slow, and symptoms may or may not be present. Treatment is aimed at increasing the heart rate and improving AV conduction.

There are two possible criteria for AV blocks. *If either of these criteria is met, there is an AV block.* Let's look at the criteria. See Table 11–2.

**TABLE 11–2   Criteria for AV Blocks**

| |
|---|
| PR interval prolonged (> 0.20 seconds) in some kind of sinus rhythm *or* |
| Some Ps not followed by a QRS; P-P interval regular |

Let's look at the AV blocks now.

## First-Degree AV Block

*First-degree AV block* is a prolonged PR interval that results from a delay in the AV node's conduction of sinus impulses to the ventricle. All the sinus impulses do get through; they just take longer than normal because the AV node is ischemic or otherwise suppressed.

| | |
|---|---|
| Rate | Can occur at any rate |
| Regularity | Depends on the underlying rhythm |
| P waves | Upright, matching; one P to each QRS |
| Intervals | PR prolonged (>0.20 secs), constant<br>QRS <0.12 secs |
| Cause | AV node ischemia, digitalis toxicity or a side effect of other medications such as beta-blockers or calcium channel blockers. This is a benign type of block, but be alert for worsening AV block. *First-degree AV block is seen only with rhythms originating in the sinus node.* |
| Adverse effects | The first-degree AV block itself usually causes no symptoms. |
| Treatment | Remove any medication causing it. Otherwise, treat the cause. |

Figure 11–3 shows QRS complexes, all shaped the same. Regularity is regular. Heart rate is 62. P waves are upright, matching, one to each QRS. PR interval is 0.28. QRS interval is 0.08. Interpretation: sinus rhythm with a first-degree AV block.

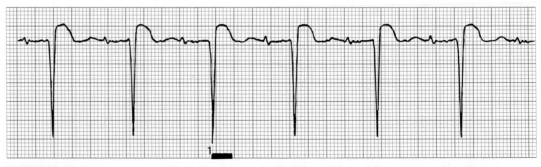

**FIGURE 11–3**

**First-degree AV block.**

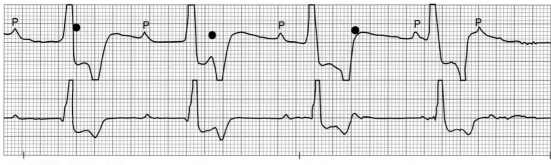

**FIGURE 11–4**

**Where are the hidden P waves?**

Before we move on to the second and third degree AV blocks, we must discuss a critical skill—finding hidden P waves.

## Footprints in the Sand

You're walking on the beach and step into a puddle of water. Your footprints, which have been regularly spaced, disappear in the water, then re-emerge once past the puddle. You know that your footprints continue through the puddle even though those footprints are not visible. In second and third degree AV blocks the P waves, like your footprints, are regular. But they may not be visible at times if something (like a QRS complex or T wave) is in the way, blocking the Ps from view.

The trick to finding hidden P waves is to march out the P waves you **do** see so as to predict where the other ones **should** be. See Figure 11–4. There are four QRS complexes, each preceded by a P wave. That P-P interval is long. Do you see the P wave following the last QRS? It is visible at the end of the T wave. The distance from this P wave to the one preceding that QRS is much shorter. That makes no sense unless there are hidden P waves. Now let's look backwards for those hidden Ps. March out the distance between those last two P waves and measure out that same distance going backwards. (If you use calipers, put the points of the calipers on those two P waves, then swing the calipers around to find the other P waves). You should now see that there are P waves hidden in the first three T waves. These Ps are not visible because the T wave is blocking them from view. (The T wave is our puddle here). On this strip there are eight P waves. The hidden Ps are marked by a dot. Did you find them all? Remember—in all AV blocks, the P waves are regularly spaced.

Now let's move on to second and third degree AV blocks.

## Mobitz I Second-Degree AV Block (Wenckebach)

*Wenckebach* (as Mobitz I is usually called) is usually a transient block, lasting only a few days. It occurs when the AV node becomes progressively weaker and less able to conduct the sinus impulses until finally it is unable to send the impulse down to the ventricle at all. As a result, the PR intervals grow progressively longer until there is a P wave not followed by a QRS.

| | |
|---|---|
| Rate | Atrial rate usually 60 to 100; ventricular rate less than the atrial rate due to nonconducted beats |
| Regularity | Usually irregular. A hallmark of Wenckebach is groups of beats, then a pause. |

| P waves | Normal sinus P waves. All Ps except the blocked P are followed by a QRS. P-P interval is regular. There may be P waves that are hidden in the QRS complex or the T wave (Look for the footprints in the sand). |
|---|---|
| Intervals | PR gradually prolongs until a QRS is dropped. QRS <0.12 secs |
| Cause | Myocardial infarction (MI), digitalis toxicity, medication side effects |
| Adverse effects | Usually no ill effects. Watch for worsening block. |
| Treatment | Prepare for transcutaneous pacing if signs of decreased cardiac output exist. Administer atropine if a pacemaker is not immediately available and the patient is symptomatic. Most patients with Wenckebach require nothing more than cautious observation |

Figure 11–5 shows QRS complexes, all shaped the same. Regularity is irregular. Heart rate is 50 to 83, with a mean rate of 70. P waves are matching, upright, some not followed by a QRS. Some Ps are at the end of the T waves. P-P interval is regular. Atrial rate is 83. PR interval varies from 0.04 to 0.28. Note the relatively short PR of the first beat on the strip. Compare this to the third beat. The PR interval prolongs from beat to beat until the fourth P wave does not conduct through to the ventricle at all. We know it doesn't get through to the ventricle because that P wave is not followed by a QRS complex. The cycle then repeats, with prolonging PR intervals, until the eighth P wave is not conducted. QRS interval is 0.10. Interpretation: Mobitz I second-degree AV block (Wenckebach).

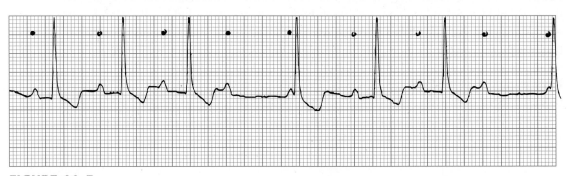

**FIGURE 11–5**

**Wenckebach.**

## chapter CHECKUP

We're about halfway through this chapter. To evaluate your understanding of the material thus far, answer the following questions. If you have trouble with them, review the material again before continuing.

Mrs. Uhura had a heart attack yesterday. Today the nurse notices her rhythm has changed. Her PR intervals are prolonging and then a QRS is dropped. This is happening in cycles. Her blood pressure is fine and she has no symptoms.

1. What is this new rhythm?
2. Is this an emergency?
3. What treatment, if any, is required?

# Mobitz II Second-Degree AV Block

*Mobitz II* is a block caused by an intermittent block at the AV node or the bundle branches, preventing some sinus impulses from getting to the ventricles. *With AV node block, the resultant QRS complexes will be narrow. With block at the bundle branches, the QRS will be wide.* Usually, Mobitz II patients already have a bundle branch block, meaning that one of their bundle branches does not let impulses through. They are therefore dependent on the other bundle branch to conduct the impulses through to the ventricles. If that other bundle branch becomes suddenly blocked, then none of the sinus impulses can get through. Sinus P waves therefore conduct through to the ventricles when the one bundle branch is open, but they don't get through at all when both bundle branches are blocked. When the impulses do get through, they do so with an unchanging PR interval every time. Bottom line: *Mobitz II second-degree AV block looks like a sinus rhythm with all P waves in place, but with some QRS-Ts removed.*

| | |
|---|---|
| Rate | Atrial rate usually 60 to 100; ventricular rate less than atrial rate due to dropped beats |
| Regularity | May be regular, irregular, or regular but interrupted |
| P waves | Normal sinus P waves. All Ps except the blocked Ps have a QRS behind them. P-P interval is regular. Some P waves may be hidden inside QRS complexes or T waves. Look for the footprints in the sand. |
| Intervals | PR constant on the conducted beats QRS <0.12 secs if the block is at the AV node; ≥0.12 secs if the block is at the bundle branches |
| Cause | MI, conduction system lesion, medication side effect, hypoxia |
| Adverse effects | Because the heart rate can be very slow, the patient may have signs of decreased cardiac output. Mobitz II can progress to third-degree block if untreated. |
| Treatment | Immediate transcutaneous pacing if symptomatic. Start oxygen. May try atropine or an epinephrine or dopamine infusion first if a pacemaker is not readily available. Depending on where the block is, atropine may not work. Atropine speeds up the rate of sinus node firing and improves AV node conduction. If the block is at the AV node, atropine will improve conduction, and the impulse will travel on down the pathway unimpeded. If the block is at the bundle branches, however, the impulse will blast through the AV node and head down the pathway only to find that both bundle branches are still blocked. Atropine has no effect on the bundle branches. So bottom line: *With Mobitz II and narrow QRS (<0.12 secs), atropine should work. With wide QRS (≥0.12 secs), epinephrine may be a better choice.* |

Figure 11–6 shows QRS complexes, all the same shape. Regularity is regular. Heart rate is 44. P waves are upright, matching, some not followed by a QRS. P-P interval is regular. Atrial rate is 137. PR interval is constant at 0.12. QRS interval is 0.12. Interpretation: Mobitz II second-degree AV block and a wide QRS, indicating a likely bundle branch block.

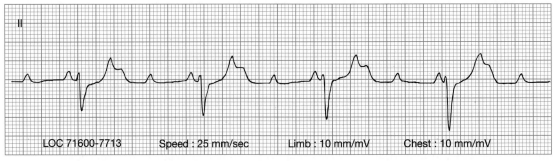

**FIGURE 11–6**

Mobitz II second-degree AV block.

## 2:1 AV Block

*2:1 AV block* is a type of second-degree block in which there are two P waves to each QRS complex. The first P wave in each pair of P waves is blocked (not followed by a QRS). 2:1 AV block can be caused by either Wenckebach or Mobitz II. To differentiate between Wenchebach and Mobitz II, at least two sequential P-QRS-T cycles must be present before any beats are dropped (to determine whether the PR intervals prolong [as in Wenchebach] or stay the same [as in Mobitz II]). With this rhythm the sequence is P-P-QRS-T, so differentiation can go no further and it's just called 2:1 AV block.

| | |
|---|---|
| Rate | Atrial rate 60 to 100; ventricular rate half the atrial rate |
| Regularity | Regular |
| P waves | Normal sinus P waves; two Ps to each QRS; P-P interval regular |
| Intervals | PR constant on the conducted beats QRS <0.12 secs if the block is at the AV node; ≥0.12 secs if the block is at the bundle branches |
| Cause | Same as Wenckebach or Mobitz II |
| Adverse effects | Decreased cardiac output if the heart rate is too slow |
| Treatment | Transcutaneous pacing if the patient has symptoms of decreased cardiac output. May try atropine or an epinephrine or dopamine infusion first if a pacemaker is not readily available. Start oxygen |

Figure 11–7 shows QRS complexes, all the same shape. Regularity is regular. Heart rate is 37. Atrial rate is 75. P waves are upright and matching, two to each QRS. P-P interval is regular. PR interval is 0.16. QRS interval is 0.08. Interpretation: 2:1 AV block.

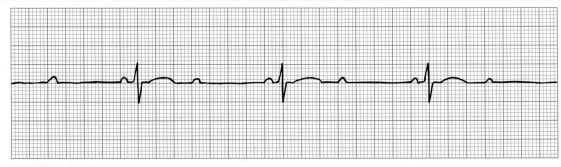

**FIGURE 11–7**

2:1 AV block.

# Third-Degree AV Block (Complete Heart Block)

In *third-degree AV block*, the sinus node sends out its impulses as usual, *but none of them ever get to the ventricles* because there is a complete block at the AV node or the bundle branches. Meanwhile, the AV node and the ventricle are waiting patiently for the sinus impulses to reach them. When it's obvious that the sinus impulse isn't coming, one of the lower pacemakers escapes and assumes pacemaking control to provide a QRS complex. If the block is at the AV node, a lower spot in the AV junction should take over as pacemaker and provide a heart rate of 40 to 60. If the block is at the bundle branches, the ventricle should then assume control with a heart rate of 20 to 40. Even though the lower pacemaker has assumed control of providing the QRS complex, the sinus node continues firing out its impulses as usual, providing regularly spaced P waves.

| | |
|---|---|
| Rate | Atrial rate usually 60 to 100; ventricular rate usually 20 to 60 |
| Regularity | Regular |
| P waves | Normal sinus P waves; P-P interval is regular; P waves may be hidden inside QRS complexes or T waves (look for the footprints in the sand). P waves are not associated with any of the QRS complexes, even though there may at times appear to be a relationship. This is called **AV dissociation**, and it is a hallmark of third-degree block. AV dissociation means that the sinus node is firing at its normal rate, and the lower pacemaker is firing at its slower rate, and the two have nothing to do with each other. AV dissociation results in independent beating of the atria and the ventricles. |
| | Imagine the lower pacemaker that controls the ventricles as an old man jogging around a circular racetrack at 2 miles per hour. The sinus node is an 18-year-old boy sprinting at 4 miles per hour. Because the boy is going faster than the old man, he will periodically catch up with him and then pass him. An onlooker might see the boy at the split second he's side by side with the old man and assume they are together and that there is a relationship between the two. There isn't, of course. Their being side by side was just coincidence, just as its coincidence that a sinus P wave might land right in front of a QRS in third-degree AV block and make it seem as though there is a relationship there. |
| Intervals | PR varies. QRS narrow (<0.12 secs) or wide (≥0.12 secs) depending on the location of the block. If the block is at the AV node, the AV junction should become the pacemaker and the QRS will be narrow. If the block is at the bundle branches, the ventricle will become the pacemaker, with a wide QRS. |
| Cause | MI, conduction system lesion, medication side effects, hypoxia |

| Adverse effects | Signs of low cardiac output may occur if the heart rate is slow enough. |
| Treatment | Transcutaneous pacing if the patient is symptomatic (and if a transvenous pacemaker cannot be emergently inserted). Atropine, epinephrine, or dopamine can be given until a more permanent transvenous pacemaker can be inserted. Start oxygen |

Figure 11–8 shows QRS complexes, all shaped the same. Regularity is regular. Heart rate is 37. P waves are upright and matching. Atrial rate is 60. P-P interval is regular. One P wave is hidden in the ST segment of the third QRS complex. PR interval varies. QRS interval is 0.20. Interpretation: third-degree AV block with a ventricular escape rhythm. Because the QRS is wide, we know the ventricle is the pacemaker. If the AV junction had been the pacemaker, the QRS would have been narrow and the heart rate a bit faster.

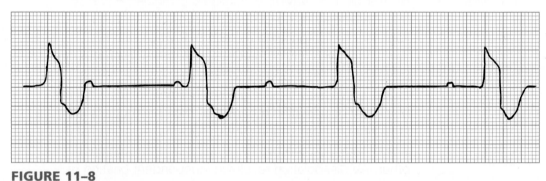

**FIGURE 11–8**

**Third-degree AV block.**

Before we get started on our practice strips, let's look at an algorithm (flow chart) to help identify second- and third-degree AV blocks. (First-degree AV blocks are easier to identify because there are no dropped beats). See Figure 11–9. It includes the algorithm and a practice example.

On the practice example, are there any P waves not followed by a QRS? Yes, lots of them. Is the P-P interval regular? Yes, the Ps are all about the same distance apart from one another. We've answered yes to both, so we follow the arrow. There's a second- or third-degree AV block present. Does the PR interval vary (does it change throughout the strip)? For this we look at the P wave right in front of the QRS. Yes, it varies quite a bit. See where the P wave is in front of the second QRS? Now look at the third QRS. See that hump at the beginning of the QRS? That's the start of a P wave. Both those P waves have different PR intervals. So we've again answered yes to the question, so we follow the yes arrow (if we'd answered no we would follow the no arrow). Is the R-R interval regular? Yes, the QRS complexes are evenly spaced. We follow the yes arrow and it takes us to the answer—third-degree AV block.

Now practice some strips on your own. Use the algorithm if you wish, but be sure to do it without as well, to be sure you know the criteria.

See Table 11–3 and Figure 11–10 for a review of AV blocks.

## 2nd and 3rd Degree AV Block Algorithm

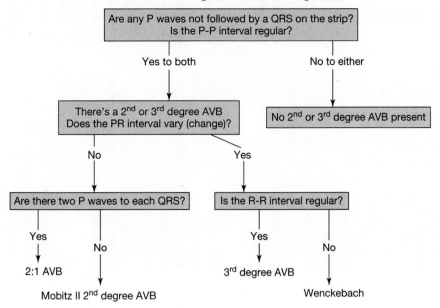

Are any P waves not followed by a QRS on the strip?
Is the P-P interval regular?

Yes to both — There's a 2nd or 3rd degree AVB. Does the PR interval vary (change)?

No to either — No 2nd or 3rd degree AVB present

No → Are there two P waves to each QRS?
- Yes → 2:1 AVB
- No → Mobitz II 2nd degree AVB

Yes → Is the R-R interval regular?
- Yes → 3rd degree AVB
- No → Wenckebach

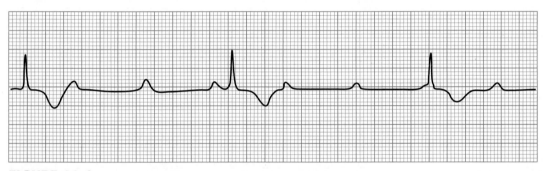

**FIGURE 11–9**

**Second- and third-degree AV block algorithm.**

**TABLE 11–3  Rhythm Summary: AV Blocks**

| | Rate | Regularity | P Wave | PR Interval | QRS Interval | Cause | Adverse Effects | Treatment |
|---|---|---|---|---|---|---|---|---|
| First-degree AV block | Can occur at any rate | Depends on underlying rhythm | Normal; one per QRS; all shaped the same | >0.20; constant | <0.12 | AV node ischemia, prolonged bundle branch depolarization time, digitalis toxicity, other medication side effects | Usually no ill effects | Remove the cause |
| Mobitz I second-degree AV block (Wenckebach) | Atria: 60–100; ventricle: less than atrial rate | Regular but interrupted or irregular; groups of beats, then a pause | Normal; one not followed by a QRS; all shaped the same | Gradually prolongs until a QRS is dropped | QRS <0.12 | MI, digitalis toxicity, medication side effects | Usually well tolerated, but watch for worsening AV block | Pacemaker, atropine, epinephrine or dopamine if symptoms from low HR |
| Mobitz II second-degree AV block | Atria: 60–100; ventricle: less than atrial rate | Regular, regular but interrupted, or irregular | Normal; some not followed by a QRS | Constant on the conducted beats | <0.12 if block at AV node; ≥0.12 if block at bundle branches | MI, conduction system lesion, hypoxia, medication side effects | Decreased cardiac output if HR slow | Pacemaker, atropine, epinephrine or dopamine, O$_2$ |
| 2:1 AVB | Atria: 60–100; ventricle: half the atrial rate | Regular | Normal; 2 Ps to each QRS | Constant on the conducted beats | <0.12 if block at AV node; ≥0.12 if block at bundle branches | Same as Wenckebach and Mobitz II | Decreased cardiac output if HR slow | Pacemaker, atropine, epinephrine or dopamine, consider O$_2$ |
| Third-degree AV block | Atria: 60–100; ventricle: 20–60 | Regular | Normal; dissociated from QRS | Varies | <0.12 if AV node is the pacemaker; >0.12 if ventricle is the pacemaker | MI, conduction system lesion, hypoxia, medication side effect | Decreased cardiac output if HR slow | Pacemaker, atropine, epinephrine or dopamine, O$_2$ |

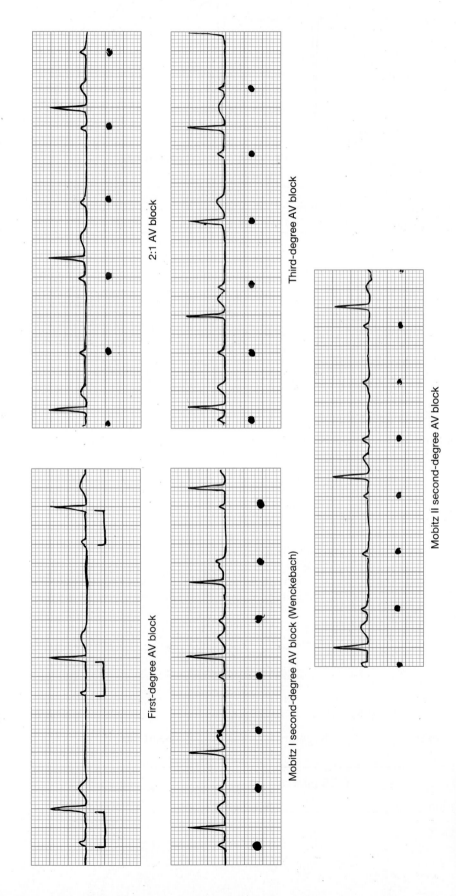

First-degree AV block

2:1 AV block

Mobitz I second-degree AV block (Wenckebach)

Third-degree AV block

Mobitz II second-degree AV block

**FIGURE 11–10**

**AV Blocks Pictorial Review.**

## Practice Strips: AV Blocks

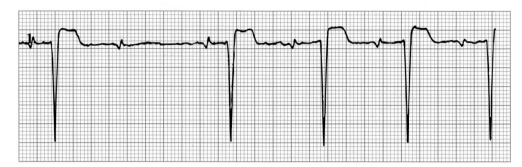

1. QRS complexes _____ Regularity _____ Heart rate _____

   P waves _____

   PR interval _____ QRS interval _____

   Interpretation (name of rhythm) _____

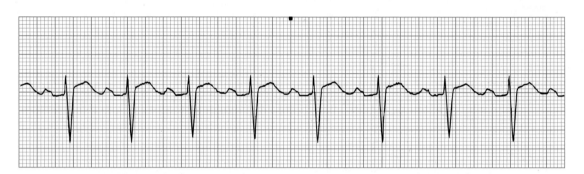

2. QRS complexes _____ Regularity _____ Heart rate _____

   P waves _____

   PR interval _____ QRS interval _____

   Interpretation _____

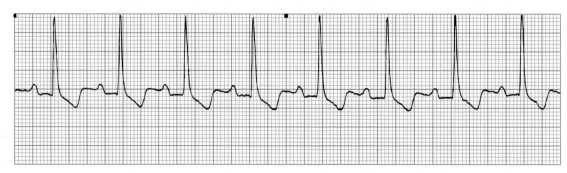

3. QRS complexes _____ Regularity _____ Heart rate _____

   P waves _____

   PR interval _____ QRS interval _____

   Interpretation _____

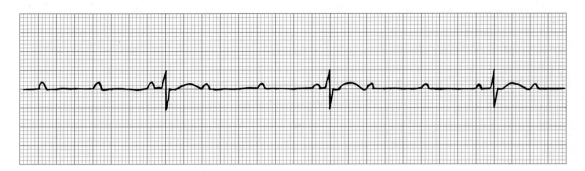

**4.** QRS complexes _____ Regularity _____ Heart rate _____

P waves _____

PR interval _____ QRS interval _____

Interpretation _____

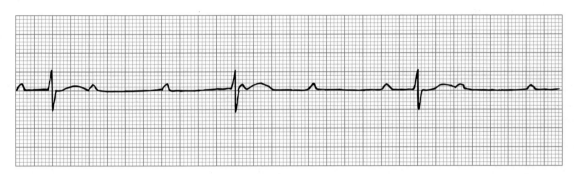

**5.** QRS complexes _____ Regularity _____ Heart rate _____

P waves _____

PR interval _____ QRS interval _____

Interpretation _____

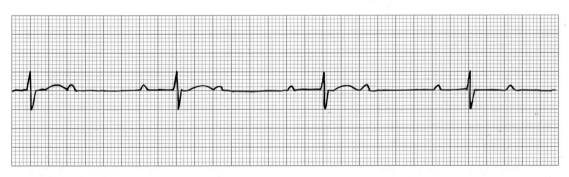

**6.** QRS complexes _____ Regularity _____ Heart rate _____

P waves _____

PR interval _____ QRS interval _____

Interpretation _____

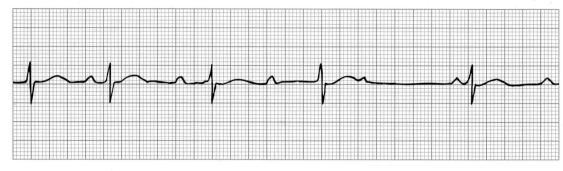

7. QRS complexes _____ Regularity _____ Heart rate _____

P waves _____

PR interval _____ QRS interval _____

Interpretation _____

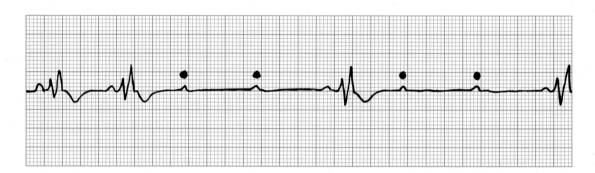

8. QRS complexes _____ Regularity _____ Heart rate _____

P waves _____

PR interval _____ QRS interval _____

Interpretation _____

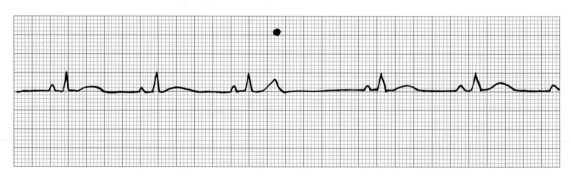

9. QRS complexes _____ Regularity _____ Heart rate _____

P waves _____

PR interval _____ QRS interval _____

Interpretation _____

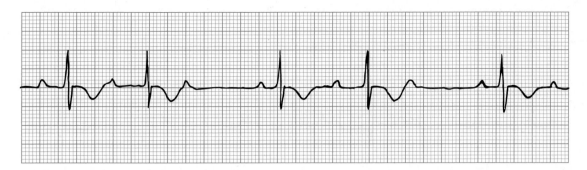

**10.** QRS complexes _____ Regularity _____ Heart rate _____

P waves _____

PR interval _____ QRS interval _____

Interpretation _____

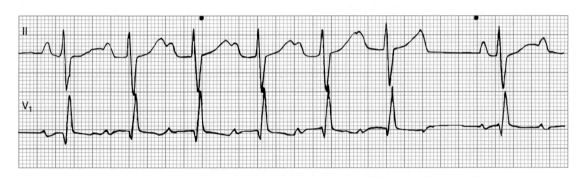

**11.** QRS complexes _____ Regularity _____ Heart rate _____

P waves _____

PR interval _____ QRS interval _____

Interpretation _____

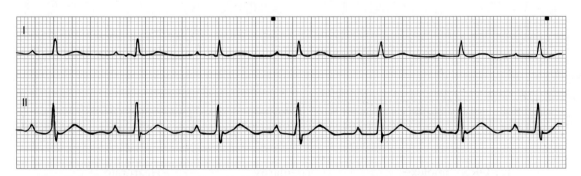

**12.** QRS complexes _____ Regularity _____ Heart rate _____

P waves _____

PR interval _____ QRS interval _____

Interpretation _____

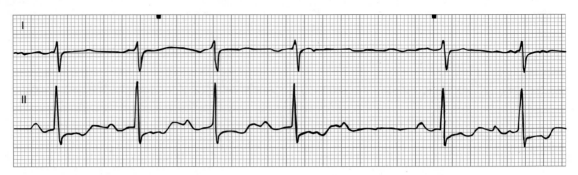

13. QRS complexes _____ Regularity _____ Heart rate _____

P waves _____

PR interval _____ QRS interval _____

Interpretation _____

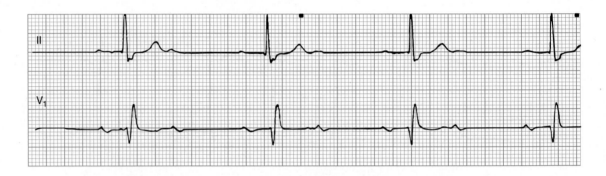

14. QRS complexes _____ Regularity _____ Heart rate _____

P waves _____

PR interval _____ QRS interval _____

Interpretation _____

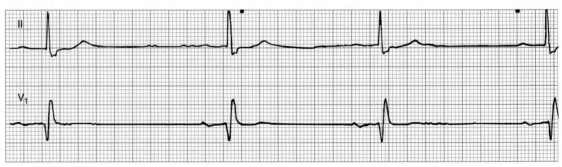

15. QRS complexes _____ Regularity _____ Heart rate _____

P waves _____

PR interval _____ QRS interval _____

Interpretation _____

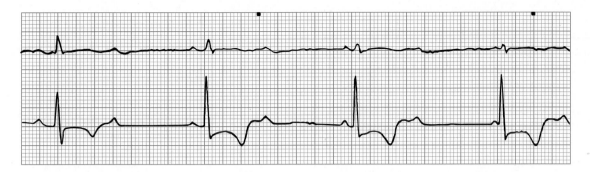

**16.** QRS complexes _____ Regularity _____ Heart rate _____

P waves _____

PR interval _____ QRS interval _____

Interpretation _____

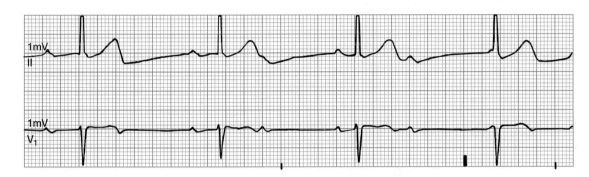

**17.** QRS complexes _____ Regularity _____ Heart rate _____

P waves _____

PR interval _____ QRS interval _____

Interpretation _____

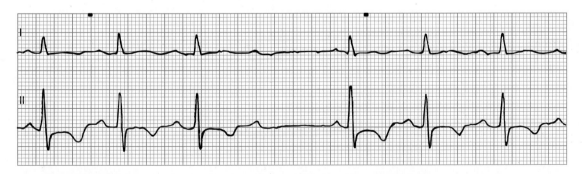

**18.** QRS complexes _____ Regularity _____ Heart rate _____

P waves _____

PR interval _____ QRS interval _____

Interpretation _____

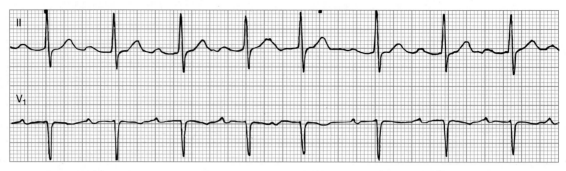

**19.** QRS complexes _____ Regularity _____ Heart rate _____

P waves _____

PR interval _____ QRS interval _____

Interpretation _____

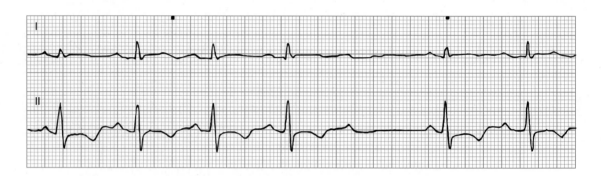

**20.** QRS complexes _____ Regularity _____ Heart rate _____

P waves _____

PR interval _____ QRS interval _____

Interpretation _____

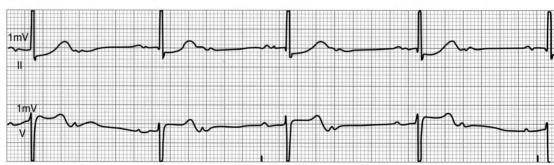

**21.** QRS complexes _____ Regularity _____ Heart rate _____

P waves _____

PR interval _____ QRS interval _____

Interpretation _____

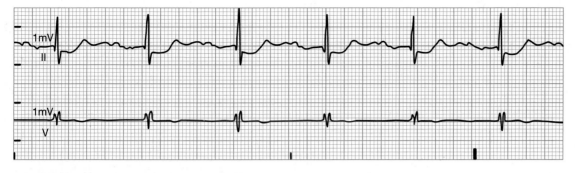

22. QRS complexes _____ Regularity _____ Heart rate _____

    P waves _____

    PR interval _____ QRS interval _____

    Interpretation _____


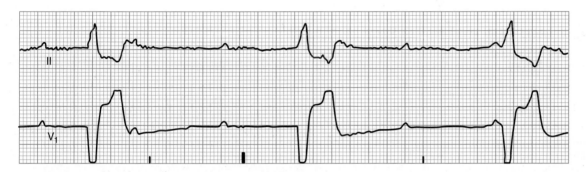

23. QRS complexes _____ Regularity _____ Heart rate _____

    P waves _____

    PR interval _____ QRS interval _____

    Interpretation _____


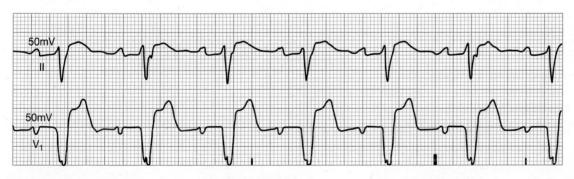

24. QRS complexes _____ Regularity _____ Heart rate _____

    P waves _____

    PR interval _____ QRS interval _____

    Interpretation _____

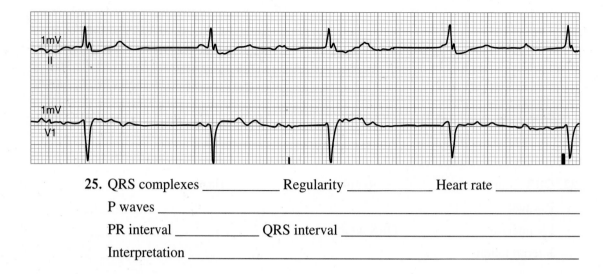

25. QRS complexes _____ Regularity _____ Heart rate _____

    P waves _____

    PR interval _____ QRS interval _____

    Interpretation _____

## chapter eleven notes TO SUM IT ALL UP . . .

- **Three degrees of AV blocks:**
  - *First degree*—Delay in impulse transmission between atria and ventricles. All impulses do make it through.
  - *Second degree*—Some impulses get through to ventricles; some don't.
  - *Third degree*—No impulses make it through from atria to ventricles. A lower pacemaker has to escape to provide stimulus to ventricles.
- **All AV blocks start out as sinus rhythms.** Therefore, all P waves are sinus Ps.
- **The block can occur in the AV node or the bundle branches.**
- **First-degree AV block:**
  - *Heart rate*—Can occur at any rate
  - *Regularity*—Depends on underlying rhythm
  - *P waves*—Sinus Ps; one P per QRS
  - *Intervals*—PR >0.20 secs; QRS <0.12 secs.
  - *Causes*—AV node ischemia, digitalis toxicity, other medication side effects
  - *Adverse effects*—None
  - *Treatment*—Treat the cause
- **Mobitz I second-degree AV block (Wenckebach):**
  - *Heart rate*—Atrial rate 60–100; ventricular rate slower than atrial due to dropped beats
  - *Regularity*—Irregular or regular but interrupted in appearance
  - *P waves*—Sinus P waves; some not followed by a QRS
  - *Intervals*—PR varies, gradually prolonging until a QRS is dropped; QRS <0.12 secs
  - *Causes*—MI, digitalis toxicity, medication side effects
  - Adverse effects: Usually none because heart rate is usually good
  - *Treatment*—Usually none needed; watch for worsening block; oxygen, atropine, pacemaker if symptomatic from low heart rate
- **Mobitz II second-degree AV block:**
  - *Heart rate*—Atrial rate 60–100; ventricular rate slower due to dropped beats

- *Regularity*—Regular, irregular, or regular but interrupted in appearance
- *P waves*—Sinus Ps; some Ps not followed by a QRS
- *Intervals*—PR 0.12–0.20 secs constant on the conducted beats. QRS <0.12 secs if the block is at the AV node; ≥0.12 secs if the block is at the bundle branches
- *Causes*—MI, conduction system lesion, medications, hypoxia
- *Adverse effects*—Decreased cardiac output
- *Treatment*—Oxygen, pacemaker if symptomatic; atropine, epinephrine, or dopamine infusions can be used while awaiting transvenous pacemaker arrival.

- **2:1 AV block:**
  - *Heart rate*—Atrial rate 60–100; ventricular rate half of atrial rate
  - *Regularity*—Regular
  - *P waves*—Sinus Ps; every other P not followed by a QRS
  - *Intervals*—PR 0.12–0.20 secs constant on conducted beats. QRS <0.12 secs if the block is at the AV node; ≥0.12 secs if the block is at the bundle branches.
  - *Causes*—Same as Wenckebach or Mobitz II
  - *Adverse effects*—Decreased cardiac output if heart rate too slow
  - *Treatment*—Oxygen, pacemaker if symptomatic, atropine, epinephrine, or dopamine infusion

- **Third-degree AV block:**
  - *Heart rate*—Atrial rate 60–100; ventricular rate much slower due to dropped beats
  - *Regularity*—Regular
  - *P waves*—Sinus Ps; some not followed by a QRS
  - *Intervals*—PR varies. QRS <0.12 secs if the block is at the AV node; ≥0.12 secs if the block is at the bundle branches.
  - *Causes*—MI, conduction system lesion, medication side effects, hypoxia
  - *Adverse effects*—Decreased cardiac output
  - *Treatment*—Pacemaker, oxygen. May use atropine, epinephrine, or dopamine infusion while awaiting pacemaker arrival.

## Practice Quiz

1. Name the two typical locations of the block in AV blocks. _____

_____

2. True or false: People with a first-degree AV block need a pacemaker inserted.

3. Wenckebach is another name for which kind of block? _____

_____

4. AV dissociation is a hallmark of which kind of AV block? _____

_____

_____

5. True or false: Atropine is effective in all types of AV blocks, whether the block is at the AV node or the bundle branches.

6. The AV block that merely results in a prolonged PR interval is _____

_____

7. What is atropine's mode of action? _____

_____

8. The most dangerous type of AV block is _____

9. The least dangerous type of AV block is _____

10. True or false: All AV blocks require atropine or epinephrine to increase the heart rate.

## Putting It All Together—Critical Thinking Exercises

These exercises may consist of diagrams to label, scenarios to analyze, brain-stumping questions to ponder, or other challenging exercises to boost your understanding of the chapter material.

Let's play with AV blocks a bit. The following scenario will provide you with information about a fictional patient and will ask you to analyze the situation, answer questions, and decide on appropriate actions.

Ms. Watson, age 89, presents to her physician's office complaining of feeling weak and tired for the past 3 days. She has a history of atrial fibrillation and has been taking digoxin for years. She also takes insulin for diabetes and beta-blockers for high blood pressure. Vital signs are stable and within normal limits. Suspecting that Ms. Watson's atrial fib has again gotten out of control, the nurse records the rhythm strip below. See Figure 11–11.

1. What is the rhythm and heart rate? _____

_____

2. Does this rhythm require emergency treatment? ____

_____

Suddenly, Ms. Watson says "I feel funny," and the nurse helps her lie back on the examining table. Vital signs are still within normal limits, but her BP has dropped some. Her repeat rhythm strip is seen in Figure 11–12.

3. What has happened? _____

4. Which of Ms. Watson's medications could be responsible for this rhythm?

_____

The physician admits Ms. Watson to the telemetry floor and orders a digoxin level, which comes back elevated. Further questioning of Ms. Watson reveals that she'd doubled up on her digoxin the past three days because she thought it would help her feel better.

5. Given this latest information, what treatment is appropriate for this rhythm?

_____

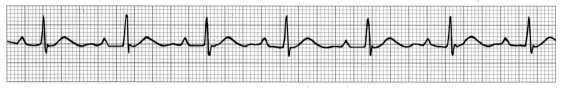

**FIGURE 11–11**

Ms. Watson's initial strip.

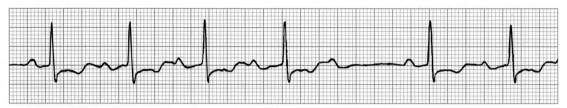

**FIGURE 11–12**

Ms. Watson's "funny" strip.

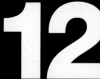

# Rhythm Practice Strips

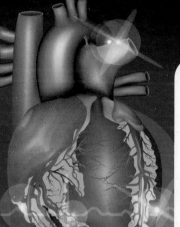

## CHAPTER 12 OBJECTIVES

Upon completion of this chapter, the student will be able to

- Correctly identify the rhythms.
- Identify any weak areas for further study.

## What It's All About

Two nurses were conferring about Mr. Cohen's rhythm. They suspect he is in third degree AV block. His heart rate is 42 and he's pale and complaining of lightheadedness, but his blood pressure is holding within his normal limits so far. One nurse puts the transcutaneous pacemaker on standby while the other readies the atropine. The cardiologist looks at the rhythm strip and agrees with the nurses that the rhythm is third-degree AV block. She calls the cath lab team in to do an emergency transvenous pacemaker and orders atropine to be given intravenously in the meantime. The next morning, with his new pacemaker working well, Mr. Cohen states he hasn't felt this good in years.

## Introduction

This chapter focuses on the interpretation of rhythm strips utilizing the five steps you learned in Chapter 6 and the rhythm descriptions in Chapters 7 through 11. The strips are in no particular order; there may be sinus rhythms next to ventricular rhythms. Some strips are easy to interpret; others are more challenging. Take your time and go step by step.

## Rhythms for Practice

Some rhythms in this chapter are on single-lead strips; others are on double-lead strips. Remember that on double-lead strips, both leads represent the same rhythm seen in different leads. Thus the heart rate, interval measurements, and other interpretation will be the same whether you assess the top lead or the bottom lead. Use either lead to do your interpretation. On the intervals, allow plus or minus 0.02 secs for your answer. (If the answer for a PR interval is listed as 0.16, for example, anywhere between 0.14 and 0.18 would still be correct. Intervals can vary just a little from beat to beat because of the sympathetic and parasympathetic nervous system's influence).

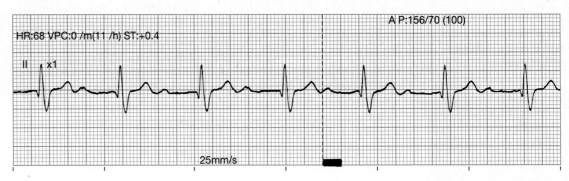

1. QRS complexes _____ Regularity _____ Heart rate _____

   P waves _____

   PR interval _____ QRS interval _____

   Interpretation _____

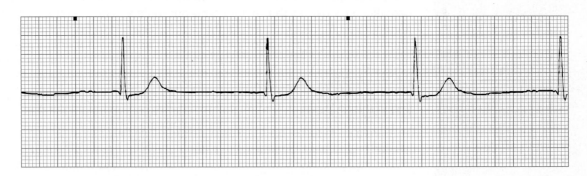

2. QRS complexes _____ Regularity _____ Heart rate _____

   P waves _____

   PR interval _____ QRS interval _____

   Interpretation _____

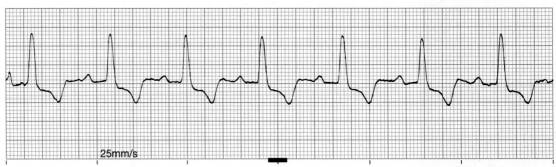

3. QRS complexes _____ Regularity _____ Heart rate _____

   P waves _____

   PR interval _____ QRS interval _____

   Interpretation _____

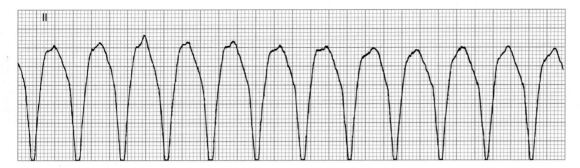

**4.** QRS complexes _____ Regularity _____ Heart rate _____

P waves _____

PR interval _____ QRS interval _____

Interpretation _____

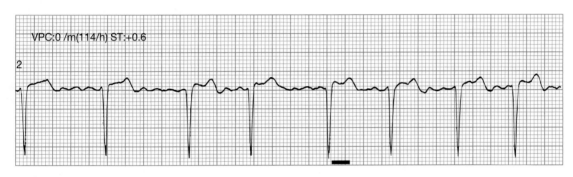

**5.** QRS complexes _____ Regularity _____ Heart rate _____

P waves _____

PR interval _____ QRS interval _____

Interpretation _____

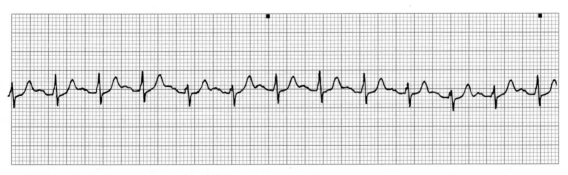

**6.** QRS complexes _____ Regularity _____ Heart rate _____

P waves _____

PR interval _____ QRS interval _____

Interpretation _____

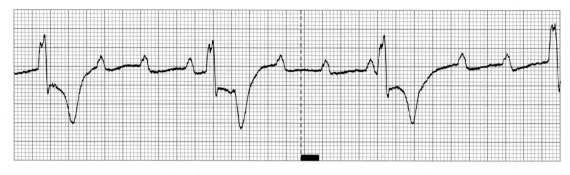

7. QRS complexes _____ Regularity _____ Heart rate _____

   P waves _____

   PR interval _____ QRS interval _____

   Interpretation _____

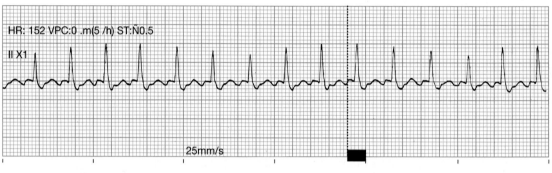

8. QRS complexes _____ Regularity _____ Heart rate _____

   P waves _____

   PR interval _____ QRS interval _____

   Interpretation _____

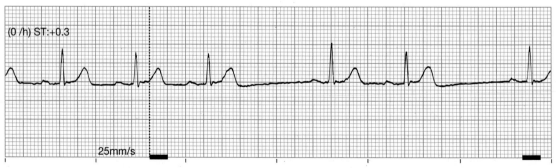

9. QRS complexes _____ Regularity _____ Heart rate _____

   P waves _____

   PR interval _____ QRS interval _____

   Interpretation _____

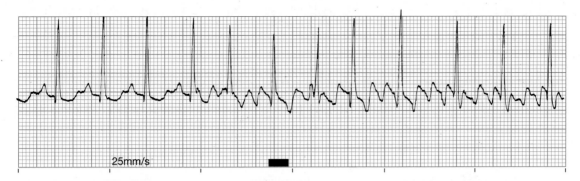

25mm/s

**10.** QRS complexes _____ Regularity _____ Heart rate _____

P waves _____

PR interval _____ QRS interval _____

Interpretation _____

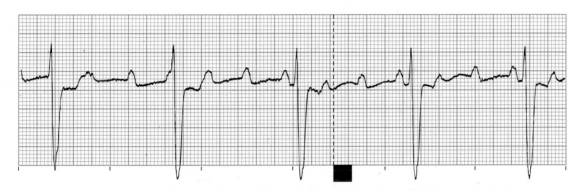

**11.** QRS complexes _____ Regularity _____ Heart rate _____

P waves _____

PR interval _____ QRS interval _____

Interpretation _____

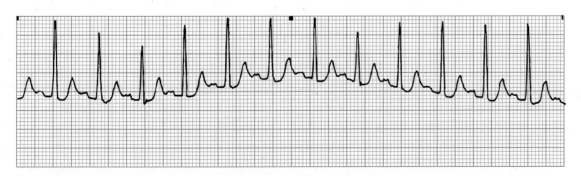

**12.** QRS complexes _____ Regularity _____ Heart rate _____

P waves _____

PR interval _____ QRS interval _____

Interpretation _____

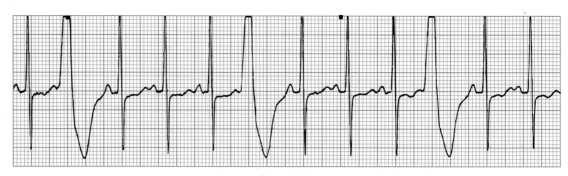

**13.** QRS complexes _____ Regularity _____ Heart rate _____

P waves _____

PR interval _____ QRS interval _____

Interpretation _____

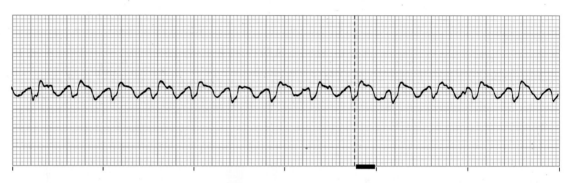

**14.** QRS complexes _____ Regularity _____ Heart rate _____

P waves _____

PR interval _____ QRS interval _____

Interpretation _____

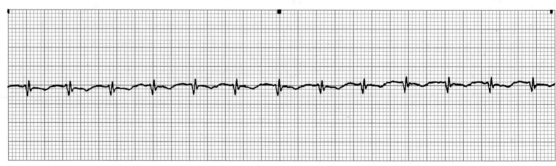

**15.** QRS complexes _____ Regularity _____ Heart rate _____

P waves _____

PR interval _____ QRS interval _____

Interpretation _____

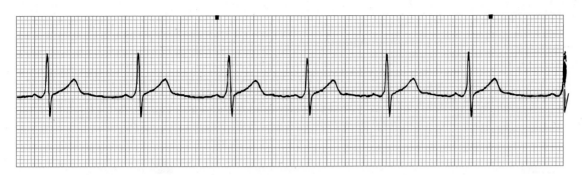

**16.** QRS complexes _____ Regularity _____ Heart rate _____

P waves _____

PR interval _____ QRS interval _____

Interpretation _____

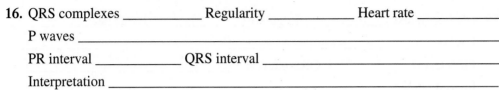

**17.** QRS complexes _____ Regularity _____ Heart rate _____

P waves _____

PR interval _____ QRS interval _____

Interpretation _____

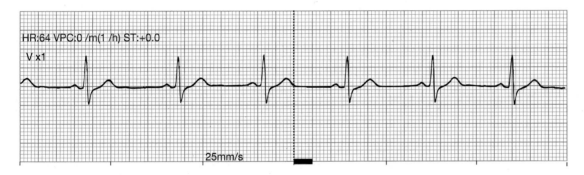

**18.** QRS complexes _____ Regularity _____ Heart rate _____

P waves _____

PR interval _____ QRS interval _____

Interpretation _____

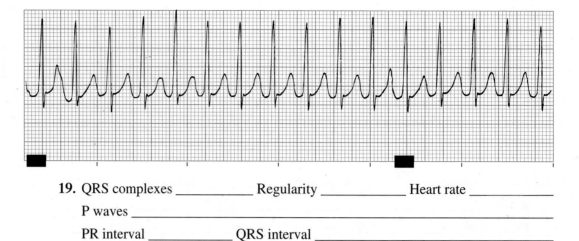

**19.** QRS complexes _____ Regularity _____ Heart rate _____

P waves _____

PR interval _____ QRS interval _____

Interpretation _____

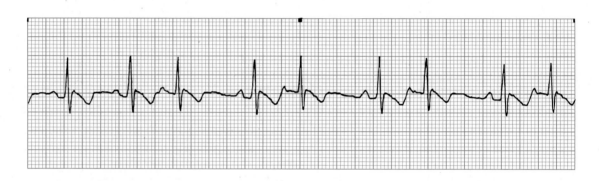

**20.** QRS complexes _____ Regularity _____ Heart rate _____

P waves _____

PR interval _____ QRS interval _____

Interpretation _____

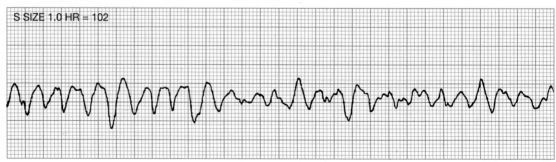

S SIZE 1.0 HR = 102

**21.** QRS complexes _____ Regularity _____ Heart rate _____

P waves _____

PR interval _____ QRS interval _____

Interpretation _____

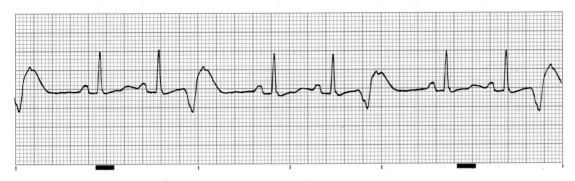

**22.** QRS complexes ＿＿＿＿＿ Regularity ＿＿＿＿＿ Heart rate ＿＿＿＿＿

P waves ＿＿＿＿＿＿＿＿＿＿＿＿＿＿＿＿＿＿＿＿＿＿＿＿＿＿＿＿＿＿＿

PR interval ＿＿＿＿＿ QRS interval ＿＿＿＿＿＿＿＿＿＿＿＿＿＿＿

Interpretation ＿＿＿＿＿＿＿＿＿＿＿＿＿＿＿＿＿＿＿＿＿＿＿＿＿＿

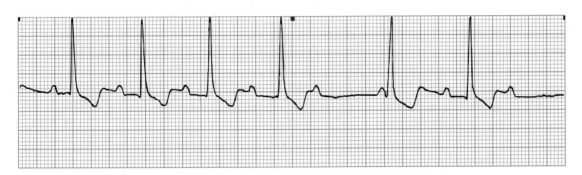

**23.** QRS complexes ＿＿＿＿＿ Regularity ＿＿＿＿＿ Heart rate ＿＿＿＿＿

P waves ＿＿＿＿＿＿＿＿＿＿＿＿＿＿＿＿＿＿＿＿＿＿＿＿＿＿＿＿＿＿＿

PR interval ＿＿＿＿＿ QRS interval ＿＿＿＿＿＿＿＿＿＿＿＿＿＿＿

Interpretation ＿＿＿＿＿＿＿＿＿＿＿＿＿＿＿＿＿＿＿＿＿＿＿＿＿＿

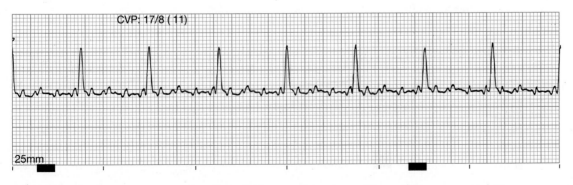

**24.** QRS complexes ＿＿＿＿＿ Regularity ＿＿＿＿＿ Heart rate ＿＿＿＿＿

P waves ＿＿＿＿＿＿＿＿＿＿＿＿＿＿＿＿＿＿＿＿＿＿＿＿＿＿＿＿＿＿＿

PR interval ＿＿＿＿＿ QRS interval ＿＿＿＿＿＿＿＿＿＿＿＿＿＿＿

Interpretation ＿＿＿＿＿＿＿＿＿＿＿＿＿＿＿＿＿＿＿＿＿＿＿＿＿＿

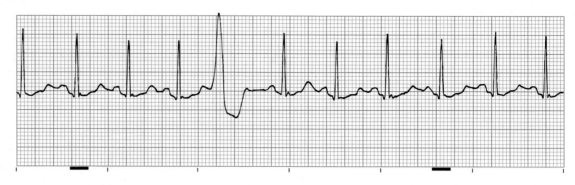

**25.** QRS complexes _____ Regularity _____ Heart rate _____

P waves _____

PR interval _____ QRS interval _____

Interpretation _____

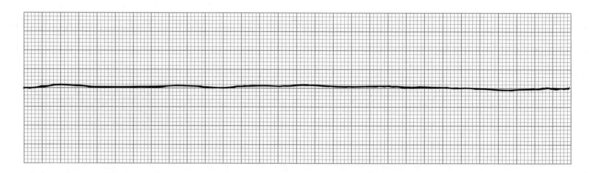

**26.** QRS complexes _____ Regularity _____ Heart rate _____

P waves _____

PR interval _____ QRS interval _____

Interpretation _____

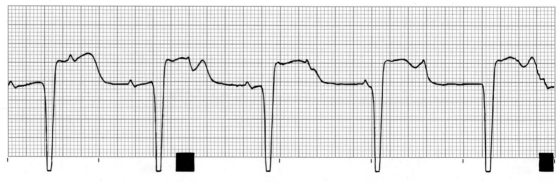

**27.** QRS complexes _____ Regularity _____ Heart rate _____

P waves _____

PR interval _____ QRS interval _____

Interpretation _____

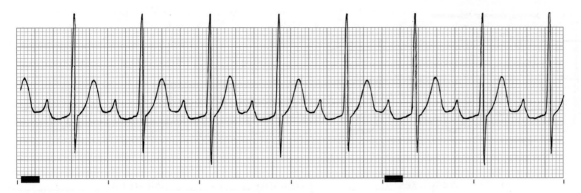

**28.** QRS complexes _____ Regularity _____ Heart rate _____

P waves _____

PR interval _____ QRS interval _____

Interpretation _____

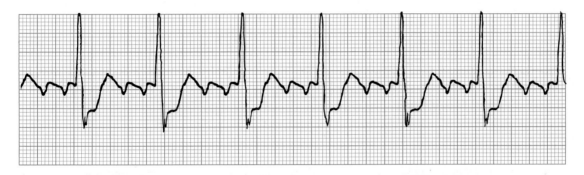

**29.** QRS complexes _____ Regularity _____ Heart rate _____

P waves _____

PR interval _____ QRS interval _____

Interpretation _____

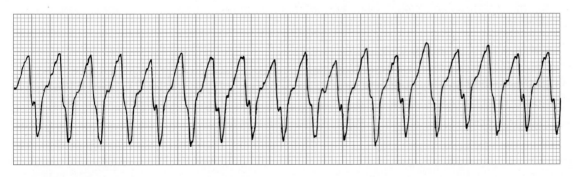

**30.** QRS complexes _____ Regularity _____ Heart rate _____

P waves _____

PR interval _____ QRS interval _____

Interpretation _____

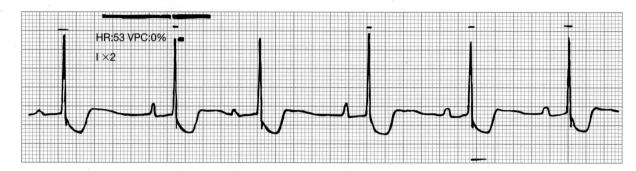

**31.** QRS complexes _____ Regularity _____ Heart rate _____

P waves _____

PR interval _____ QRS interval _____

Interpretation _____

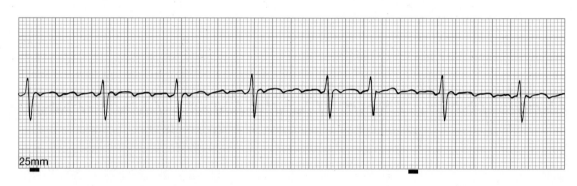

**32.** QRS complexes _____ Regularity _____ Heart rate _____

P waves _____

PR interval _____ QRS interval _____

Interpretation _____

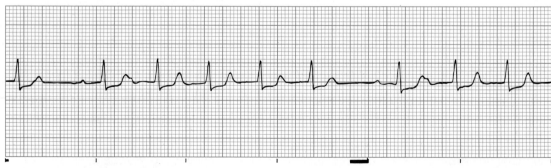

**33.** QRS complexes _____ Regularity _____ Heart rate _____

P waves _____

PR interval _____ QRS interval _____

Interpretation _____

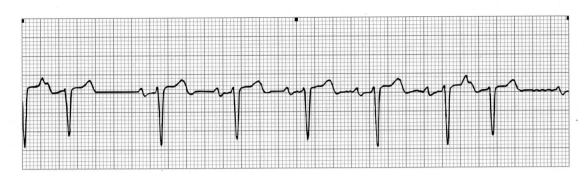

**34.** QRS complexes _____ Regularity _____ Heart rate _____

P waves _____

PR interval _____ QRS interval _____

Interpretation _____

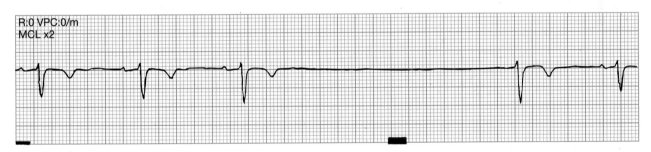

**35.** QRS complexes _____ Regularity _____ Heart rate _____

P waves _____

PR interval _____ QRS interval _____

Interpretation _____

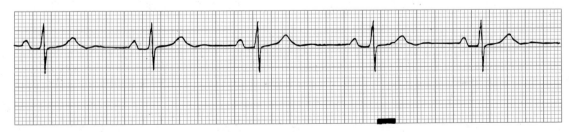

**36.** QRS complexes _____ Regularity _____ Heart rate _____

P waves _____

PR interval _____ QRS interval _____

Interpretation _____

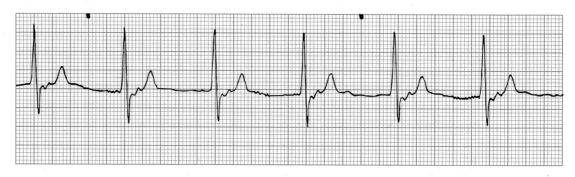

37. QRS complexes _____ Regularity _____ Heart rate _____

    P waves _____

    PR interval _____ QRS interval _____

    Interpretation _____

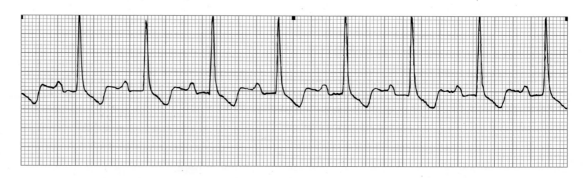

38. QRS complexes _____ Regularity _____ Heart rate _____

    P waves _____

    PR interval _____ QRS interval _____

    Interpretation _____

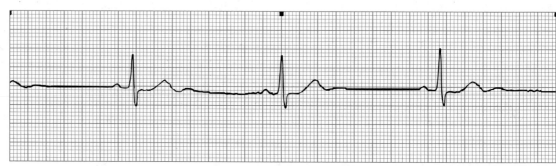

39. QRS complexes _____ Regularity _____ Heart rate _____

    P waves _____

    PR interval _____ QRS interval _____

    Interpretation _____

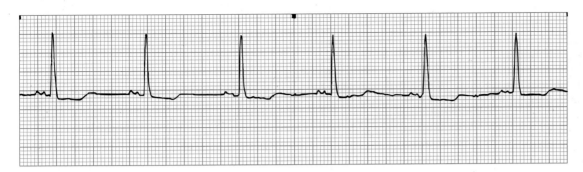

**40.** QRS complexes _____ Regularity _____ Heart rate _____

P waves _____

PR interval _____ QRS interval _____

Interpretation _____

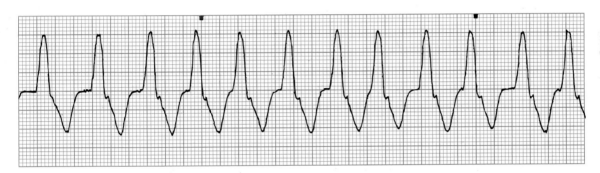

**41.** QRS complexes _____ Regularity _____ Heart rate _____

P waves _____

PR interval _____ QRS interval _____

Interpretation _____

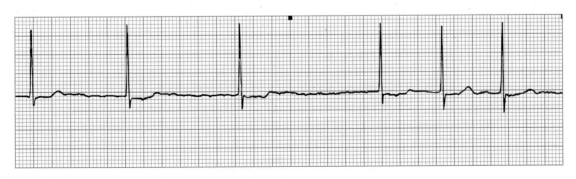

**42.** QRS complexes _____ Regularity _____ Heart rate _____

P waves _____

PR interval _____ QRS interval _____

Interpretation _____

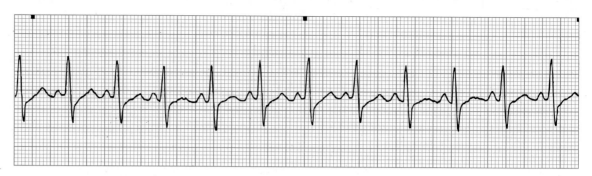

**43.** QRS complexes _____ Regularity _____ Heart rate _____

P waves _____

PR interval _____ QRS interval _____

Interpretation _____

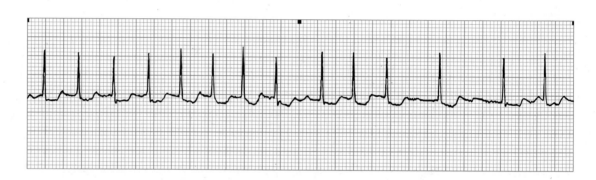

**44.** QRS complexes _____ Regularity _____ Heart rate _____

P waves _____

PR interval _____ QRS interval _____

Interpretation _____

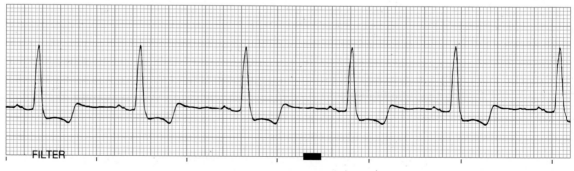

**45.** QRS complexes _____ Regularity _____ Heart rate _____

P waves _____

PR interval _____ QRS interval _____

Interpretation _____

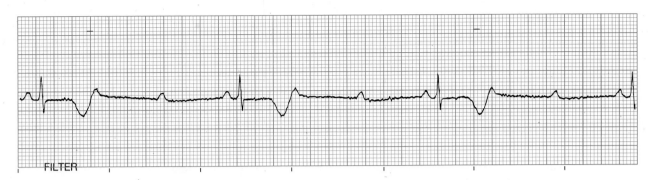

**46.** QRS complexes _____ Regularity _____ Heart rate _____

P waves _____

PR interval _____ QRS interval _____

Interpretation _____

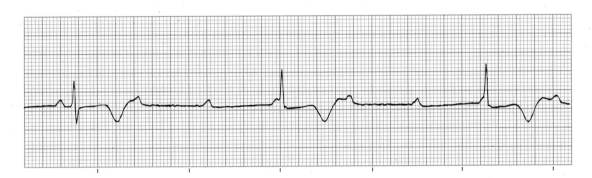

**47.** QRS complexes _____ Regularity _____ Heart rate _____

P waves _____

PR interval _____ QRS interval _____

Interpretation _____

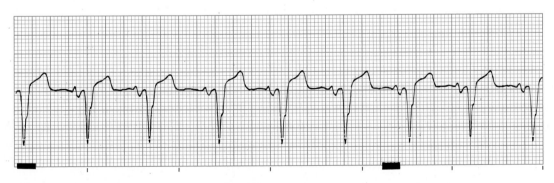

**48.** QRS complexes _____ Regularity _____ Heart rate _____

P waves _____

PR interval _____ QRS interval _____

Interpretation _____

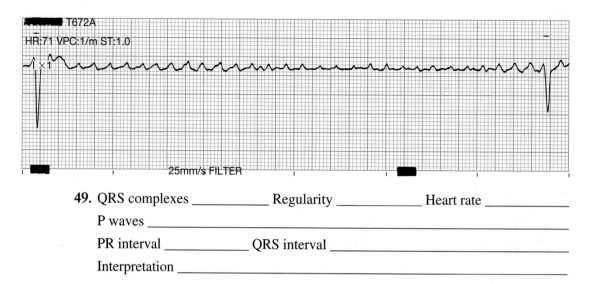

**49.** QRS complexes _____ Regularity _____ Heart rate _____

P waves _____

PR interval _____ QRS interval _____

Interpretation _____

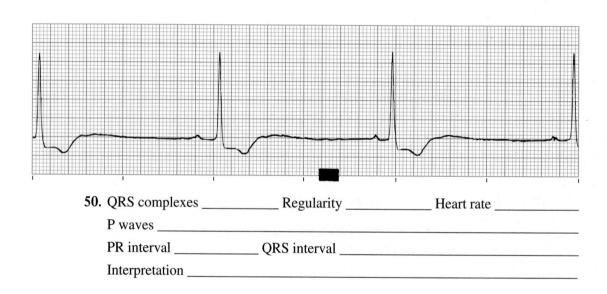

**50.** QRS complexes _____ Regularity _____ Heart rate _____

P waves _____

PR interval _____ QRS interval _____

Interpretation _____

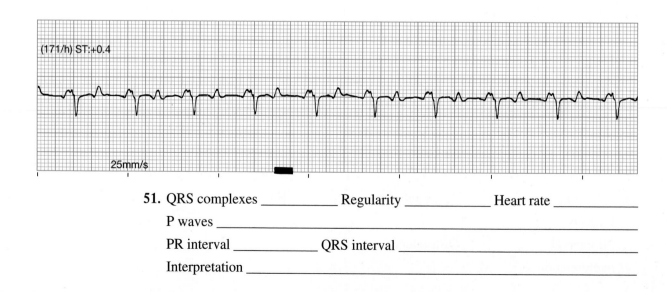

**51.** QRS complexes _____ Regularity _____ Heart rate _____

P waves _____

PR interval _____ QRS interval _____

Interpretation _____

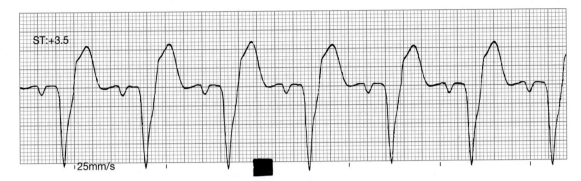

**52.** QRS complexes _____ Regularity _____ Heart rate _____

P waves _____

PR interval _____ QRS interval _____

Interpretation _____

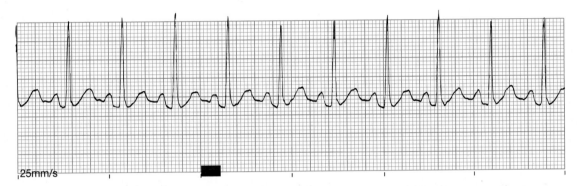

**53.** QRS complexes _____ Regularity _____ Heart rate _____

P waves _____

PR interval _____ QRS interval _____

Interpretation _____

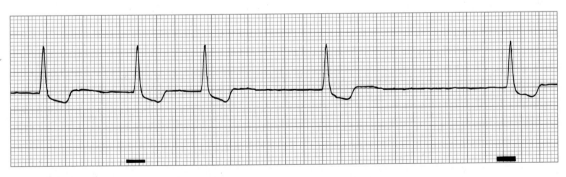

**54.** QRS complexes _____ Regularity _____ Heart rate _____

P waves _____

PR interval _____ QRS interval _____

Interpretation _____

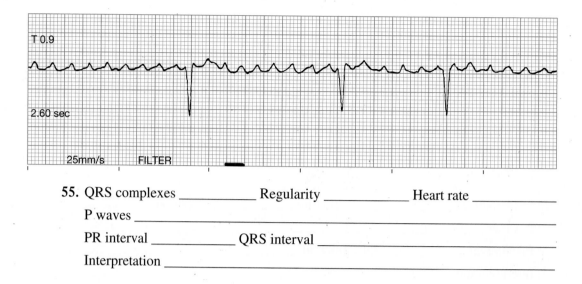

**55.** QRS complexes _____ Regularity _____ Heart rate _____

P waves _____

PR interval _____ QRS interval _____

Interpretation _____

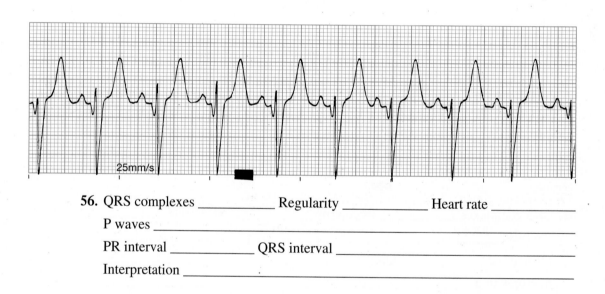

**56.** QRS complexes _____ Regularity _____ Heart rate _____

P waves _____

PR interval _____ QRS interval _____

Interpretation _____

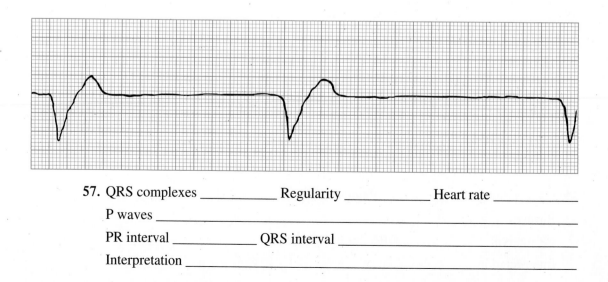

**57.** QRS complexes _____ Regularity _____ Heart rate _____

P waves _____

PR interval _____ QRS interval _____

Interpretation _____

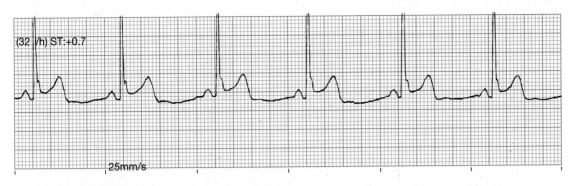

(32 /h) ST:+0.7

25mm/s

**58.** QRS complexes _____ Regularity _____ Heart rate _____

   P waves _____

   PR interval _____ QRS interval _____

   Interpretation _____

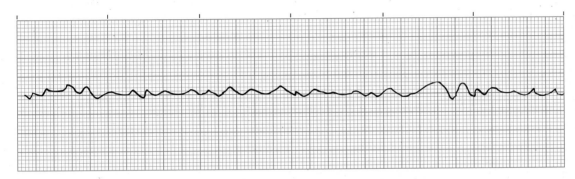

**59.** QRS complexes _____ Regularity _____ Heart rate _____

   P waves _____

   PR interval _____ QRS interval _____

   Interpretation _____

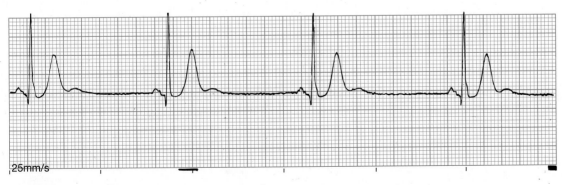

25mm/s

**60.** QRS complexes _____ Regularity _____ Heart rate _____

   P waves _____

   PR interval _____ QRS interval _____

   Interpretation _____

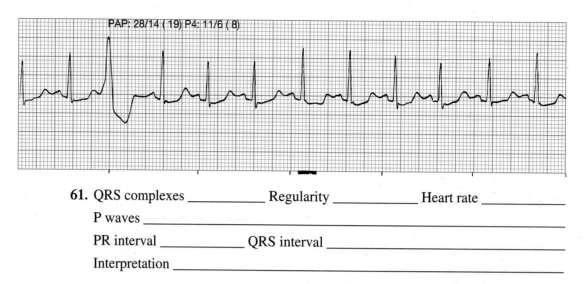

PAP: 28/14 ( 19) P4: 11/6 ( 8)

**61.** QRS complexes _____ Regularity _____ Heart rate _____

P waves _____

PR interval _____ QRS interval _____

Interpretation _____

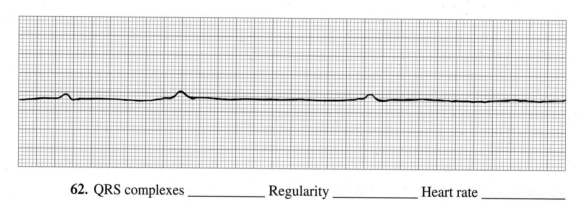

**62.** QRS complexes _____ Regularity _____ Heart rate _____

P waves _____

PR interval _____ QRS interval _____

Interpretation _____

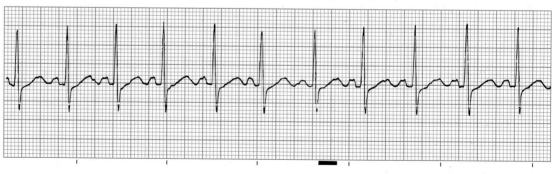

**63.** QRS complexes _____ Regularity _____ Heart rate _____

P waves _____

PR interval _____ QRS interval _____

Interpretation _____

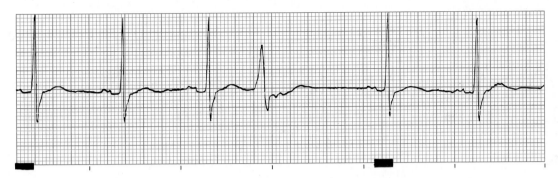

**64.** QRS complexes _____ Regularity _____ Heart rate _____

P waves _____

PR interval _____ QRS interval _____

Interpretation _____

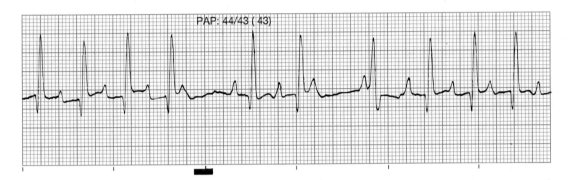

**65.** QRS complexes _____ Regularity _____ Heart rate _____

P waves _____

PR interval _____ QRS interval _____

Interpretation _____

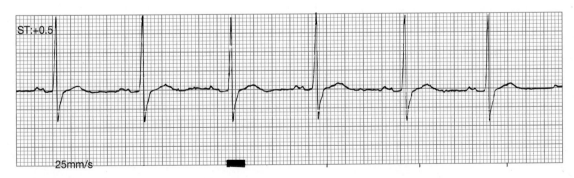

**66.** QRS complexes _____ Regularity _____ Heart rate _____

P waves _____

PR interval _____ QRS interval _____

Interpretation _____

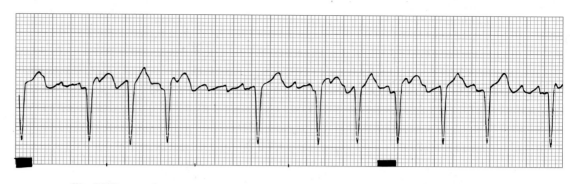

**67.** QRS complexes _____ Regularity _____ Heart rate _____

P waves _____

PR interval _____ QRS interval _____

Interpretation _____

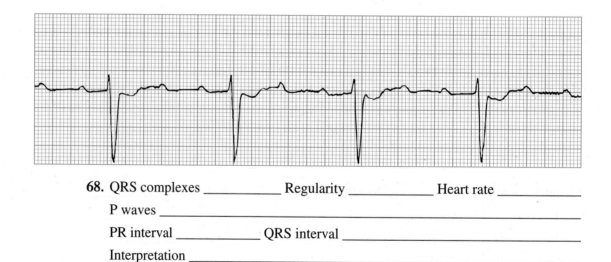

**68.** QRS complexes _____ Regularity _____ Heart rate _____

P waves _____

PR interval _____ QRS interval _____

Interpretation _____

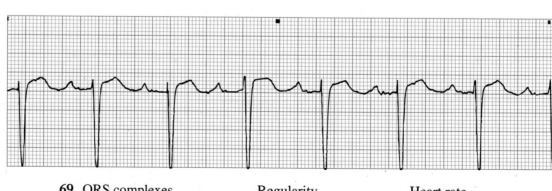

**69.** QRS complexes _____ Regularity _____ Heart rate _____

P waves _____

PR interval _____ QRS interval _____

Interpretation _____

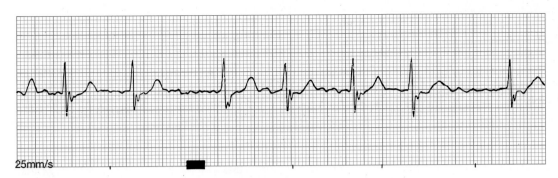

25mm/s

**70.** QRS complexes _____ Regularity _____ Heart rate _____

   P waves _____

   PR interval _____ QRS interval _____

   Interpretation _____

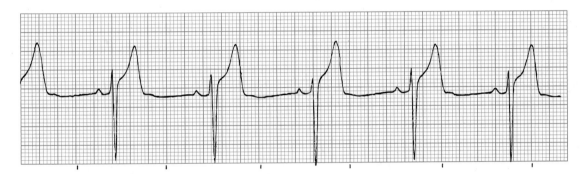

**71.** QRS complexes _____ Regularity _____ Heart rate _____

   P waves _____

   PR interval _____ QRS interval _____

   Interpretation _____

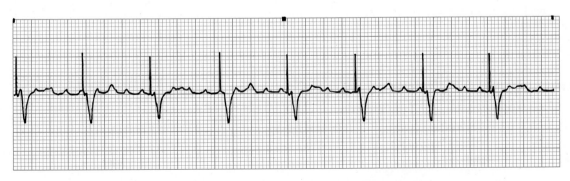

**72.** QRS complexes _____ Regularity _____ Heart rate _____

   P waves _____

   PR interval _____ QRS interval _____

   Interpretation _____

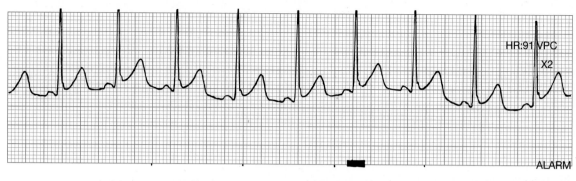

**73.** QRS complexes _____ Regularity _____ Heart rate _____

P waves _____

PR interval _____ QRS interval _____

Interpretation _____

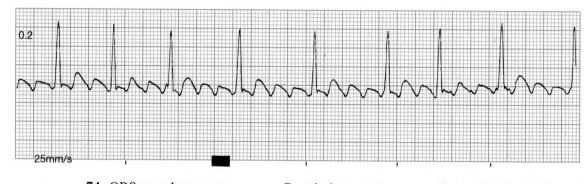

**74.** QRS complexes _____ Regularity _____ Heart rate _____

P waves _____

PR interval _____ QRS interval _____

Interpretation _____

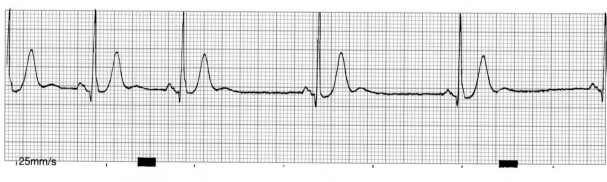

**75.** QRS complexes _____ Regularity _____ Heart rate _____

P waves _____

PR interval _____ QRS interval _____

Interpretation _____

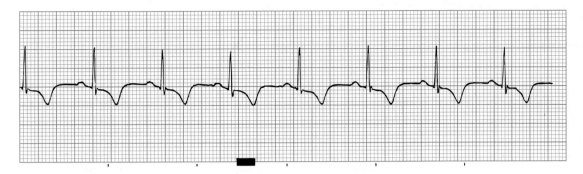

**76.** QRS complexes _____ Regularity _____ Heart rate _____

P waves _____

PR interval _____ QRS interval _____

Interpretation _____

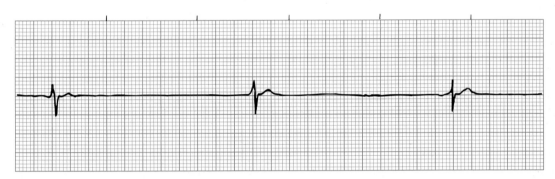

**77.** QRS complexes _____ Regularity _____ Heart rate _____

P waves _____

PR interval _____ QRS interval _____

Interpretation _____

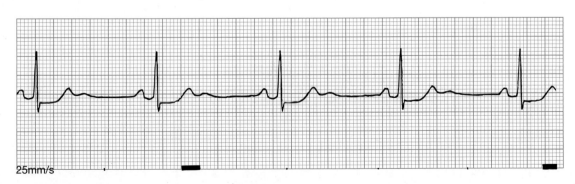

25mm/s

**78.** QRS complexes _____ Regularity _____ Heart rate _____

P waves _____

PR interval _____ QRS interval _____

Interpretation _____

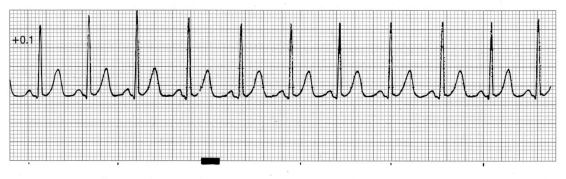

**79.** QRS complexes _____ Regularity _____ Heart rate _____

P waves _____

PR interval _____ QRS interval _____

Interpretation _____

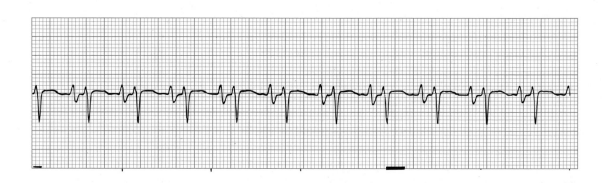

**80.** QRS complexes _____ Regularity _____ Heart rate _____

P waves _____

PR interval _____ QRS interval _____

Interpretation _____

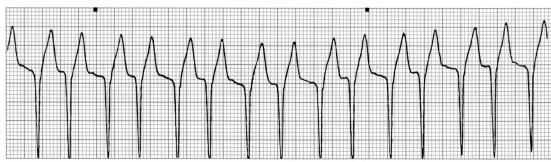

**81.** QRS complexes _____ Regularity _____ Heart rate _____

P waves _____

PR interval _____ QRS interval _____

Interpretation _____

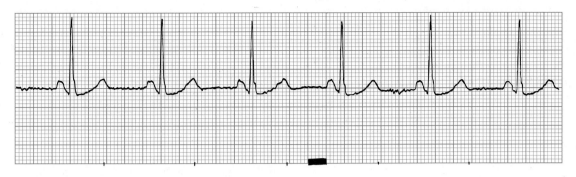

**82.** QRS complexes _____ Regularity _____ Heart rate _____

P waves _____

PR interval _____ QRS interval _____

Interpretation _____

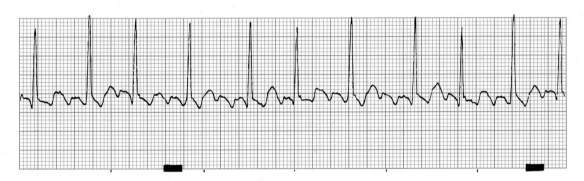

**83.** QRS complexes _____ Regularity _____ Heart rate _____

P waves _____

PR interval _____ QRS interval _____

Interpretation _____

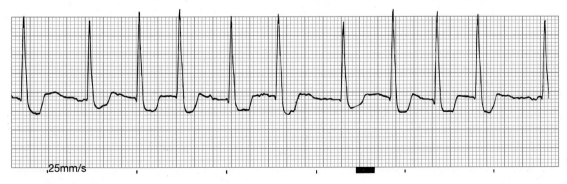

,25mm/s

**84.** QRS complexes _____ Regularity _____ Heart rate _____

P waves _____

PR interval _____ QRS interval _____

Interpretation _____

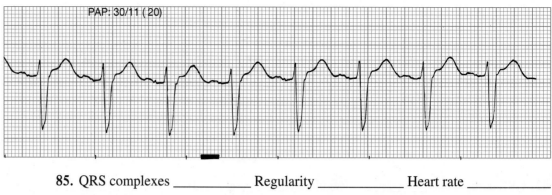

**85.** QRS complexes _____ Regularity _____ Heart rate _____

P waves _____

PR interval _____ QRS interval _____

Interpretation _____

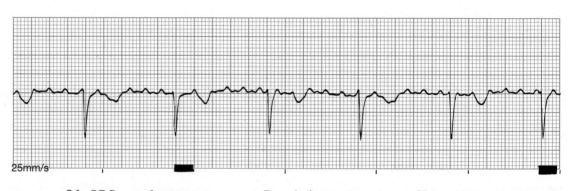

**86.** QRS complexes _____ Regularity _____ Heart rate _____

P waves _____

PR interval _____ QRS interval _____

Interpretation _____

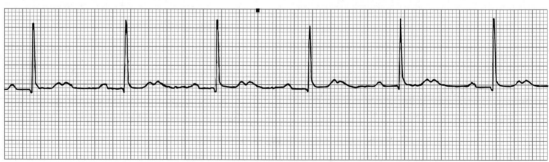

**87.** QRS complexes _____ Regularity _____ Heart rate _____

P waves _____

PR interval _____ QRS interval _____

Interpretation _____

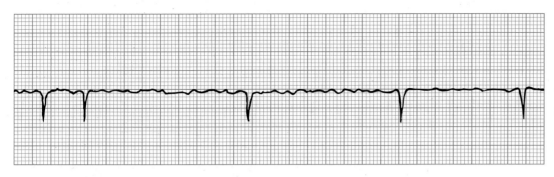

**88.** QRS complexes _____ Regularity _____ Heart rate _____

P waves _____

PR interval _____ QRS interval _____

Interpretation _____

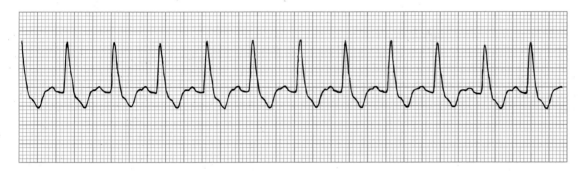

**89.** QRS complexes _____ Regularity _____ Heart rate _____

P waves _____

PR interval _____ QRS interval _____

Interpretation _____

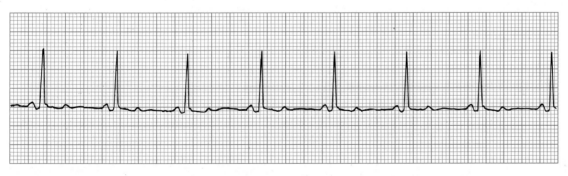

**90.** QRS complexes _____ Regularity _____ Heart rate _____

P waves _____

PR interval _____ QRS interval _____

Interpretation _____

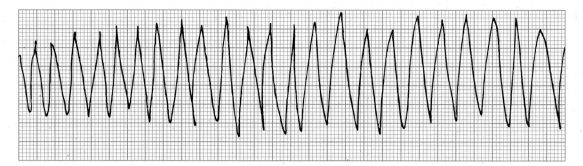

**91.** QRS complexes _____ Regularity _____ Heart rate _____

P waves _____

PR interval _____ QRS interval _____

Interpretation _____

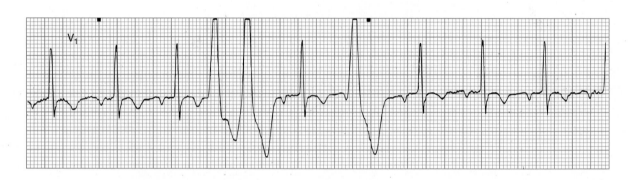

**92.** QRS complexes _____ Regularity _____ Heart rate _____

P waves _____

PR interval _____ QRS interval _____

Interpretation _____

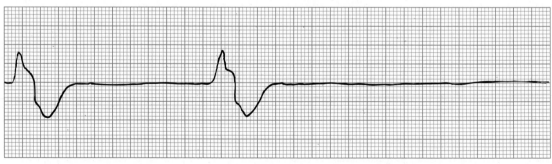

**93.** QRS complexes _____ Regularity _____ Heart rate _____

P waves _____

PR interval _____ QRS interval _____

Interpretation _____

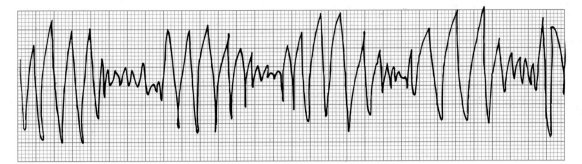

**94.** QRS complexes _____ Regularity _____ Heart rate _____

P waves _____

PR interval _____ QRS interval _____

Interpretation _____

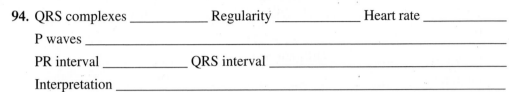

**95.** QRS complexes _____ Regularity _____ Heart rate _____

P waves _____

PR interval _____ QRS interval _____

Interpretation _____

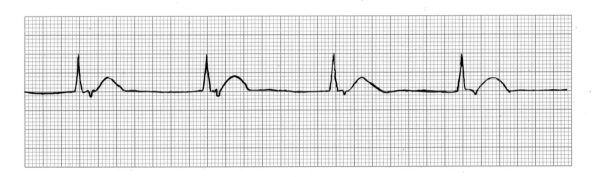

**96.** QRS complexes _____ Regularity _____ Heart rate _____

P waves _____

PR interval _____ QRS interval _____

Interpretation _____

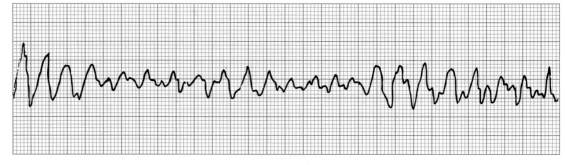

**97.** QRS complexes _____ Regularity _____ Heart rate _____

P waves _____

PR interval _____ QRS interval _____

Interpretation _____

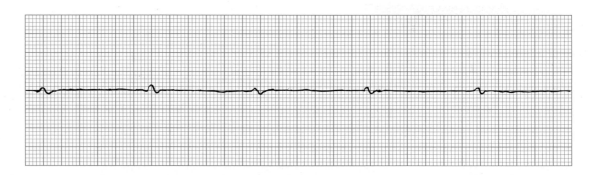

**98.** QRS complexes _____ Regularity _____ Heart rate _____

P waves _____

PR interval _____ QRS interval _____

Interpretation _____

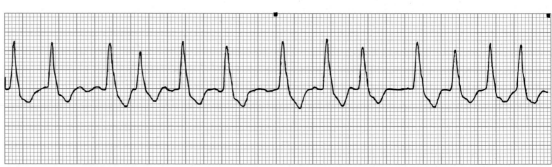

**99.** QRS complexes _____ Regularity _____ Heart rate _____

P waves _____

PR interval _____ QRS interval _____

Interpretation _____

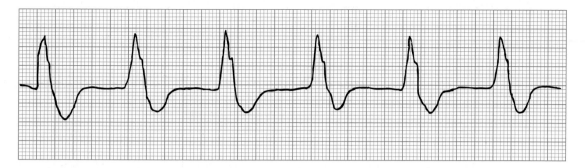

**100.** QRS complexes _____ Regularity _____ Heart rate _____

P waves _____

PR interval _____ QRS interval _____

Interpretation _____

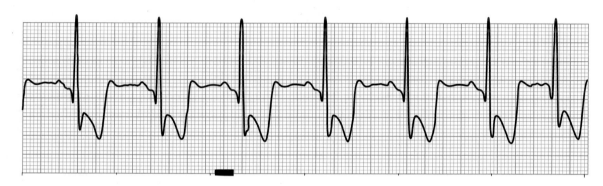

**101.** QRS complexes _____ Regularity _____ Heart rate _____

P waves _____

PR interval _____ QRS interval _____

Interpretation _____

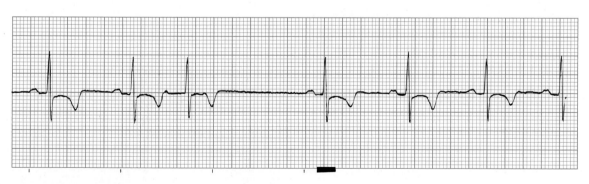

**102.** QRS complexes _____ Regularity _____ Heart rate _____

P waves _____

PR interval _____ QRS interval _____

Interpretation _____

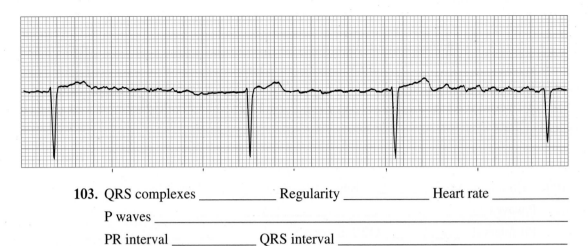

**103.** QRS complexes _____ Regularity _____ Heart rate _____

P waves _____

PR interval _____ QRS interval _____

Interpretation _____

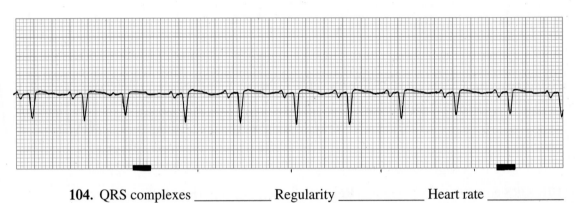

**104.** QRS complexes _____ Regularity _____ Heart rate _____

P waves _____

PR interval _____ QRS interval _____

Interpretation _____

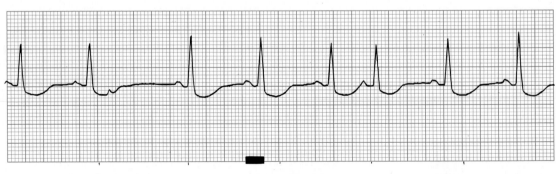

**105.** QRS complexes _____ Regularity _____ Heart rate _____

P waves _____

PR interval _____ QRS interval _____

Interpretation _____

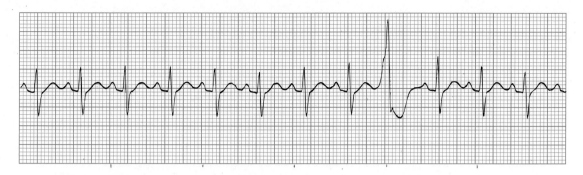

**106.** QRS complexes _____ Regularity _____ Heart rate _____

P waves _____

PR interval _____ QRS interval _____

Interpretation _____

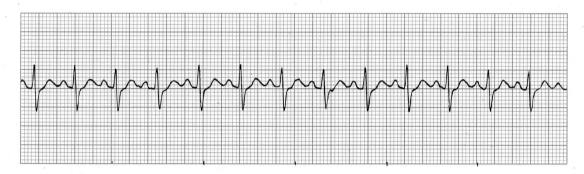

**107.** QRS complexes _____ Regularity _____ Heart rate _____

P waves _____

PR interval _____ QRS interval _____

Interpretation _____

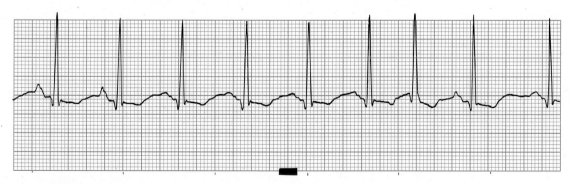

**108.** QRS complexes _____ Regularity _____ Heart rate _____

P waves _____

PR interval _____ QRS interval _____

Interpretation _____

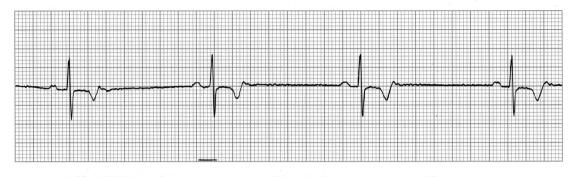

**109.** QRS complexes _____ Regularity _____ Heart rate _____

P waves _____

PR interval _____ QRS interval _____

Interpretation _____

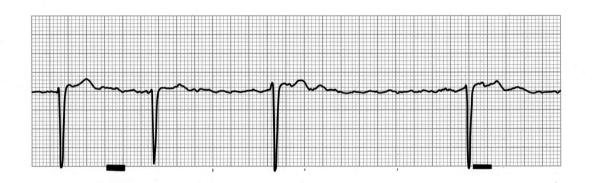

**110.** QRS complexes _____ Regularity _____ Heart rate _____

P waves _____

PR interval _____ QRS interval _____

Interpretation _____

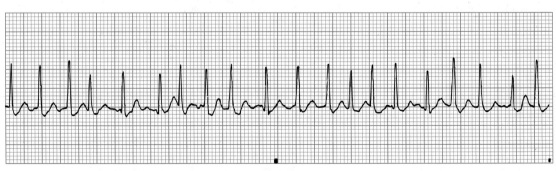

**111.** QRS complexes _____ Regularity _____ Heart rate _____

P waves _____

PR interval _____ QRS interval _____

Interpretation _____

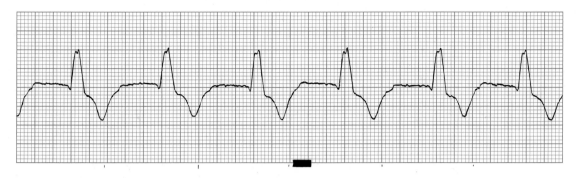

**112.** QRS complexes _____ Regularity _____ Heart rate _____

P waves _____

PR interval _____ QRS interval _____

Interpretation _____

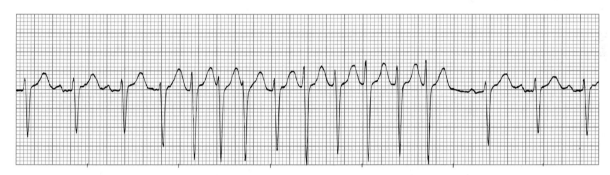

**113.** QRS complexes _____ Regularity _____ Heart rate _____

P waves _____

PR interval _____ QRS interval _____

Interpretation _____

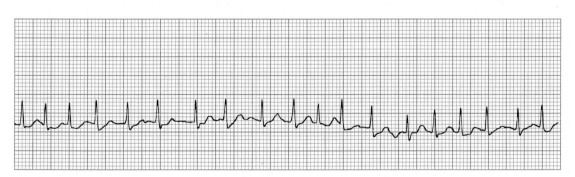

**114.** QRS complexes _____ Regularity _____ Heart rate _____

P waves _____

PR interval _____ QRS interval _____

Interpretation _____

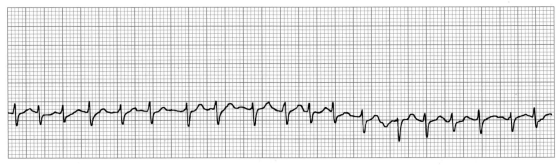

**115.** QRS complexes _____ Regularity _____ Heart rate _____

P waves _____

PR interval _____ QRS interval _____

Interpretation _____

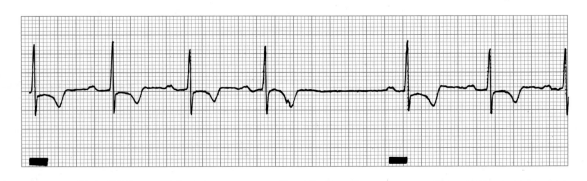

**116.** QRS complexes _____ Regularity _____ Heart rate _____

P waves _____

PR interval _____ QRS interval _____

Interpretation _____

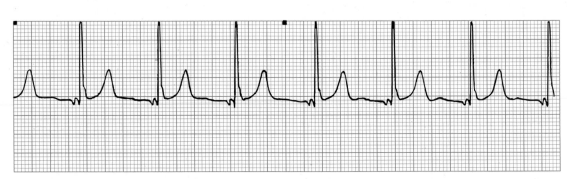

**117.** QRS complexes _____ Regularity _____ Heart rate _____

P waves _____

PR interval _____ QRS interval _____

Interpretation _____

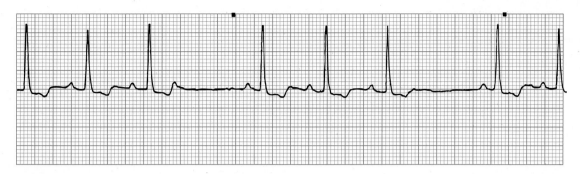

**118.** QRS complexes _____ Regularity _____ Heart rate _____

P waves _____

PR interval _____ QRS interval _____

Interpretation _____

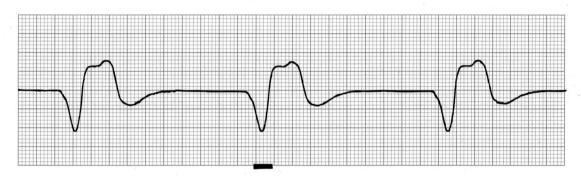

**119.** QRS complexes _____ Regularity _____ Heart rate _____

P waves _____

PR interval _____ QRS interval _____

Interpretation _____

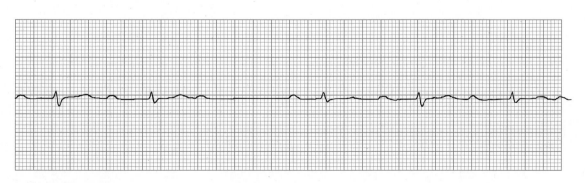

**120.** QRS complexes _____ Regularity _____ Heart rate _____

P waves _____

PR interval _____ QRS interval _____

Interpretation _____

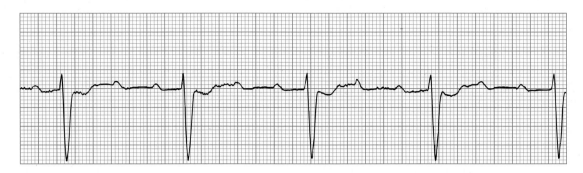

**121.** QRS complexes _____ Regularity _____ Heart rate _____

P waves _____

PR interval _____ QRS interval _____

Interpretation _____

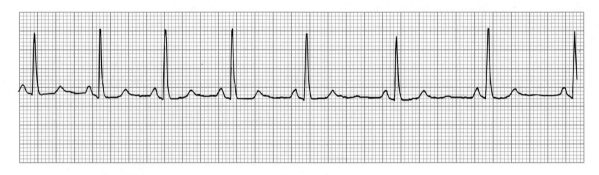

**122.** QRS complexes _____ Regularity _____ Heart rate _____

P waves _____

PR interval _____ QRS interval _____

Interpretation _____

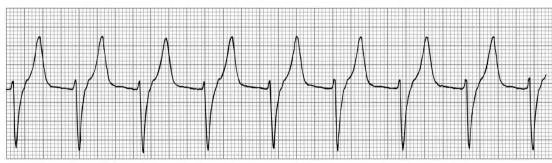

**123.** QRS complexes _____ Regularity _____ Heart rate _____

P waves _____

PR interval _____ QRS interval _____

Interpretation _____

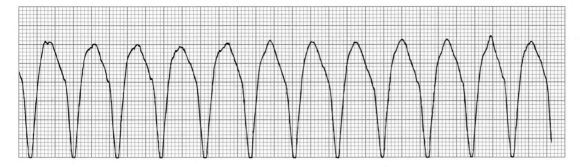

**124.** QRS complexes _____ Regularity _____ Heart rate _____

P waves _____

PR interval _____ QRS interval _____

Interpretation _____

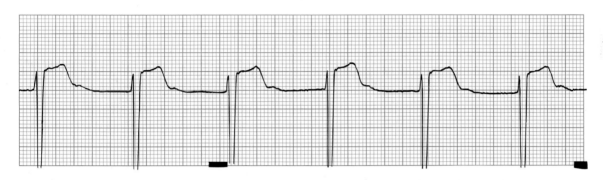

**125.** QRS complexes _____ Regularity _____ Heart rate _____

P waves _____

PR interval _____ QRS interval _____

Interpretation _____

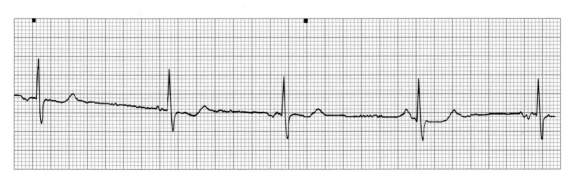

**126.** QRS complexes _____ Regularity _____ Heart rate _____

P waves _____

PR interval _____ QRS interval _____

Interpretation _____

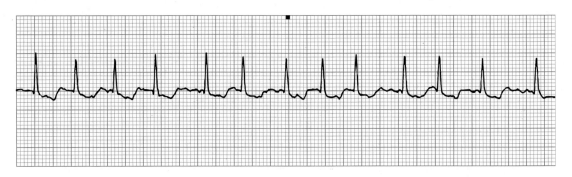

**127.** QRS complexes _____ Regularity _____ Heart rate _____

P waves _____

PR interval _____ QRS interval _____

Interpretation _____

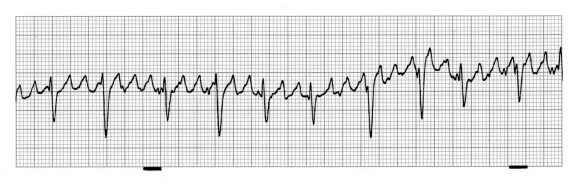

**128.** QRS complexes _____ Regularity _____ Heart rate _____

P waves _____

PR interval _____ QRS interval _____

Interpretation _____

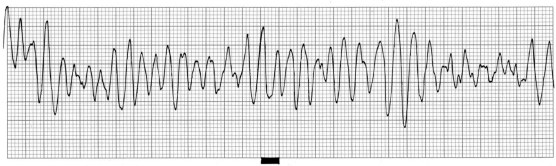

**129.** QRS complexes _____ Regularity _____ Heart rate _____

P waves _____

PR interval _____ QRS interval _____

Interpretation _____

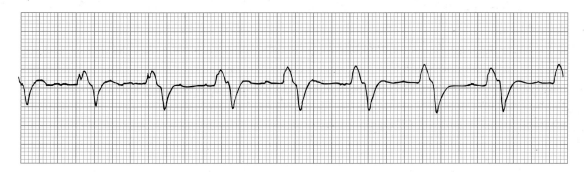

**130.** QRS complexes _____ Regularity _____ Heart rate _____

P waves _____

PR interval _____ QRS interval _____

Interpretation _____

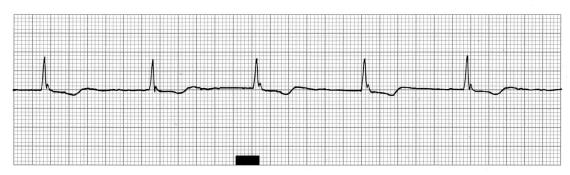

**131.** QRS complexes _____ Regularity _____ Heart rate _____

P waves _____

PR interval _____ QRS interval _____

Interpretation _____

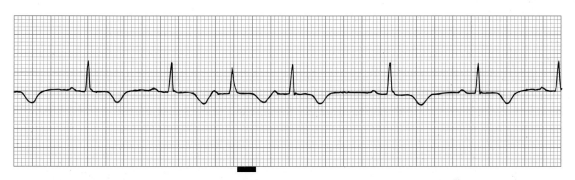

**132.** QRS complexes _____ Regularity _____ Heart rate _____

P waves _____

PR interval _____ QRS interval _____

Interpretation _____

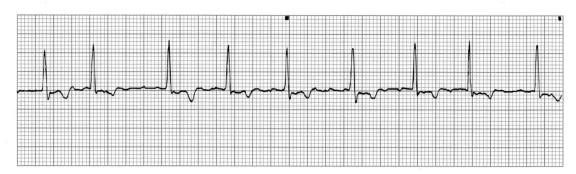

**133.** QRS complexes _____ Regularity _____ Heart rate _____

P waves _____

PR interval _____ QRS interval _____

Interpretation _____

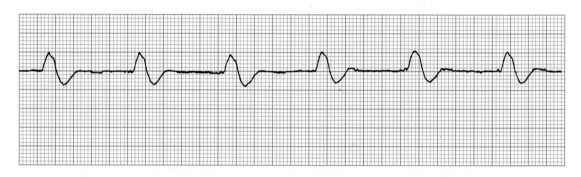

**134.** QRS complexes _____ Regularity _____ Heart rate _____

P waves _____

PR interval _____ QRS interval _____

Interpretation _____

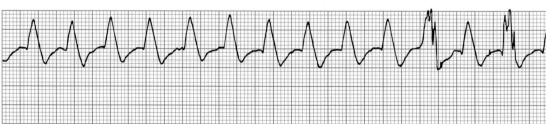

**135.** QRS complexes _____ Regularity _____ Heart rate _____

P waves _____

PR interval _____ QRS interval _____

Interpretation _____

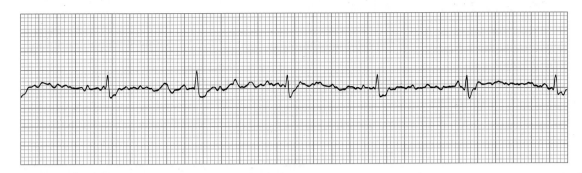

**136.** QRS complexes _____ Regularity _____ Heart rate _____

P waves _____

PR interval _____ QRS interval _____

Interpretation _____

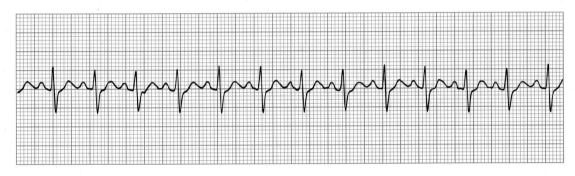

**137.** QRS complexes _____ Regularity _____ Heart rate _____

P waves _____

PR interval _____ QRS interval _____

Interpretation _____

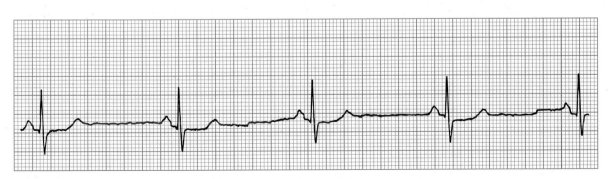

**138.** QRS complexes _____ Regularity _____ Heart rate _____

P waves _____

PR interval _____ QRS interval _____

Interpretation _____

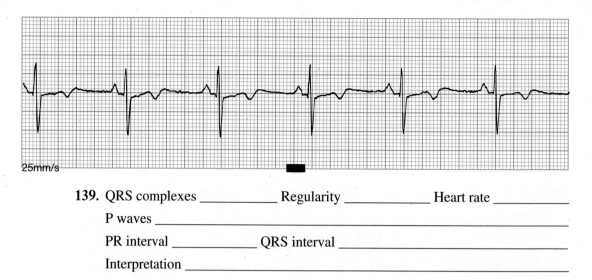

25mm/s

**139.** QRS complexes _____ Regularity _____ Heart rate _____

P waves _____

PR interval _____ QRS interval _____

Interpretation _____

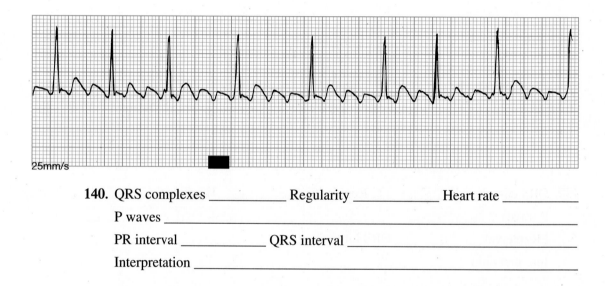

25mm/s

**140.** QRS complexes _____ Regularity _____ Heart rate _____

P waves _____

PR interval _____ QRS interval _____

Interpretation _____

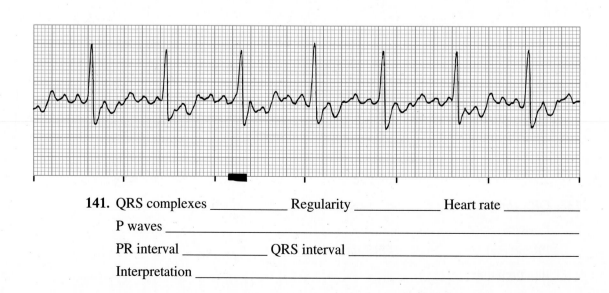

**141.** QRS complexes _____ Regularity _____ Heart rate _____

P waves _____

PR interval _____ QRS interval _____

Interpretation _____

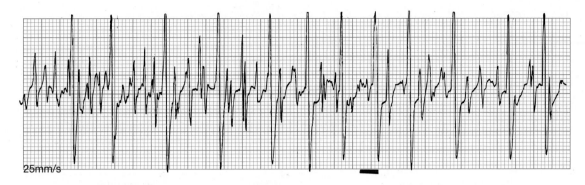

25mm/s

**142.** QRS complexes _____ Regularity _____ Heart rate _____

P waves _____

PR interval _____ QRS interval _____

Interpretation _____

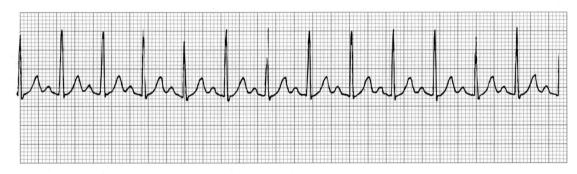

**143.** QRS complexes _____ Regularity _____ Heart rate _____

P waves _____

PR interval _____ QRS interval _____

Interpretation _____

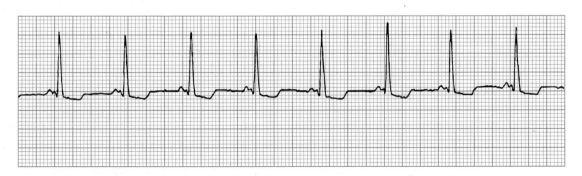

**144.** QRS complexes _____ Regularity _____ Heart rate _____

P waves _____

PR interval _____ QRS interval _____

Interpretation _____

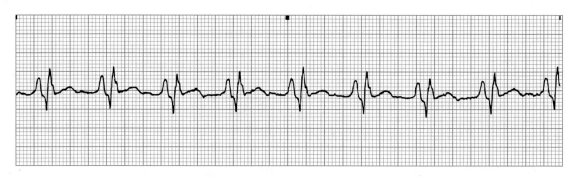

**145.** QRS complexes _____ Regularity _____ Heart rate _____

P waves _____

PR interval _____ QRS interval _____

Interpretation _____

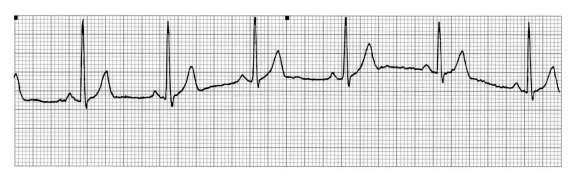

**146.** QRS complexes _____ Regularity _____ Heart rate _____

P waves _____

PR interval _____ QRS interval _____

Interpretation _____

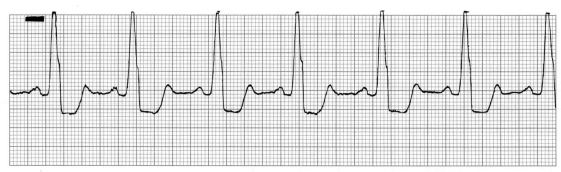

**147.** QRS complexes _____ Regularity _____ Heart rate _____

P waves _____

PR interval _____ QRS interval _____

Interpretation _____

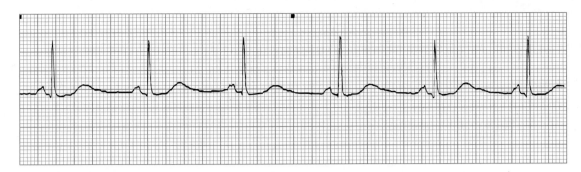

**148.** QRS complexes _____ Regularity _____ Heart rate _____

P waves _____

PR interval _____ QRS interval _____

Interpretation _____

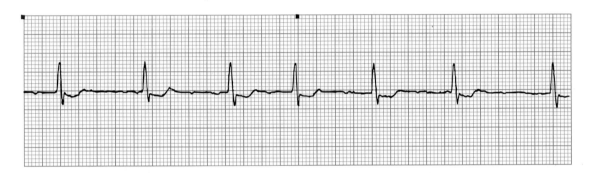

**149.** QRS complexes _____ Regularity _____ Heart rate _____

P waves _____

PR interval _____ QRS interval _____

Interpretation _____

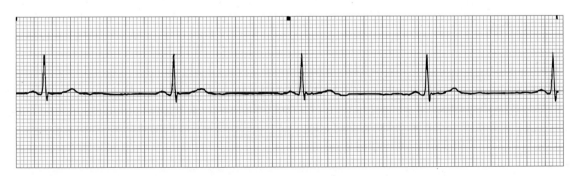

**150.** QRS complexes _____ Regularity _____ Heart rate _____

P waves _____

PR interval _____ QRS interval _____

Interpretation _____

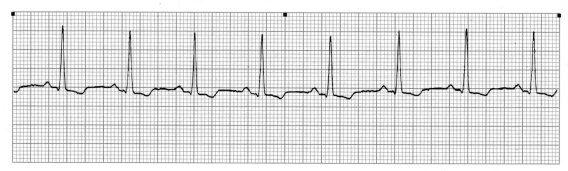

**151.** QRS complexes _____ Regularity _____ Heart rate _____

P waves _____

PR interval _____ QRS interval _____

Interpretation _____

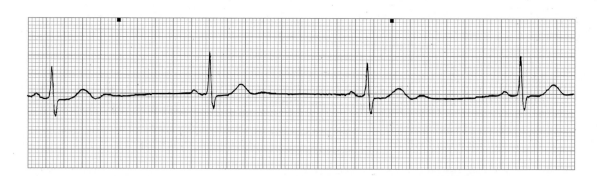

**152.** QRS complexes _____ Regularity _____ Heart rate _____

P waves _____

PR interval _____ QRS interval _____

Interpretation _____

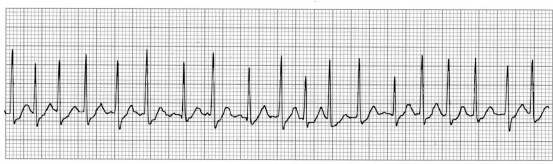

**153.** QRS complexes _____ Regularity _____ Heart rate _____

P waves _____

PR interval _____ QRS interval _____

Interpretation _____

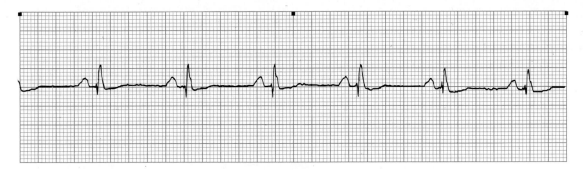

**154.** QRS complexes _____ Regularity _____ Heart rate _____

P waves _____

PR interval _____ QRS interval _____

Interpretation _____

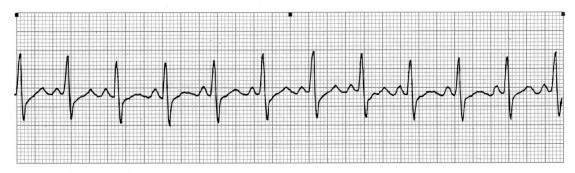

**155.** QRS complexes _____ Regularity _____ Heart rate _____

P waves _____

PR interval _____ QRS interval _____

Interpretation _____

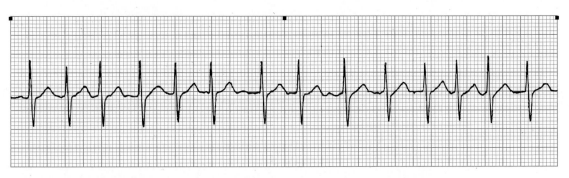

**156.** QRS complexes _____ Regularity _____ Heart rate _____

P waves _____

PR interval _____ QRS interval _____

Interpretation _____

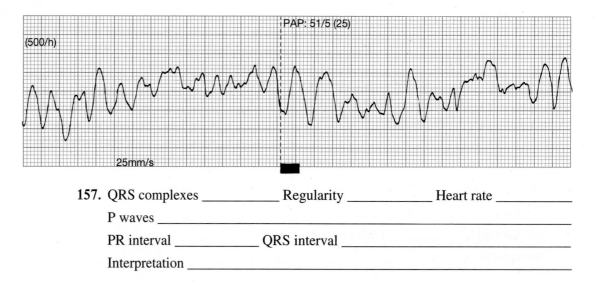

**157.** QRS complexes _____ Regularity _____ Heart rate _____

P waves _____

PR interval _____ QRS interval _____

Interpretation _____

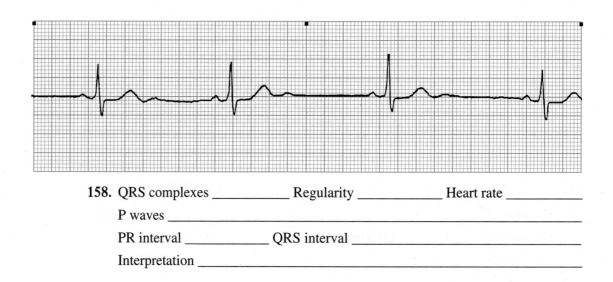

**158.** QRS complexes _____ Regularity _____ Heart rate _____

P waves _____

PR interval _____ QRS interval _____

Interpretation _____

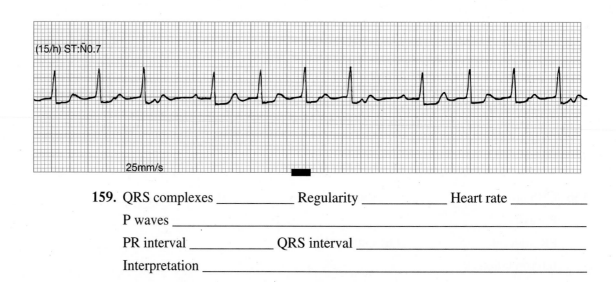

**159.** QRS complexes _____ Regularity _____ Heart rate _____

P waves _____

PR interval _____ QRS interval _____

Interpretation _____

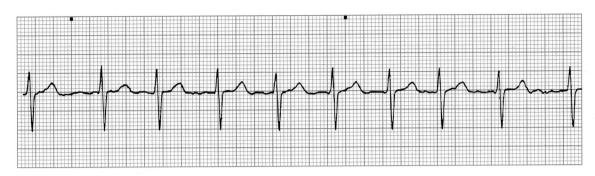

**160.** QRS complexes _____ Regularity _____ Heart rate _____

P waves _____

PR interval _____ QRS interval _____

Interpretation _____

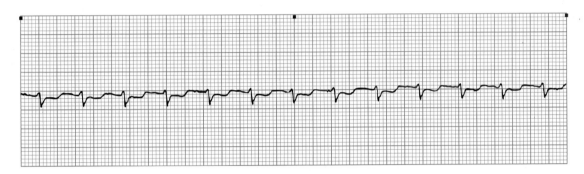

**161.** QRS complexes _____ Regularity _____ Heart rate _____

P waves _____

PR interval _____ QRS interval _____

Interpretation _____

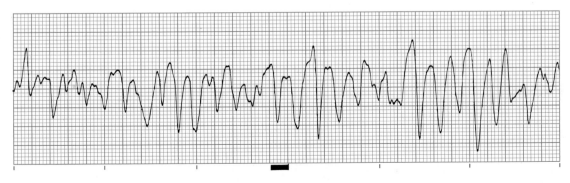

**162.** QRS complexes _____ Regularity _____ Heart rate _____

P waves _____

PR interval _____ QRS interval _____

Interpretation _____

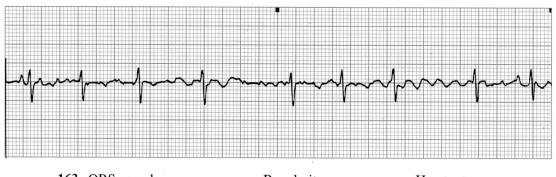

**163.** QRS complexes _____ Regularity _____ Heart rate _____

P waves _____

PR interval _____ QRS interval _____

Interpretation _____

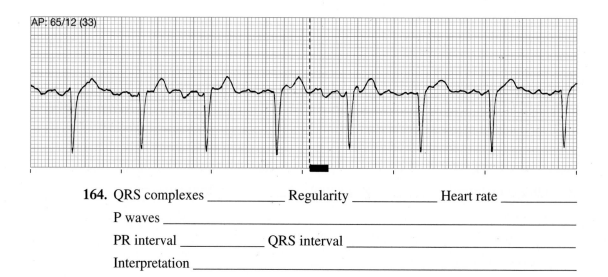

**164.** QRS complexes _____ Regularity _____ Heart rate _____

P waves _____

PR interval _____ QRS interval _____

Interpretation _____

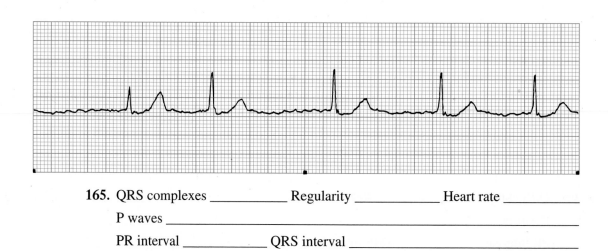

**165.** QRS complexes _____ Regularity _____ Heart rate _____

P waves _____

PR interval _____ QRS interval _____

Interpretation _____

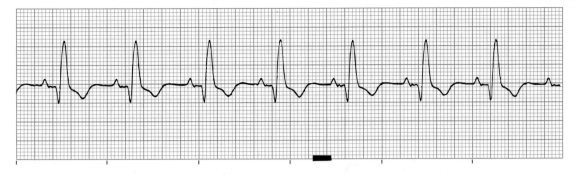

166. QRS complexes _____ Regularity _____ Heart rate _____

P waves _____

PR interval _____ QRS interval _____

Interpretation _____

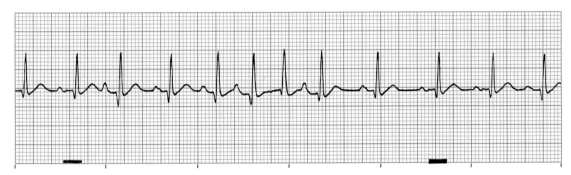

167. QRS complexes _____ Regularity _____ Heart rate _____

P waves _____

PR interval _____ QRS interval _____

Interpretation _____

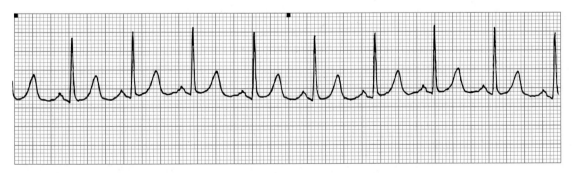

168. QRS complexes _____ Regularity _____ Heart rate _____

P waves _____

PR interval _____ QRS interval _____

Interpretation _____

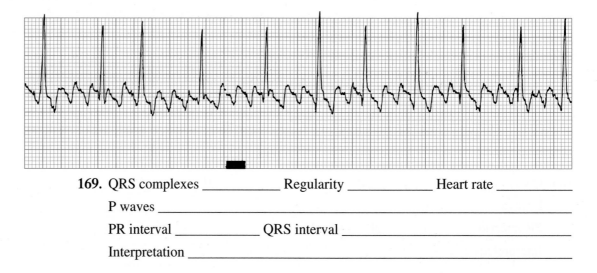

**169.** QRS complexes _____ Regularity _____ Heart rate _____

P waves _____

PR interval _____ QRS interval _____

Interpretation _____

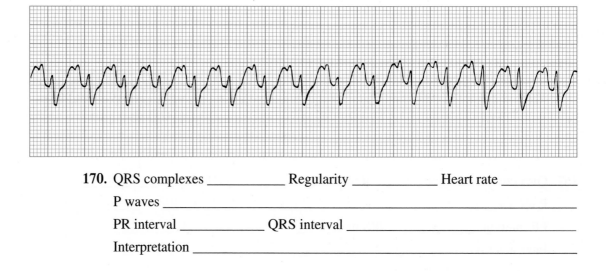

**170.** QRS complexes _____ Regularity _____ Heart rate _____

P waves _____

PR interval _____ QRS interval _____

Interpretation _____

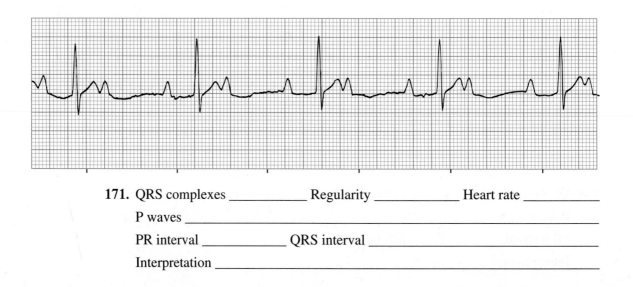

**171.** QRS complexes _____ Regularity _____ Heart rate _____

P waves _____

PR interval _____ QRS interval _____

Interpretation _____

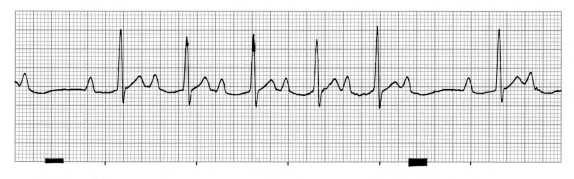

**172.** QRS complexes _____ Regularity _____ Heart rate _____

P waves _____

PR interval _____ QRS interval _____

Interpretation _____

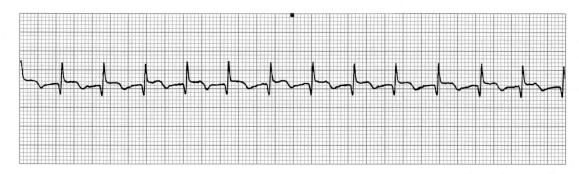

**173.** QRS complexes _____ Regularity _____ Heart rate _____

P waves _____

PR interval _____ QRS interval _____

Interpretation _____

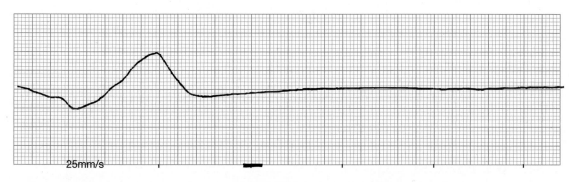

**174.** QRS complexes _____ Regularity _____ Heart rate _____

P waves _____

PR interval _____ QRS interval _____

Interpretation _____

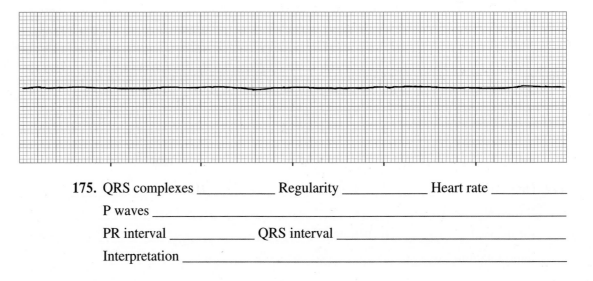

**175.** QRS complexes _____ Regularity _____ Heart rate _____

P waves _____

PR interval _____ QRS interval _____

Interpretation _____

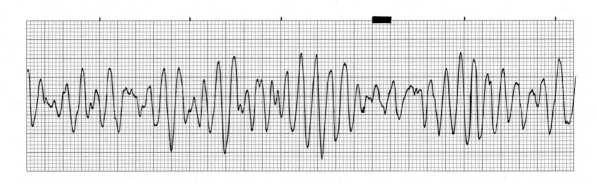

**176.** QRS complexes _____ Regularity _____ Heart rate _____

P waves _____

PR interval _____ QRS interval _____

Interpretation _____

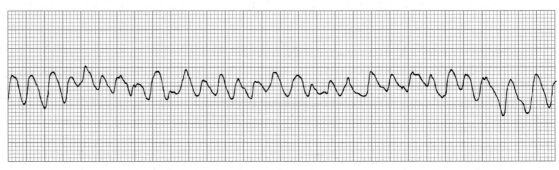

**177.** QRS complexes _____ Regularity _____ Heart rate _____

P waves _____

PR interval _____ QRS interval _____

Interpretation _____

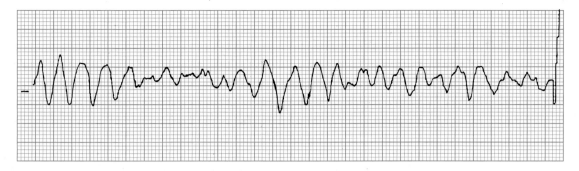

**178.** QRS complexes _____ Regularity _____ Heart rate _____

P waves _____

PR interval _____ QRS interval _____

Interpretation _____

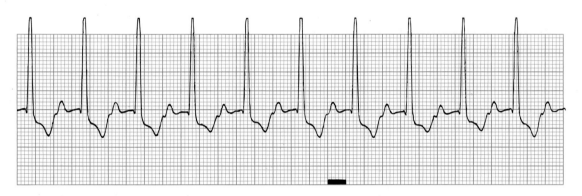

**179.** QRS complexes _____ Regularity _____ Heart rate _____

P waves _____

PR interval _____ QRS interval _____

Interpretation _____

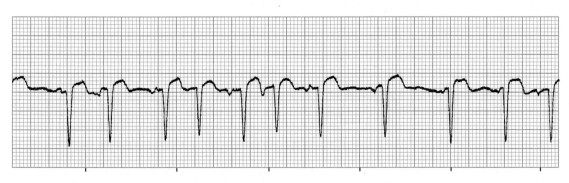

**180.** QRS complexes _____ Regularity _____ Heart rate _____

P waves _____

PR interval _____ QRS interval _____

Interpretation _____

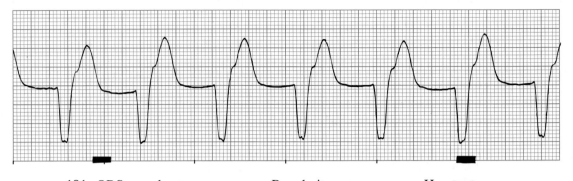

**181.** QRS complexes _____ Regularity _____ Heart rate _____

P waves _____

PR interval _____ QRS interval _____

Interpretation _____

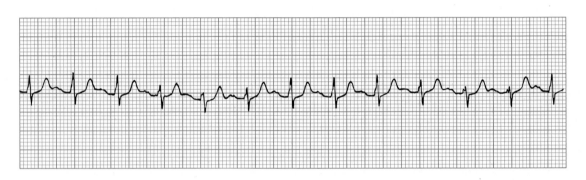

**182.** QRS complexes _____ Regularity _____ Heart rate _____

P waves _____

PR interval _____ QRS interval _____

Interpretation _____

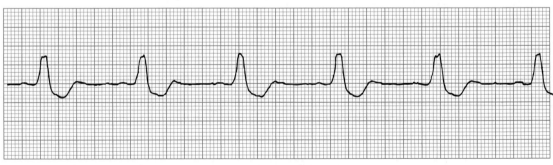

**183.** QRS complexes _____ Regularity _____ Heart rate _____

P waves _____

PR interval _____ QRS interval _____

Interpretation _____

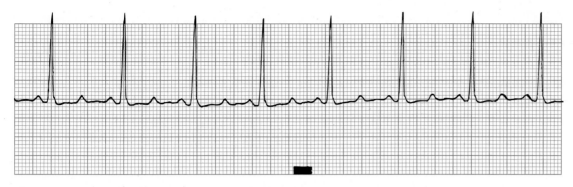

**184.** QRS complexes _____ Regularity _____ Heart rate _____

P waves _____

PR interval _____ QRS interval _____

Interpretation _____

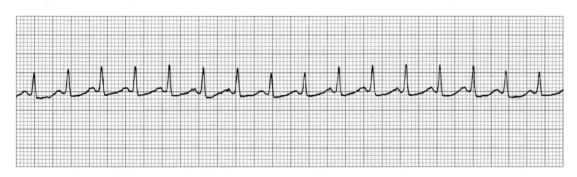

**185.** QRS complexes _____ Regularity _____ Heart rate _____

P waves _____

PR interval _____ QRS interval _____

Interpretation _____

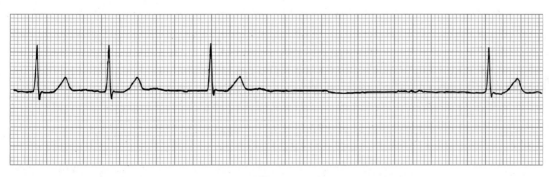

**186.** QRS complexes _____ Regularity _____ Heart rate _____

P waves _____

PR interval _____ QRS interval _____

Interpretation _____

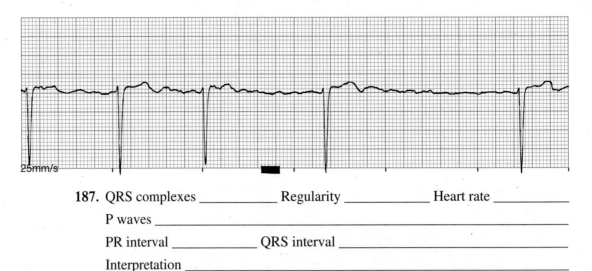

25mm/s

**187.** QRS complexes _____ Regularity _____ Heart rate _____

P waves _____

PR interval _____ QRS interval _____

Interpretation _____

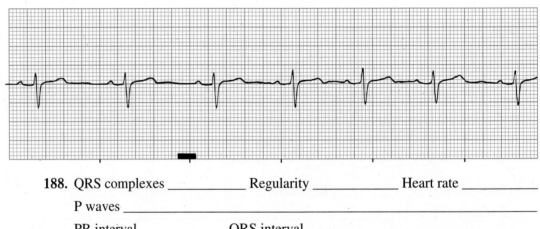

**188.** QRS complexes _____ Regularity _____ Heart rate _____

P waves _____

PR interval _____ QRS interval _____

Interpretation _____

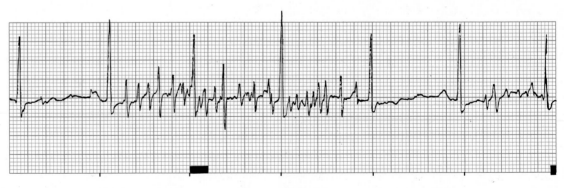

**189.** QRS complexes _____ Regularity _____ Heart rate _____

P waves _____

PR interval _____ QRS interval _____

Interpretation _____

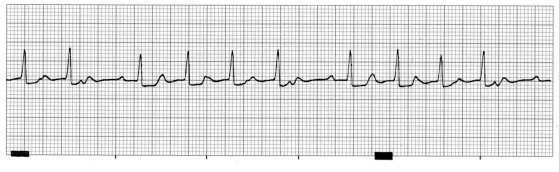

**190.** QRS complexes _____ Regularity _____ Heart rate _____

P waves _____

PR interval _____ QRS interval _____

Interpretation _____

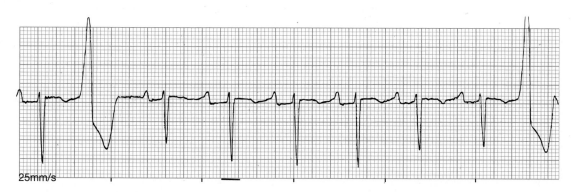

**191.** QRS complexes _____ Regularity _____ Heart rate _____

P waves _____

PR interval _____ QRS interval _____

Interpretation _____

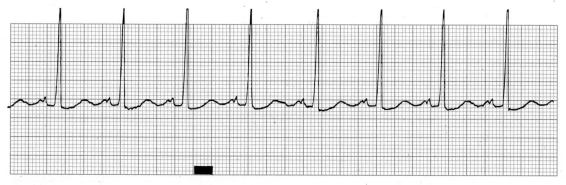

**192.** QRS complexes _____ Regularity _____ Heart rate _____

P waves _____

PR interval _____ QRS interval _____

Interpretation _____

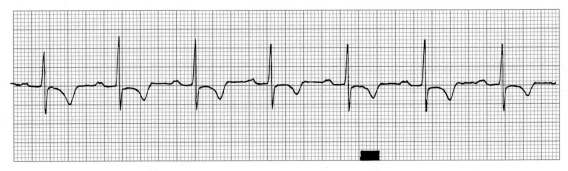

**193.** QRS complexes _____ Regularity _____ Heart rate _____

P waves _____

PR interval _____ QRS interval _____

Interpretation _____

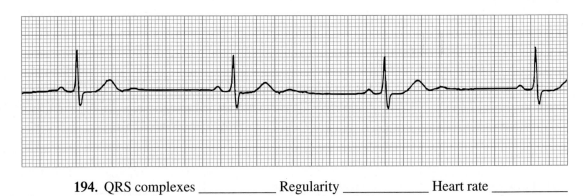

**194.** QRS complexes _____ Regularity _____ Heart rate _____

P waves _____

PR interval _____ QRS interval _____

Interpretation _____

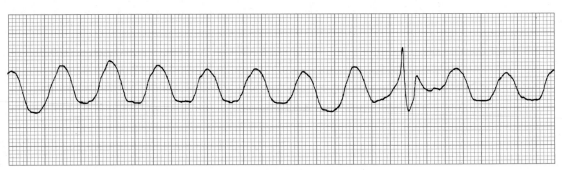

**195.** QRS complexes _____ Regularity _____ Heart rate _____

P waves _____

PR interval _____ QRS interval _____

Interpretation _____

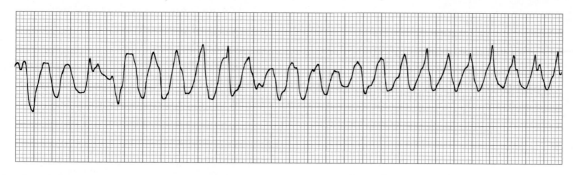

**196.** QRS complexes _____ Regularity _____ Heart rate _____

P waves _____

PR interval _____ QRS interval _____

Interpretation _____

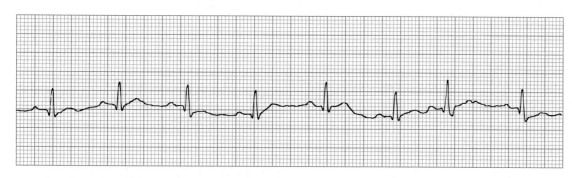

**197.** QRS complexes _____ Regularity _____ Heart rate _____

P waves _____

PR interval _____ QRS interval _____

Interpretation _____

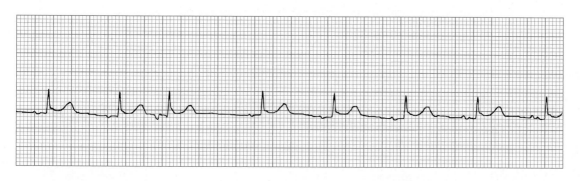

**198.** QRS complexes _____ Regularity _____ Heart rate _____

P waves _____

PR interval _____ QRS interval _____

Interpretation _____

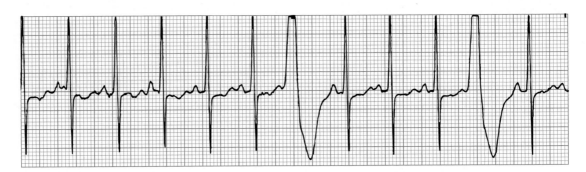

**199.** QRS complexes _____ Regularity _____ Heart rate _____

P waves _____

PR interval _____ QRS interval _____

Interpretation _____

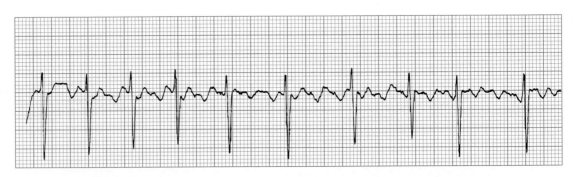

**200.** QRS complexes _____ Regularity _____ Heart rate _____

P waves _____

PR interval _____ QRS interval _____

Interpretation _____

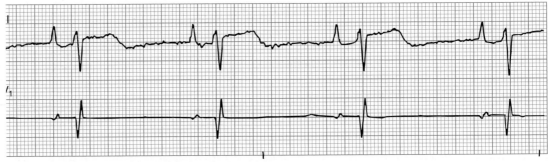

**201.** QRS complexes _____ Regularity _____ Heart rate _____

P waves _____

PR interval _____ QRS interval _____

Interpretation _____

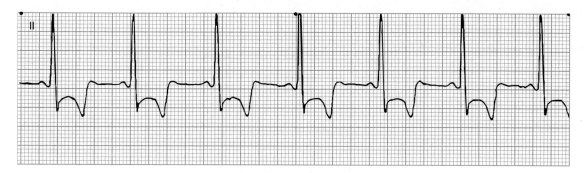

**202.** QRS complexes _____ Regularity _____ Heart rate _____

P waves _____

PR interval _____ QRS interval _____

Interpretation _____

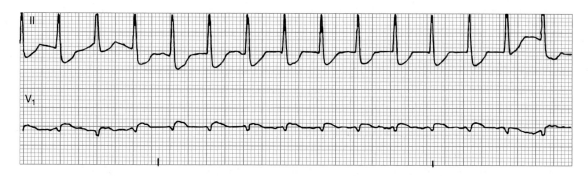

**203.** QRS complexes _____ Regularity _____ Heart rate _____

P waves _____

PR interval _____ QRS interval _____

Interpretation _____

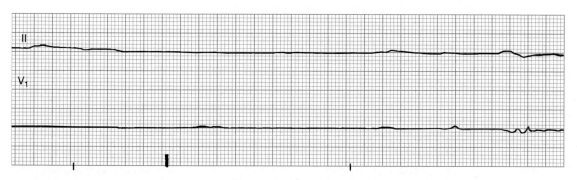

**204.** QRS complexes _____ Regularity _____ Heart rate _____

P waves _____

PR interval _____ QRS interval _____

Interpretation _____

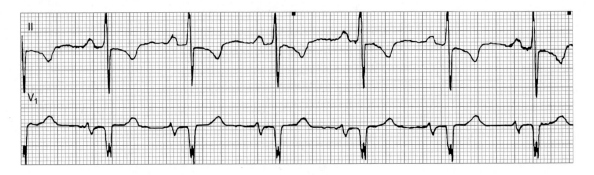

**205.** QRS complexes _____ Regularity _____ Heart rate _____

P waves _____

PR interval _____ QRS interval _____

Interpretation _____

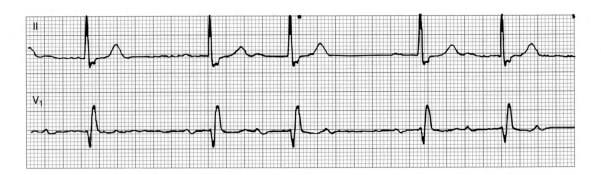

**206.** QRS complexes _____ Regularity _____ Heart rate _____

P waves _____

PR interval _____ QRS interval _____

Interpretation _____

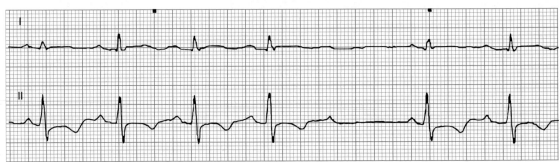

**207.** QRS complexes _____ Regularity _____ Heart rate _____

P waves _____

PR interval _____ QRS interval _____

Interpretation _____

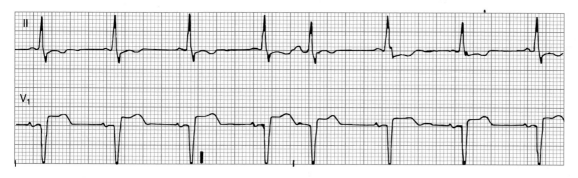

**208.** QRS complexes _____ Regularity _____ Heart rate _____

P waves _____

PR interval _____ QRS interval _____

Interpretation _____

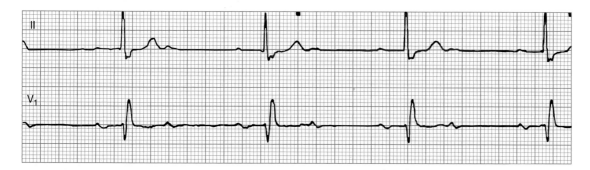

**209.** QRS complexes _____ Regularity _____ Heart rate _____

P waves _____

PR interval _____ QRS interval _____

Interpretation _____

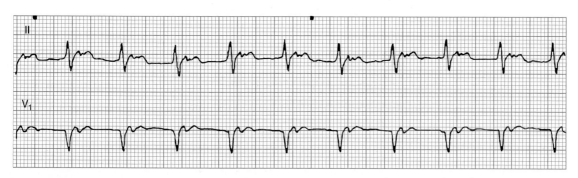

**210.** QRS complexes _____ Regularity _____ Heart rate _____

P waves _____

PR interval _____ QRS interval _____

Interpretation _____

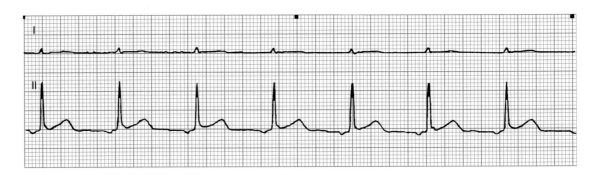

**211.** QRS complexes _____ Regularity _____ Heart rate _____

P waves _____

PR interval _____ QRS interval _____

Interpretation _____

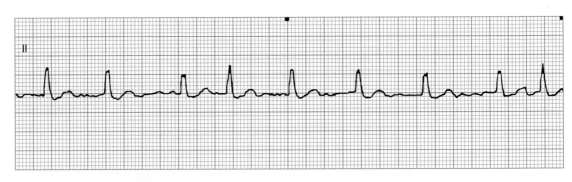

**212.** QRS complexes _____ Regularity _____ Heart rate _____

P waves _____

PR interval _____ QRS interval _____

Interpretation _____

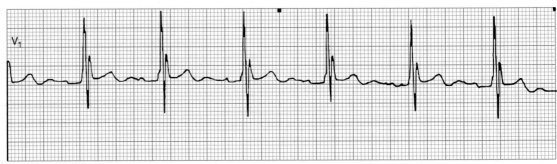

**213.** QRS complexes _____ Regularity _____ Heart rate _____

P waves _____

PR interval _____ QRS interval _____

Interpretation _____

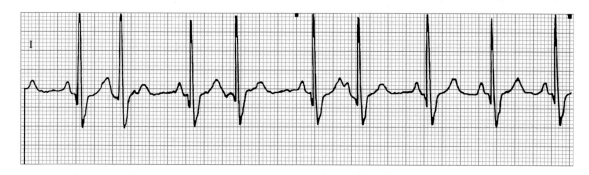

**214.** QRS complexes _____ Regularity _____ Heart rate _____

P waves _____

PR interval _____ QRS interval _____

Interpretation _____

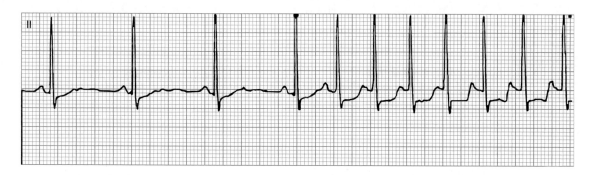

**215.** QRS complexes _____ Regularity _____ Heart rate _____

P waves _____

PR interval _____ QRS interval _____

Interpretation _____

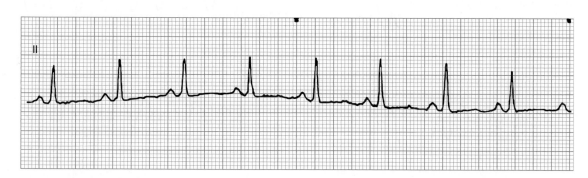

**216.** QRS complexes _____ Regularity _____ Heart rate _____

P waves _____

PR interval _____ QRS interval _____

Interpretation _____

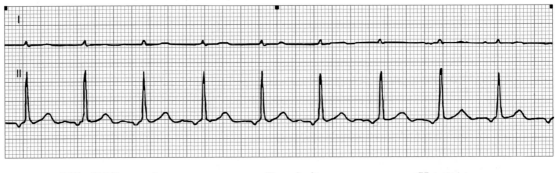

**217.** QRS complexes _____ Regularity _____ Heart rate _____

P waves _____

PR interval _____ QRS interval _____

Interpretation _____

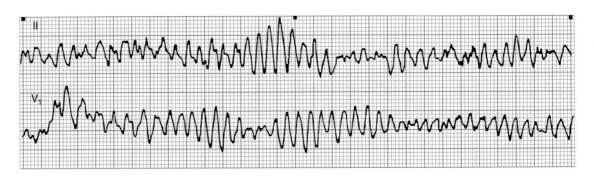

**218.** QRS complexes _____ Regularity _____ Heart rate _____

P waves _____

PR interval _____ QRS interval _____

Interpretation _____

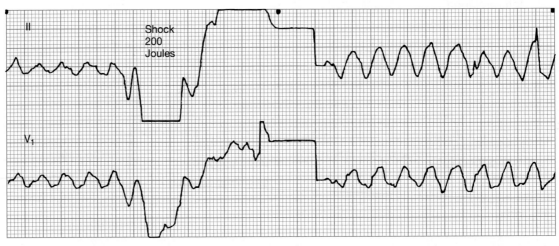

**219.** QRS complexes _____ Regularity _____ Heart rate _____

P waves _____

PR interval _____ QRS interval _____

Interpretation _____

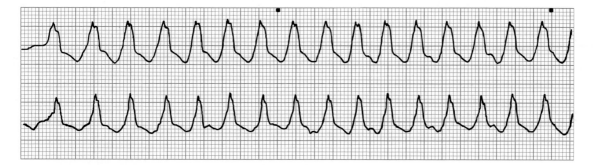

**220.** QRS complexes _____ Regularity _____ Heart rate _____

P waves _____

PR interval _____ QRS interval _____

Interpretation _____

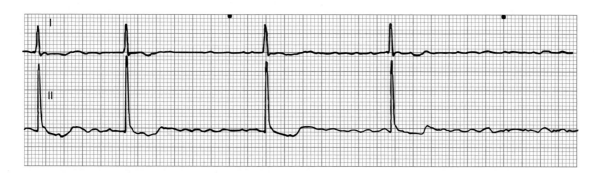

**221.** QRS complexes _____ Regularity _____ Heart rate _____

P waves _____

PR interval _____ QRS interval _____

Interpretation _____

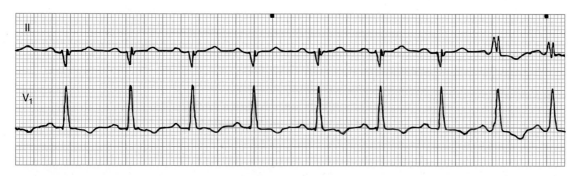

**222.** QRS complexes _____ Regularity _____ Heart rate _____

P waves _____

PR interval _____ QRS interval _____

Interpretation _____

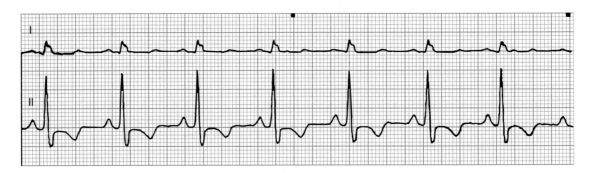

**223.** QRS complexes _____ Regularity _____ Heart rate _____

P waves _____

PR interval _____ QRS interval _____

Interpretation _____

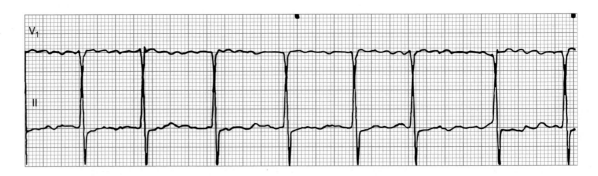

**224.** QRS complexes _____ Regularity _____ Heart rate _____

P waves _____

PR interval _____ QRS interval _____

Interpretation _____

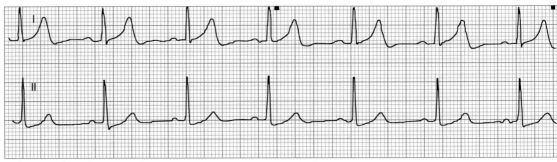

**225.** QRS complexes _____ Regularity _____ Heart rate _____

P waves _____

PR interval _____ QRS interval _____

Interpretation _____

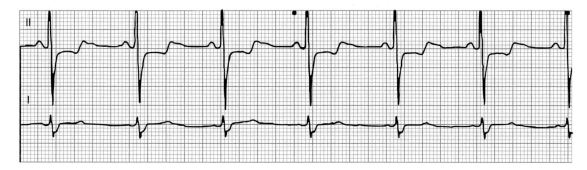

**226.** QRS complexes _____ Regularity _____ Heart rate _____

P waves _____

PR interval _____ QRS interval _____

Interpretation _____

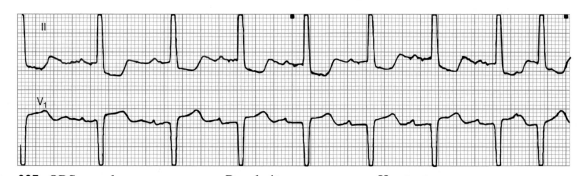

**227.** QRS complexes _____ Regularity _____ Heart rate _____

P waves _____

PR interval _____ QRS interval _____

Interpretation _____

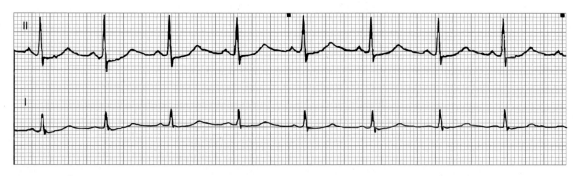

**228.** QRS complexes _____ Regularity _____ Heart rate _____

P waves _____

PR interval _____ QRS interval _____

Interpretation _____

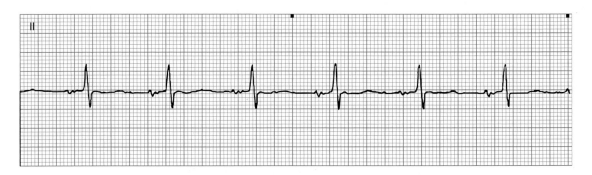

**229.** QRS complexes _____ Regularity _____ Heart rate _____

P waves _____

PR interval _____ QRS interval _____

Interpretation _____

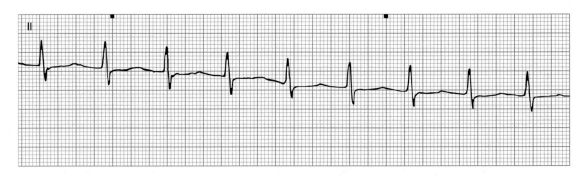

**230.** QRS complexes _____ Regularity _____ Heart rate _____

P waves _____

PR interval _____ QRS interval _____

Interpretation _____

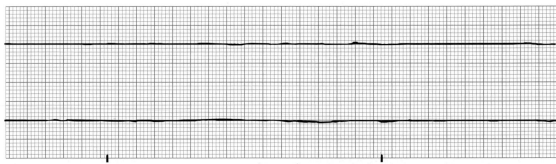

**231.** QRS complexes _____ Regularity _____ Heart rate _____

P waves _____

PR interval _____ QRS interval _____

Interpretation _____

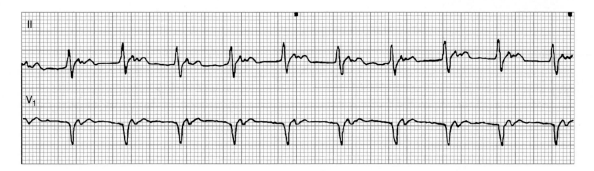

**232.** QRS complexes _____ Regularity _____ Heart rate _____

P waves _____

PR interval _____ QRS interval _____

Interpretation _____

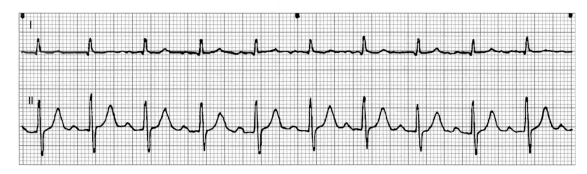

**233.** QRS complexes _____ Regularity _____ Heart rate _____

P waves _____

PR interval _____ QRS interval _____

Interpretation _____

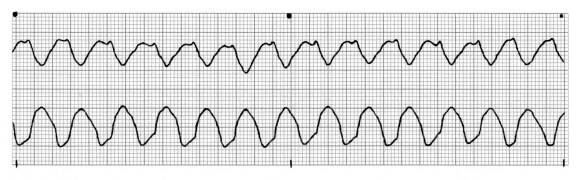

**234.** QRS complexes _____ Regularity _____ Heart rate _____

P waves _____

PR interval _____ QRS interval _____

Interpretation _____

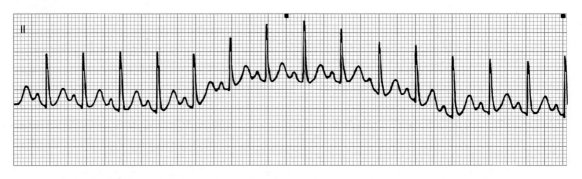

**235.** QRS complexes _____ Regularity _____ Heart rate _____

P waves _____

PR interval _____ QRS interval _____

Interpretation _____

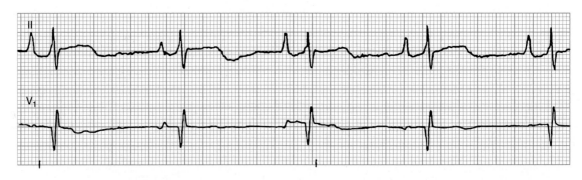

**236.** QRS complexes _____ Regularity _____ Heart rate _____

P waves _____

PR interval _____ QRS interval _____

Interpretation _____

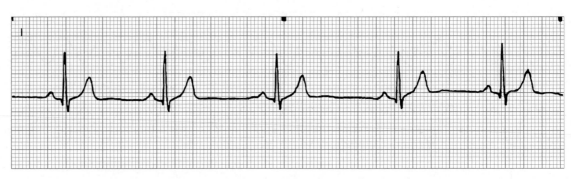

**237.** QRS complexes _____ Regularity _____ Heart rate _____

P waves _____

PR interval _____ QRS interval _____

Interpretation _____

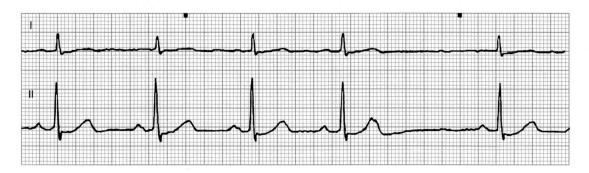

**238.** QRS complexes _____ Regularity _____ Heart rate _____

P waves _____

PR interval _____ QRS interval _____

Interpretation _____

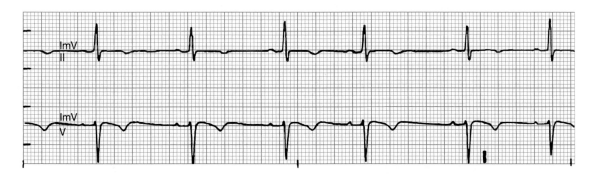

**239.** QRS complexes _____ Regularity _____ Heart rate _____

P waves _____

PR interval _____ QRS interval _____

Interpretation _____

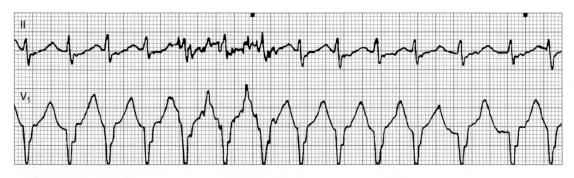

**240.** QRS complexes _____ Regularity _____ Heart rate _____

P waves _____

PR interval _____ QRS interval _____

Interpretation _____

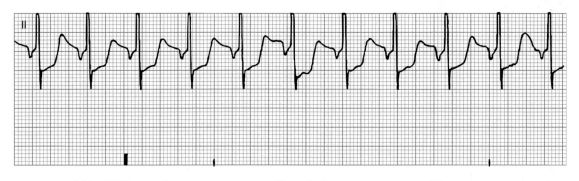

**241.** QRS complexes _____ Regularity _____ Heart rate _____

P waves _____

PR interval _____ QRS interval _____

Interpretation _____

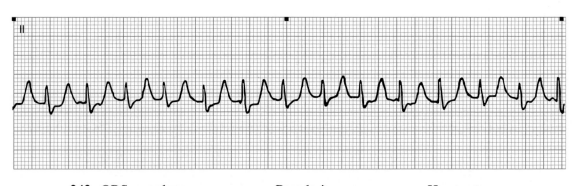

**242.** QRS complexes _____ Regularity _____ Heart rate _____

P waves _____

PR interval _____ QRS interval _____

Interpretation _____

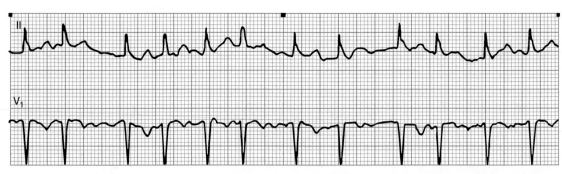

**243.** QRS complexes _____ Regularity _____ Heart rate _____

P waves _____

PR interval _____ QRS interval _____

Interpretation _____

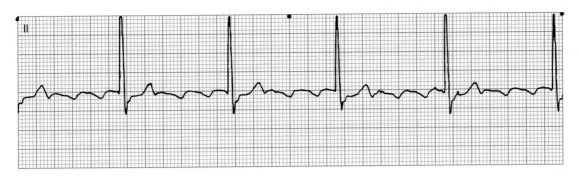

**244.** QRS complexes _____ Regularity _____ Heart rate _____

P waves _____

PR interval _____ QRS interval _____

Interpretation _____

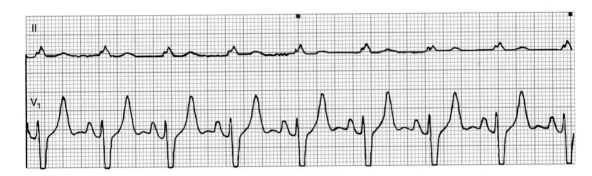

**245.** QRS complexes _____ Regularity _____ Heart rate _____

P waves _____

PR interval _____ QRS interval _____

Interpretation _____

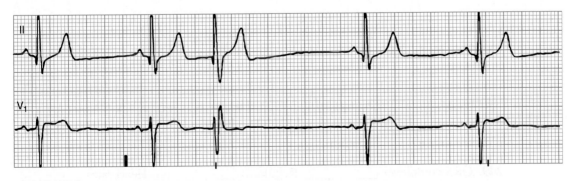

**246.** QRS complexes _____ Regularity _____ Heart rate _____

P waves _____

PR interval _____ QRS interval _____

Interpretation _____

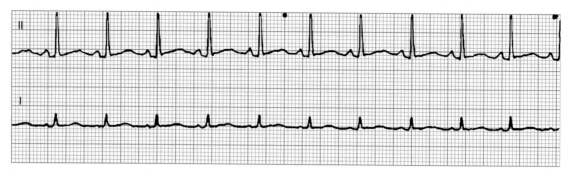

**247.** QRS complexes _____ Regularity _____ Heart rate _____

P waves _____

PR interval _____ QRS interval _____

Interpretation _____

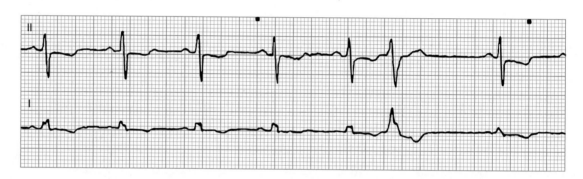

**248.** QRS complexes _____ Regularity _____ Heart rate _____

P waves _____

PR interval _____ QRS interval _____

Interpretation _____

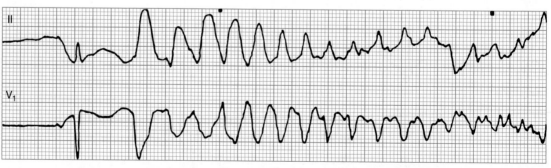

**249.** QRS complexes _____ Regularity _____ Heart rate _____

P waves _____

PR interval _____ QRS interval _____

Interpretation _____

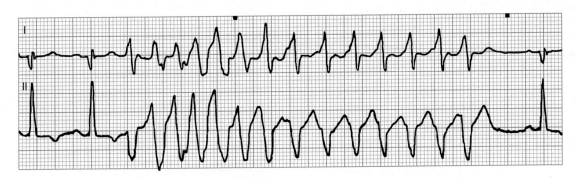

**250.** QRS complexes _____ Regularity _____ Heart rate _____

P waves _____

PR interval _____ QRS interval _____

Interpretation _____

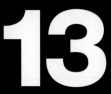

# Diagnostic Electrocardiography

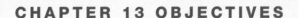

## CHAPTER 13 OBJECTIVES

Upon completion of this chapter, the student will be able to

- Explain the use for signal-averaged EKG.
- Define *stress testing.*
- State the goal of stress testing.
- Define *MET.*
- Describe the indications for stress testing.
- Describe the relative and absolute contraindications for stress testing.
- State how to calculate target heart rate.
- Describe how a stress test is done.
- Describe how a pharmacologic stress test is done.
- Name the three most commonly used protocols for treadmill exercise testing.
- Describe the reasons to terminate the test.

- Describe normal signs and symptoms during the stress test.
- Describe the normal EKG changes that occur during stress testing.
- Describe the EKG changes that indicate a positive stress test.
- Explain Bayes' theorem as it relates to the reliability of stress testing.
- Define *specificity* and *sensitivity.*
- Describe the indications for Holter monitoring.
- Explain why an event monitor might be superior to a Holter monitor for some patients.
- State what a positive Holter or event monitor is.

## What It's All About

Mr. Walter had been experiencing dizziness for a few weeks and went to the doctor to see what was wrong. "I'm scared to drive a car because I'm afraid I'll pass out at the wheel," he explained to his physician. Dr. Friedman did a 12-lead EKG and saw no abnormality, so he suggested a Holter monitor to determine if there are any heart rhythm abnormalties that could be causing his symptoms. Twenty-four hours later, Mr. Walter returned to the doctor's office where he learned that he had had several long runs of a potentially dangerous arrhythmia. His doctor suggested he see a cardiologist to evaluate the need for medications or an implantable defibrillator that could provide a small internal shock to the heart to abolish the arrhythmia. Mr. Walter was pleased at the possibilities for treatment and made an appointment with a cardiologist. He was started on medications and did well.

## Introduction

Diagnostic electrocardiography involves an EKG done to rule out disease. It can involve a resting EKG, a signal-averaged EKG (SAEKG), a stress test, or ambulatory monitoring such as Holter monitoring. We've talked about resting EKGs in depth in prior chapters. Let's look at the other three now.

## Signal-Averaged EKG

Unlike a resting EKG, which requires only a few seconds, the signal-averaged EKG takes up to 20 minutes, as the machine must collect about 250 consecutive QRS complexes and then analyze/average them together—a procedure called signal averaging. The signal-averaged EKG has been "cleansed" of background noise and

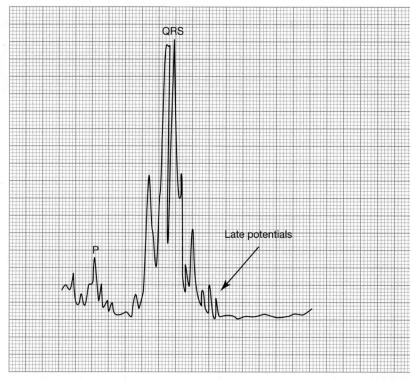

**FIGURE 13–1**

**Signal-averaged EKG.**

artifact, while true cardiac signals are strengthened. This type of EKG is done on either a special SAEKG machine or a standard EKG machine with special signal-averaging software. The SAEKG recording yields a single, averaged, very large QRS complex (see Figure 13–1) upon which the software performs calculations to uncover small variations in the final portion of the QRS complex. These late potentials, as those end-of-QRS variations are called, arise from damaged or scarred myocardial tissue, and can be useful in predicting the risk of potentially dangerous ventricular arrhythmias such as V-tach and V-fib. Preparation for the test is the same as for a standard 12-lead EKG. Patients should lie supine and be silent during the procedure to minimize artifact.

## Stress Testing

Stress testing is a diagnostic procedure done to determine the likelihood of coronary artery disease (CAD). The heart is stressed by physical exertion, usually on a bicycle or a treadmill, or by administration of medication that causes increased heart rate and thus stresses the heart. The patient's symptoms and EKG during the stress test give vital information regarding the *patency* (openness) of his or her coronary arteries. Figure 13–2 shows a treadmill stress test in progress.

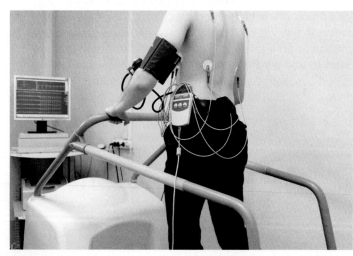

**FIGURE 13–2**

**Treadmill stress test**
(Pavel L Photo and Video/
Shutterstock).

## Goal of Stress Testing

*The goal of stress testing, whether exercise or pharmacologic, is to increase the heart rate to a maximal level that increases myocardial oxygen demand and to evaluate the EKG and subjective responses of the patient.* Decreased flow through narrowed coronary arteries will usually become evident as the test progresses. In other words, are there EKG changes that signal ischemia or infarction? Does the patient experience chest pain or arrhythmias with this stress? The test is concluded when the patient's symptoms (chest pain, fatigue, or ST segment changes) preclude continuing or, for submaximal tests, when a target heart rate is reached.

## Indications for Stress Testing

Stress testing is usually done to search for coronary artery disease in a patient having suspicious symptoms. But there are other indications as well. Here are a few:

- *Post-CABG (coronary artery bypass graft) or* postangioplasty evaluation.   The patient has had bypass surgery or a balloon procedure to open up blocked coronary arteries. The stress test is a way to determine if those procedures have improved coronary flow.
- *Diagnosis or treatment of exercise-induced arrhythmias.*   Some patients have arrhythmias only on exertion. The stress test is a safe way to induce those arrhythmias in a controlled environment so that they can be identified and treated.
- *Follow-up to cardiac rehab.*   The post-MI patient has gradually worked up to more normal exercise levels. The stress test helps determine if his or her heart is tolerating this increased exertion.
- *Family history of heart disease.*   The individual with a family history of heart disease and two or more of the recognized heart disease risk factors is advised to have a stress test at age 40 and periodically thereafter. If CAD is detected, treatment can begin early.

## Absolute Contraindications

Who is *not* a candidate for stress testing under any circumstances? For people with the following conditions, the risks of the test greatly outweigh the potential benefits. Testing these people could have serious or fatal consequences.

- *Acute MI less than 48 hours old.*   The heart is too unstable to tolerate exertion. Stress testing could cause the infarcted area to extend.
- *Uncontrolled symptomatic heart failure.*   The heart cannot tolerate the extra stress.
- *Unstable angina not previously stabilized on medications.*   Patients with unstable angina will likely not tolerate stress. It could cause them to infarct.
- *Uncontrolled cardiac arrhythmias accompanied by signs of decreased cardiac output.*   The rhythm could deteriorate to V-fib.
- *Symptomatic severe aortic stenosis.*   As a result of a narrowed aortic valve opening, cardiac output is low, and stressing these patients could cause them to faint or suffer cardiac arrest.
- *Dissecting aneurysm.*   This is a ballooning out of the wall of an artery. Stress causes an increase in blood pressure, which could cause the aneurysm to blow.
- *Acute myocarditis or pericarditis.*   The inflamed tissue may produce ST segment elevation, mimicking an MI.
- *Acute pulmonary embolus (PE).*   This is a blood clot in a lung artery. PEs result in low blood oxygen levels and require the patient to be on bed rest for a time. Exertion could move the embolus farther into the artery, causing more damage.

### Relative Contraindications

Some individuals should have a stress test *only* if the benefits outweigh the risks. In other words, it must be determined that the information to be gained from the stress test is so valuable that it outweighs the risks involved to individuals with the following conditions:

- *Left main coronary artery stenosis.*   The patient could have a massive MI.
- *Mental/physical issues that render the patient unable to exercise adequately.*
- *Uncontrolled tachyarrhythmias or bradyarrhythmias.*   With the heart rate already too fast or too slow prior to the stress test, it won't take much to make the cardiac output fall.
- *Severe hypertension (systolic >200, diastolic >110)*   Stress testing could result in stroke.
- *High degree AV block (second and third degree).*   Stressing the patient can lead to worsening AV block and the need for an emergent pacemaker.
- *Electrolyte abnormalities.*   This could lead to arrhythmias such as V-tach or V-fib.
- *Moderate stenotic heart valve disease.*   A heart valve is not able to open completely, so flow through it is impeded. This can decrease cardiac output.
- *Hypertrophic cardiomyopathy (overgrown septum) or other forms of outflow obstruction.*   This causes decreased cardiac output.

### Preparation Techniques

The single most important piece of equipment in performing a stress test is a 12-lead EKG machine. The electrode patches should adhere securely to the skin, and they may be taped if necessary. Female patients are advised to wear a bra in order to decrease artifact. To prevent nausea, patients are advised not to eat a large meal for at least 4 hours prior to the test. They should wear comfortable, loose clothing and walking shoes or other appropriate footwear. They should take their routine medications as usual unless specifically instructed not to by the physician. Certain medications, such as beta-blockers and calcium channel blockers, may be held for a period of time before the test, as they may prevent the heart rate from reaching target levels. Also, nitrates might be held, as they could prevent symptoms of coronary artery disease, such as chest pain, and could thus result in a false-negative test. Likewise, caffeinated beverages might be withheld, as they can increase the heart rate and blood pressure.

### How Is It Done?

Before all stress tests, a resting EKG is done. A history is obtained, with special emphasis on a description of any symptoms the patient has been having that prompted the test (chest pain, shortness of breath, etc.). Baseline vital signs (heart rate, blood pressure, respiratory rate) are checked with the patient lying down and standing. An EKG may be done with the patient standing up hyperventilating (breathing very rapidly). ST segment and T wave changes can be caused by hyperventilation, and during the stress test it's important to know if any ST-T changes are from ischemia or simply from hyperventilating.

For the **exercise test**, the patient then exercises on a treadmill or bicycle, or uses a special arm bicycle called an arm ergometer, while a continuous EKG is run. A nurse or technician checks the patient's blood pressure at frequent intervals and asks about any symptoms the patient may be developing. The stress test is continued until at least 85% of the target heart rate is achieved or the patient develops EKG changes or symptoms that require termination of the test. *The target heart rate is 220 minus the patient's age.* A 60-year-old patient would thus have a target heart rate of 220 − 60 = 160. For the test to be valid for interpretation, a heart rate of 85% of 160, or 136, would be required. For a submaximal test following an MI, the test is concluded when 70% of the target heart rate is achieved, assuming the patient is asymptomatic. If myocardial perfusion (adequacy of blood flow to the heart muscle) is to be studied, radioisotopes such as thallium-201 can be injected during the last minute of exercise and then special X-rays done. Thallium follows potassium ions into the heart and diffuses into the tissues. Poor myocardial uptake of the thallium produces a "cold spot" on the X-ray (compared to the "hot spots" from adequate thallium uptake) and indicates impaired myocardial blood flow in the artery supplying that area. *Multiple gated acquisition* (MUGA) scans can also be done after the exercise test to check myocardial perfusion. MUGA scans are nuclear scans that use an injected radioisotope to point out areas of poor myocardial blood flow.

The **pharmacologic stress test** does not involve exercise. This kind of testing is appropriate for individuals with physical limitations that preclude exercise, such as amputations, or for the elderly who could not do enough exercise to reach the target heart rate. For this test, an IV line is started, and the patient is given an intravenous dose of medication that causes the heart rate to climb to the target level. This increased heart rate stresses the heart and should provide the same symptoms and EKG changes as an exercise test. As with the exercise test, a continuous EKG is run, vital signs are checked, and symptoms are assessed. After at least 85% of the target heart rate is achieved, the test is concluded. The most common medications used in pharmacologic stress tests are *dobutamine, dipyridamole, adenosine,* and *Regadenoson.*

### Exercise Protocols

Three main protocols are used in treadmill exercise stress tests—the Bruce, modified Bruce, and Naughton protocols. Speed and incline of the treadmill, as well as the frequency of the changes in the protocol's stages, are determined by the protocol used. The intensity of exercise is measured in metabolic equivalents (METs), which are reflections of oxygen consumption. One MET is the oxygen consumption of a person sitting down resting. Most average adults can reach a MET level of 13 with exertion. Those with coronary artery disease may have symptoms of ischemia at low MET levels, such as 4 METs. Sometimes a *double product* is calculated in order to determine the level of exercise achieved. Double product is calculated as the heart rate times the systolic blood pressure (HR · SBP = DP). A double product greater than 25,000 indicates that an acceptable level of exercise has been achieved during stress testing. Let's look at the different protocols.

- *Bruce.*    This is the most commonly used protocol for maximal testing. The treadmill's speed and incline are increased every 3 minutes up to a total of 21 minutes. Let's look at the stages of the Bruce protocol. See Table 13–1.

    As you can see in Table 13–1, the speed starts out at a comfortable walking pace at a low incline; then every 3 minutes it accelerates until by stage VII the patient is running uphill at a 22° incline. An advantage of the Bruce protocol is the relatively short duration needed to produce maximal effort in the patient. On the downside, this protocol can be very demanding and may be too ambitious for the sedentary individual.

**TABLE 13–1    Bruce Protocol Stages**

| Stage | Speed | Incline |
| --- | --- | --- |
| I | 1.7 mph | 10° |
| II | 2.5 mph | 12° |
| III | 3.4 mph | 14° |
| IV | 4.2 mph | 16° |
| V | 5.0 mph | 18° |
| VI | 5.5 mph | 20° |
| VII | 6.0 mph | 22° |

- *Modified Bruce.*   Many institutions have modified the Bruce protocol so that the initial work is less strenuous, and the stage change is in smaller increments. This is appropriate for patients who might not tolerate the standard Bruce protocol.
- *Naughton.*   This is a slower-moving submaximal test in which the settings are changed every 2 minutes. Although the settings change more quickly than in the Bruce protocol, they are more gradual and allow the individual to adjust more easily. The Naughton protocol is used most often for testing post-MI patients just before or shortly after hospital discharge.

### Termination of the Test

The stress test should be immediately stopped if any of the following occur:

- *ST segment elevation.*   This indicates severe myocardial ischemia and injury. The sudden development of ST segment elevation is an ominous sign. Continuing the test could result in irreversible cardiac damage.
- *Sustained ventricular tachycardia.*   Cardiac arrest could result if the test is not stopped.
- *Moderate to severe chest pain, especially if accompanied by ST segment depression or elevation.*   Mild chest pain unaccompanied by ST segment changes may not be indicative of significant coronary artery disease. More severe chest pain, especially that accompanied by ST segment changes, is more reflective of significant disease.
- *Drop in blood pressure more than 10 mm Hg along with other evidence of ischemia such as chest pain or ST segment depression or elevation.*   The blood pressure usually rises in response to exercise. A drop in BP can indicate pump failure.
- *Technical problems with the monitoring systems or the treadmill.*
- *Patient requests to stop.*   Before stopping, ask why the patient wants to stop the test. There may be an occasional unmotivated patient who requests to stop the test before achieving target levels. In this case, the physician might gently encourage the patient to continue, because the test that is stopped at too early a stage will be inadequate at ruling out CAD.
- *Patient becomes dizzy, begins to stumble, or feels faint.*   The patient is showing neurologic symptoms of decreased cardiac output.
- *Patient becomes diaphoretic.*   This is a sign of decreased cardiac output. The patient is not tolerating the test.

### Test Interpretation

The following EKG changes are normal on the stress test:

- *Shortened PR interval.*   AV conduction and heart rate usually accelerate with exertion.
- *Tall P waves.*   This is often a result of increased lung capacity.

- *Lower-voltage QRS complexes.* This may be due to increased volume of air in the lungs muffling the cardiac impulse as it heads toward the skin.
- *Increased heart rate (shorter R-R intervals).* The ability of the heart rate to increase with exercise is known as the chronotropic reserve. Heart rate that does not increase with stress is chronotropic incompetence.

## Normal Signs and Symptoms

The following patient signs and symptoms are normal during a stress test:

- *Decreased systemic vascular resistance due to vasodilation.* Exercise causes blood vessels to dilate, lowering the resistance to the outflow of blood from the heart and increasing cardiac output.
- *Increased respiratory rate.* Exercise causes increased oxygen demand, so the respiratory rate increases to allow more oxygen intake.
- *Sweating.*
- *Fatigue.*
- *Muscle cramping in calves or sides.* This is a common phenomenon in exercise and does not imply poor myocardial function.
- *Increased blood pressure.* The ability of the blood pressure to rise with exercise is known as inotropic reserve. Blood pressure that does not rise with exercise can imply inotropic incompetence.
- *J point depression.* The J point is the point at which the QRS joins the ST segment. J point depression means the ST segment takes off before the QRS complex has gotten back up to the baseline. Note the J point in Figure 13–3. It is below the baseline. This is J point depression.

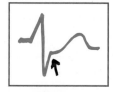

**FIGURE 13–3**

**J point depression.**

## Positive Stress Test

The following indicate a positive (abnormal) stress test:

- *ST segment depression greater than or equal to 1.0 to 1.5 mm that does not return to the baseline within 0.08 seconds (two little blocks) after the J point.* ST depression can be of 3 different types: upsloping, horizontal, and downsloping. In terms of cardiac implications, upsloping is the least indicative of coronary artery disease, horizontal is intermediate, and downsloping is the most indicative of CAD. See Figure 13–4.

Let's compare ST segments on a pre-exercise resting EKG and a stress test EKG. See Figures 13–5 and 13–6. Ignore the QRS width on these examples. In Figure 13–5, note the normal ST segments and the relatively slow heart rate. Now see Figure 13–6 for the stress test EKG. Note the normal increase in heart rate along with significant downsloping ST segment depressions in Leads II, III, and aVF. This is a positive (abnormal) stress test.

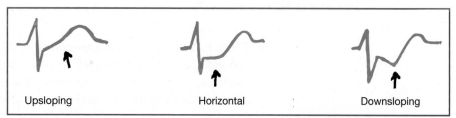

Upsloping    Horizontal    Downsloping

**FIGURE 13–4**

**Types of ST segment depression.**

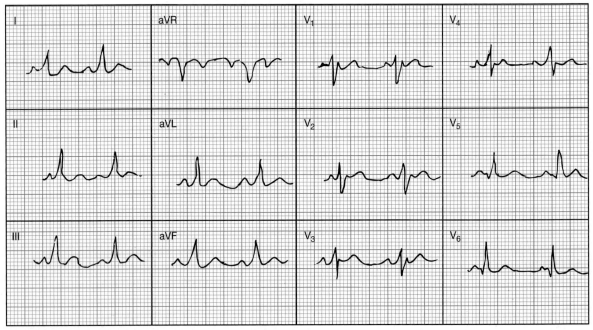

**FIGURE 13–5**

**Pre-exercise resting EKG.**

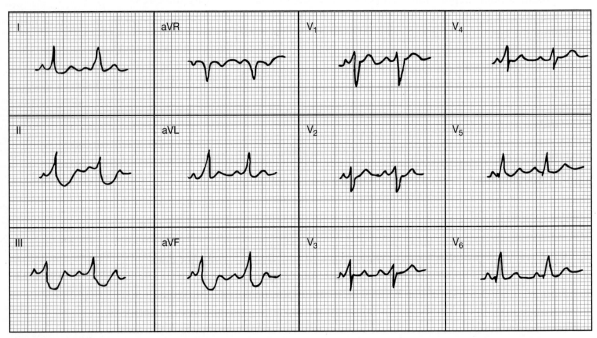

**FIGURE 13–6**

**Stress test EKG.**

- *U wave inversion or new appearance of U waves.*    Although a much less common phenomenon than ST segment changes, U wave inversion—or indeed the sudden appearance of U waves during the exercise test—is indicative of coronary ischemia. See Figure 13–7 and note the inverted U waves following the upright T waves.
- *ST segment elevation.*    Elevation of the ST segment is an indication of considerable transmural myocardial ischemia progressing to the injury phase. The stress test should be stopped immediately to prevent permanent tissue damage.

## Reliability of Stress Tests

How reliable are stress tests in diagnosing coronary artery disease? Like any medical testing, the stress test is not infallible. There can be false positives and false negatives. The validity of stress test results can be absolutely determined only by angiogram, a procedure in which dye is injected into the coronary arteries to determine if there is indeed coronary artery disease. For the stress EKG to show any diagnostic changes that indicate CAD, the coronary artery in question must be at least 75% narrowed. And conditions other than CAD can result in a positive test. To better understand the reliability of the test results, it is necessary to understand the terms *sensitivity* and *specificity*.

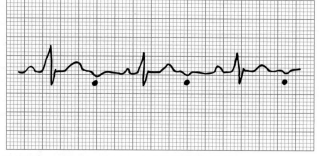

**FIGURE 13–7**

**Inverted U waves.**

Sensitivity refers to the percentage of patients who have a positive stress test and CAD as proven by angiogram. In other words, is the stress test sensitive enough to pick up those individuals who truly have coronary artery disease?

Specificity refers to the percentage of patients who have negative (normal) stress tests and normal coronary arteries as proven by angiogram. Is the stress test specific enough to exclude individuals who do not have CAD?

Thus the term *positive* refers to the test's sensitivity and *negative* refers to its specificity.

## Categories of Stress Test Results

Stress test results fall in four categories:

- *True positive.* The stress test is positive (indicating coronary artery disease) and the angiogram is also positive, confirming CAD.
- *False positive.* The stress test is positive for CAD, but the angiogram is negative, revealing normal coronary arteries.
- *True negative.* The stress test and angiogram are both negative for CAD.
- *False negative.* The stress test is negative, but the angiogram is positive for CAD.

Bayes's theorem suggests that the true predictive value of any test is not just in the accuracy (sensitivity and specificity) of the test itself, but also in the patient's probability of disease, as determined before the test was done. In other words, before the stress test is done, there should be a risk assessment, based on the patient's history, heredity, and physical exam, to predict the likelihood of that patient having CAD. If this pretest risk of CAD is low, but his or her stress test turns out to be positive, it is likely that the stress test result is a false positive. If the pretest risk is high but the stress test is negative, it's likely that the stress test is a false negative.

### After the Stress Test

What happens after the stress test? If the stress test is positive, the patient will likely be either treated with medications or scheduled for an angiogram for further diagnostic evaluation. If the test is negative, there may be no treatment indicated.

## Stress Test Assessment Practice

Let's look at a few EKGs from stress tests. On the first five, *assess the EKG and decide if the test should continue or be terminated.* Assume that each person's rhythm was sinus rhythm with a heart rate of 70 and the EKG was otherwise completely normal at the start of the stress test. Assume this EKG was done 3 minutes into the Bruce protocol.

---

**QuickTip**

The question to be answered is: Is the stress test result true or false (as proven by the angiogram results)? There are 2 steps to determining true or false, positive or negative:

- First, determine the stress test result. Is it positive or negative? Write down the word "positive" or "negative."
- Second, what is the angiogram result—positive or negative? If the stress test and angiogram results differ—if one is positive and the other is negative, for example—the stress test result will be considered false. Write "false" in front of the stress test result. If the stress test and angiogram agree (both positive or both negative), the stress test result is true. Write "true" in front of the stress test result.

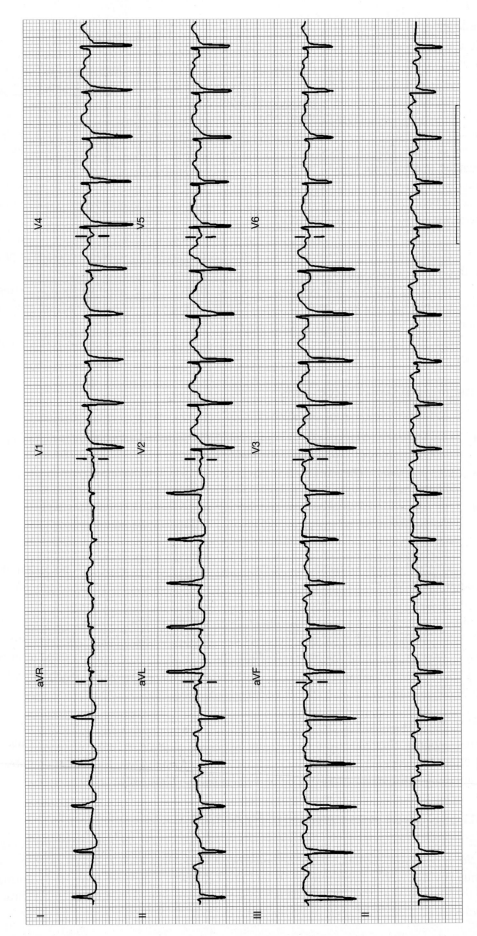

1. Continue or terminate?

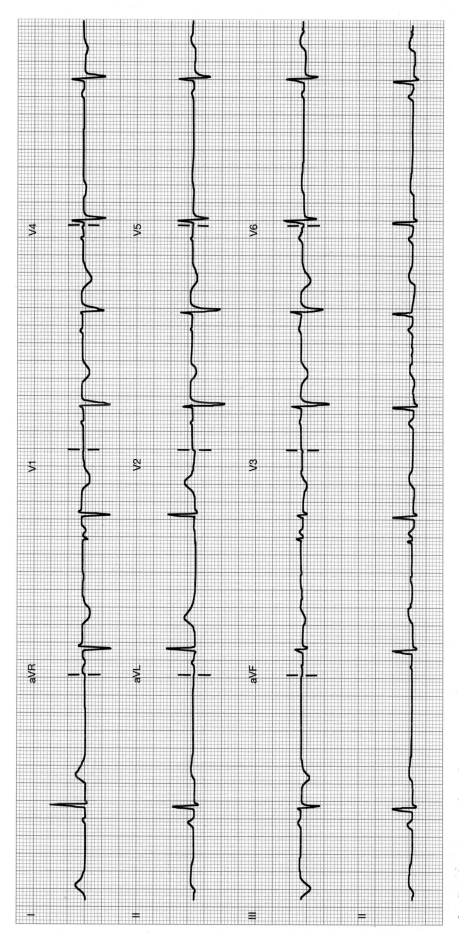

2. Continue or terminate?

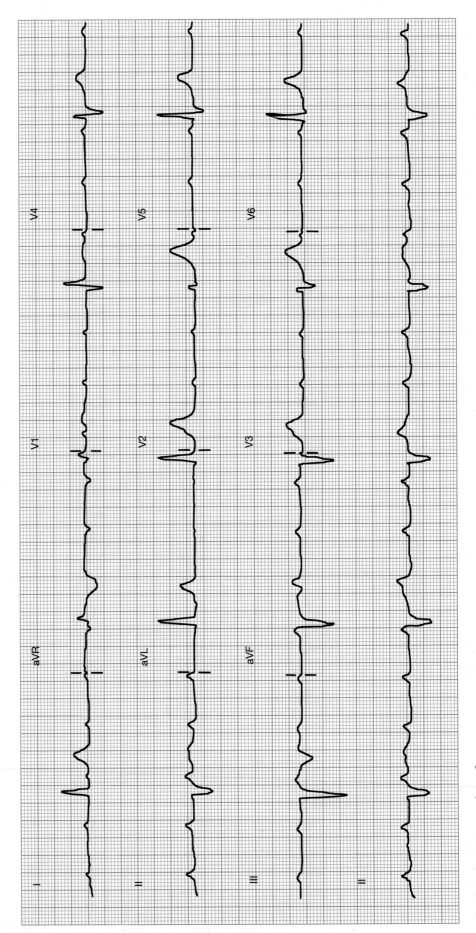

3. Continue or terminate? _____

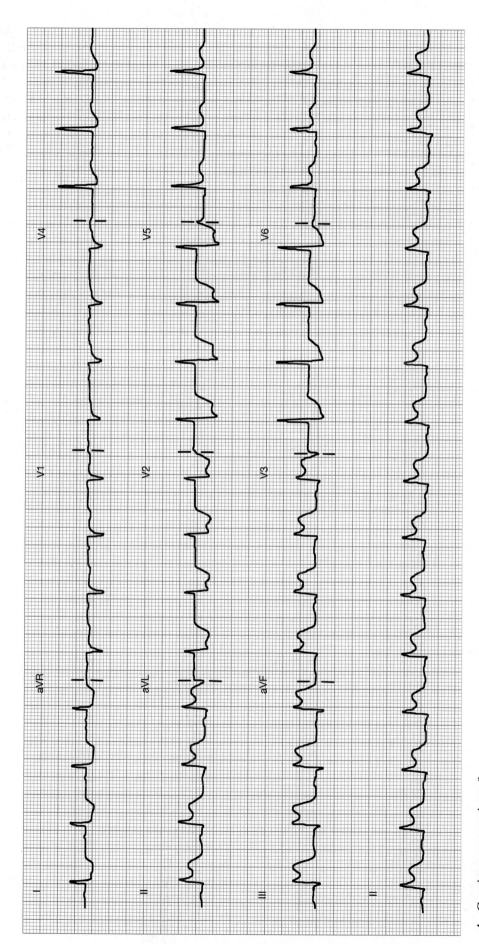

4. Continue or terminate?

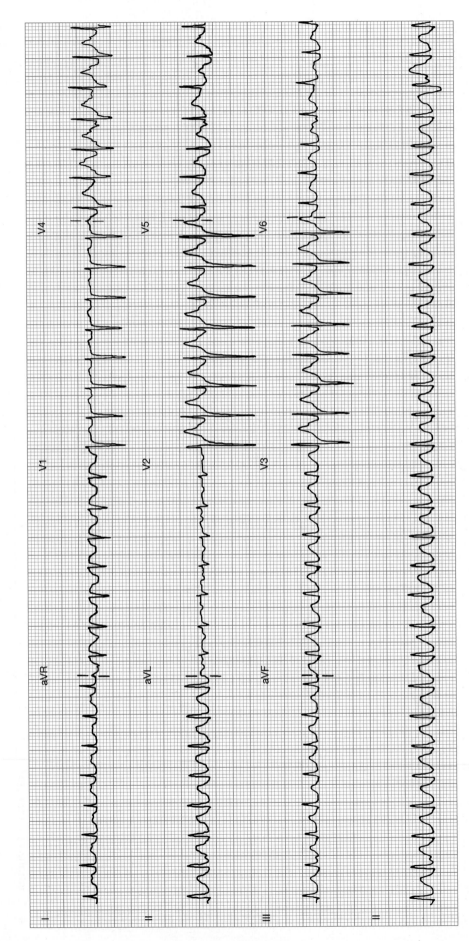

5. Continue or terminate?

On these final five, assess the EKG and determine if the stress test is positive or negative for CAD. Then *state whether the stress test is true positive, false positive, true negative, or false negative* based on the indicated angiogram results. Again, assume all pretest EKGs were normal.

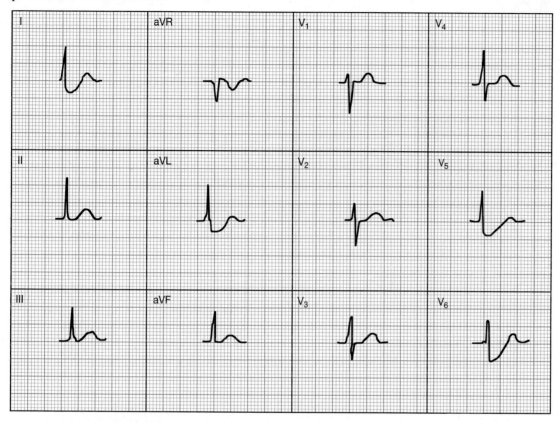

**6.** If the angiogram is negative, this stress test result is _____

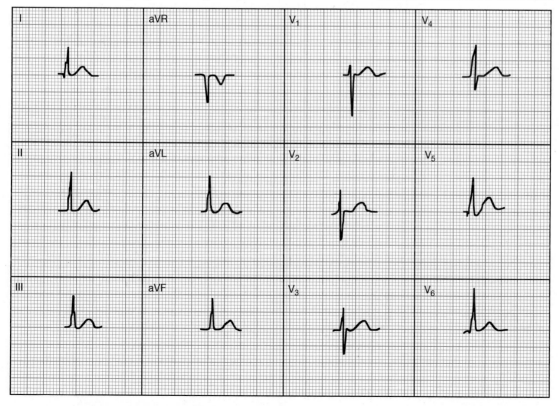

**7.** If the angiogram is positive, this stress test result is _____

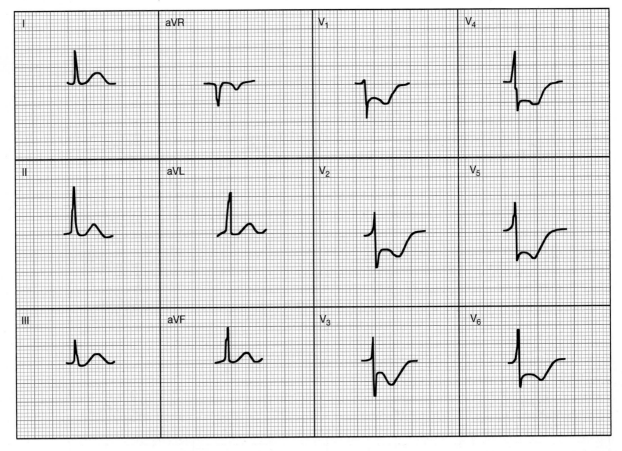

8. If the angiogram is negative, this stress test result is _____

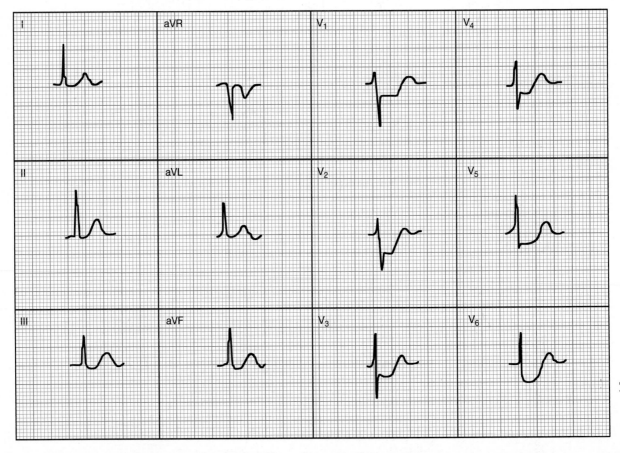

9. If the angiogram is positive, this stress test result is _____

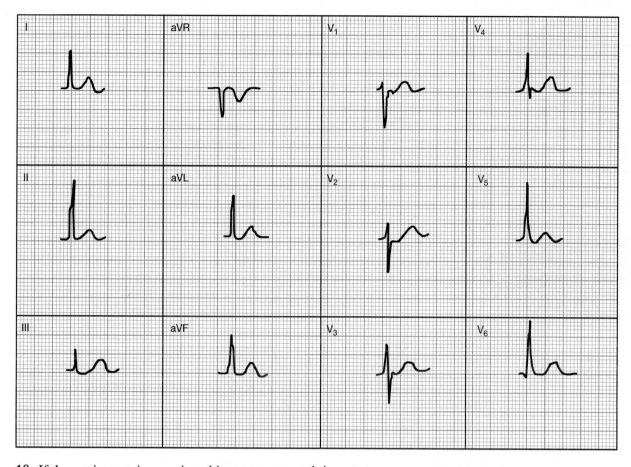

**10.** If the angiogram is negative, this stress test result is _____

## Holter Monitoring

The Holter monitor is an ambulatory EKG device used to rule out intermittent arrhythmias or cardiac ischemia that might be missed on a routine EKG. The Holter monitor consists of electrodes and a small battery-powered digital flash-memory device onto which the rhythm is recorded. The data are later uploaded into a computer that analyzes the rhythm. Technicians then review the analysis for further study. The device is small enough to be worn in a pocket or on a strap over the shoulder. It may be used as an inpatient or outpatient, although most often it is used on an outpatient basis.

### Indications for Holter Monitor Use

- *Syncope or near-syncopal episodes.*   Fainting spells could be caused by arrhythmias, which could be evident on Holter monitoring.
- *Intermittent chest pain or shortness of breath.*   These could be signs of myocardial ischemia, which could be detected with a Holter monitor.
- *Suspicion of arrhythmias.*   The patient who complains of palpitations, dizzy spells, or skipped beats may have arrhythmias that the Holter monitor would show.
- *Determination of arrhythmia treatment effectiveness.*   Holter monitoring can reveal if the rhythm being treated is still occurring and can demonstrate if a newly implanted pacemaker is functioning properly.

### Preparation Techniques

The patient is attached to five or more electrodes that are put on the trunk instead of the arms and legs in order to prevent muscle artifact. See Figure 13–8. Male patients with considerable chest hair might need the electrode sites to be clipped to allow the electrode patches to adhere properly. Female patients should have chest leads positioned beneath,

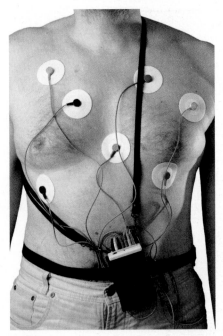

**FIGURE 13–8**

**Man with Holter monitor**
(Vadim Kozlovsky/Shutterstock).

not on top of, the breast. The skin is prepped prior to attaching the electrodes. This skin prep involves abrading the thin outer layer of skin so the electrodes adhere to the skin without losing contact. The electrodes are then taped to the skin to prevent dislodgment, because they will be on for 24 hours or longer. Typically, at least two leads are simultaneously recorded—either Leads $V_1$ and $V_5$ or Leads $V_1$ and II.

After being attached to the Holter monitor, the patient is given instructions, including not to remove the electrodes and not to take a bath or shower during the time the Holter is in use, as this could cause the electrodes to become dislodged. A careful sponge bath is permitted. The patient is otherwise instructed to go about normal daily activities. This includes work, hobbies, sex, and so on. The patient should not curtail activities just because the Holter is in use. The purpose of the Holter monitor is to catch abnormalities that show up in the course of daily activities. Curtailing those activities defeats the purpose.

The patient is advised to document any symptoms experienced while on the Holter monitor in a small diary provided for that purpose. By pressing the marker button on the Holter monitor, the patient marks the point in the EKG at which he or she feels symptoms so that this part of the EKG can be more closely examined for changes that could cause the symptoms. For example, if at 4 P.M., the patient feels dizzy, and the Holter reveals a short run of V-tach at that time, the arrhythmia would explain the dizziness. Treatment could then be started to prevent further ventricular arrhythmias. After the prescribed duration of Holter monitoring, the patient returns the Holter to the hospital or physician's office, whereupon it is entered into a computer and scanned for abnormalities.

### What Is a Positive Holter?

A positive Holter is one that reveals *abnormalities that could explain the patient's symptoms.* These abnormalities might include one or more of the following:

- Tachycardias
- Bradycardias
- Pauses
- ST segment elevation or depression

A negative Holter has no significant arrhythmias or ST changes.

## Event Monitoring

For patients whose symptoms are sporadic, a Holter monitor might not be the best choice, as the symptoms may not occur while the Holter is in use. An **event monitor** is a small device (often the size of a credit card) that the patient carries that can be programmed to record abnormalities in rhythm or ST segments or that can be activated by the patient whenever symptoms appear. Special types of event monitors can even be implanted under the skin on the chest for patients who need an even longer monitoring period.

There are two kinds of event monitors. One monitors the rhythm continuously, but only prints out abnormalities it has been preprogrammed to find. In addition, the patient can activate this recorder whenever symptoms occur. The device then records the patient's rhythm at that time and also, by way of a built-in memory, the rhythm that was present up to 5 minutes before the event. The rhythm can then be transmitted via telephone or the device turned in to the physician's office for immediate interpretation.

The second type of event monitor is not programmed to recognize abnormalities, nor does it monitor the rhythm continuously. It must be activated by the patient whenever symptoms occur. It will then record the rhythm present at that time as well as just before the event.

Unlike a Holter monitor, which is usually worn for only 24 hours, event monitors can be carried or worn for extended periods of time and are thus more likely to pick up abnormalities that are only sporadic. Like the Holter monitor, the event monitor is said to be *negative* if arrhythmias or ST-T changes are not found.

 **chapter thirteen notes** TO SUM IT ALL UP . . .

- **Diagnostic electrocardiography**—Involves an EKG done to rule out disease.
- **Signal-averaged EKG**—Averages about 250 consecutive QRS complexes—helps reveal late potentials—helps predict risk for ventricular arrhythmias.
- **Stress testing**—Involves utilizing exercise or medications to increase the heart rate and stress the heart—helps determine patency of coronary arteries.
- **Indications for stress testing:**
  - Post-cardiac surgery or post-PCI evaluation.
  - Diagnose/treat exercise-induced arrhythmias.
  - Follow-up to cardiac rehab.
  - Family history of heart disease.
- **Absolute contraindications to doing stress test:**
  - MI less than 48 hours old.
  - Uncontrolled symptomatic heart failure.
  - Unstable angina not stabilized medically.
  - Uncontrolled symptomatic cardiac arrhythmias.
  - Symptomatic severe aortic stenosis.
  - Dissecting aneurysm.
  - Acute myocarditis or pericarditis
  - Acute pulmonary embolus.
- **Relative contraindications to doing stress test:**
  - Left main coronary artery stenosis (narrowing).
  - Uncontrolled tachyarrhythmias or bradyarrhythmias.
  - Mental or physical issues that prevent adequate exercise.
  - Severe hypertension (systolic >200, diastolic >110).
  - Electrolyte abnormalities.
  - High degree AV block (second or third degree).
  - Moderate stenotic heart valve disease.
  - Hypertrophic cardiomyopathy or other forms of outflow obstruction.
- **Target heart rate**—for stress testing is calculated as 220 minus age.
- **Maximal test**—Must reach 85% of target heart rate.
- **Submaximal test**—Must reach 70% of target heart rate.
- **MET**—Metabolic equivalent—a measurement of oxygen consumption.
- **Stress testing protocols:**
  - *Bruce*—Most commonly used—treadmill speed and incline changes every 3 minutes.
  - *Modified Bruce*—Changes occur in smaller increments.
  - *Naughton*—Slower-moving submaximal test—for MI patients prior to discharge from hospital.
- **Terminate stress test when any of the following occur:**
  - ST segment elevation.
  - Sustained ventricular tachycardia.
  - Drop in systolic blood pressure >10 mm Hg.
  - Moderate to severe angina.
  - Dizziness, stumbling, feeling faint.
  - Patient's desire to stop.

- Technical problems doing the stress test.
- Patient becomes diaphoretic.
- **Normal EKG changes during stress test:**
  - Shortened PR interval.
  - Tall P waves.
  - Low-voltage QRS complexes.
  - Faster heart rate.
- **Normal signs and symptoms during stress test:**
  - Decreased systemic vascular resistance.
  - Increased respiratory rate.
  - Sweating.
  - Fatigue.
  - Muscle cramping in calves or sides.
  - Increased blood pressure.
  - Increased heart rate.
  - J-point depression.
- **Positive stress test:**
  - ST depression greater than 1–1.5 mms at 0.08 secs following the J point or,
  - U wave inversion or new U wave or,
  - ST segment elevation.
- **Sensitivity**—Percentage of patients with positive stress test and coronary artery disease proven by angiogram.
- **Specificity**—Percentage of patients with negative stress test and no coronary artery disease as proven by angiogram.
- **Categories of stress tests:**
  - *True positive*—Stress test positive, angiogram positive.
  - *False positive*—Stress test positive, angiogram negative.
  - *True negative*—Stress test negative, angiogram negative.
  - *False negative*—Stress test negative, angiogram positive.
- **Bayes's theorem**—The predictive value of any test is based not just on its accuracy but also on the patient's probability of disease.
- **Holter monitor**—Ambulatory EKG—to rule out arrhythmias or ischemic changes that could be causing the patient's symptoms.
  - Syncope or near-syncope.
  - Chest pain and/or shortness of breath.
  - Suspicion of arrhythmias.
  - Determine the effectiveness of treatment for arrhythmias.
- **Event monitor**—ambulatory EKG—to rule out very sporadic ischemia and/or arrhythmias that are unlikely to be noted on a Holter monitor—allows much longer monitoring periods; device can be implanted or carried.
- **Two kinds of event monitors:**
  - Continuously monitoring, pre-programmed to retain certain data.
  - Patient-activated—monitors only when activated by patient.
- **Indications for event monitor use**—same as for Holter.

## Practice Quiz

1. The type of monitor that is worn for 24 hours to uncover any arrhythmias or ST segment changes that might be causing the patient's symptoms is the

   _____

2. List three indications for stress testing. _____

3. What does Bayes's theorem have to say about the validity of test results? _____

   _____

4. Is ST segment elevation of 5 mm indicative of a positive stress test or a negative stress test? _____

   _____

   _____

5. True or false: Patients on medications such as beta-blockers and nitrates might be advised to avoid

taking these medications for a period of time before the stress test.

6. Target heart rate is _____

7. Event monitoring differs from Holter monitoring in what ways? _____

   _____

8. The most commonly used protocol for treadmill stress testing is the _____

   _____

9. The protocol used most often for post-MI patients just before or following hospital discharge is the

   _____

10. What is a MET? _____

## Putting It All Together—Critical Thinking Exercises

These exercises may consist of diagrams to label, scenarios to analyze, brain-stumping questions to ponder, or other challenging exercises to boost your knowledge of the chapter material.

The following scenario will provide you with information about a fictional patient and ask you to analyze the situation, answer questions, and decide on appropriate actions.

Mr. Cameron, a 46-year-old male, is having a stress test required by his new insurance company. He is 5 feet 9 inches tall and weighs 325 pounds. He smokes two packs of cigarettes daily. Aside from an occasional twinge in his chest when he mows the lawn (the only exercise he gets), he has had no chest pain. Blood pressure is 160/90 (high), respiratory rate is 22 (slightly fast). The plan is to do a maximal test using the Bruce protocol.

You explain the stress test procedure and attach Mr. Cameron to the EKG. His resting EKG is shown in Figure 13–9.

1. Do you see anything in this EKG that is of concern?

   _____

   _____

You start the Bruce protocol and all is going well, although Mr. Cameron does seem to be getting winded (slightly short of breath) quickly.

2. What in his history tells you this is nothing to be surprised about? _____

   _____

   _____

By stage II of the Bruce protocol, Mr. Cameron's heart rate is 148 and his PR intervals have shortened.

3. Should the test continue or be terminated at this point? _____

The test continues and at 7 minutes into the test, Mr. Cameron complains of fatigue and dizziness. Blood pressure is now 82/64 and his skin is diaphoretic. He looks pale but denies chest pain. You continue the test and 2 minutes later, he loses consciousness. Mr. Cameron's rhythm is seen in Figure 13–10.

4. What is this rhythm? _____

5. What is the appropriate course of action? _____

   _____

6. After appropriate treatment, Mr. Cameron is sent to the coronary care unit. Looking back on the test, what should you have done differently? _____

   _____

   _____

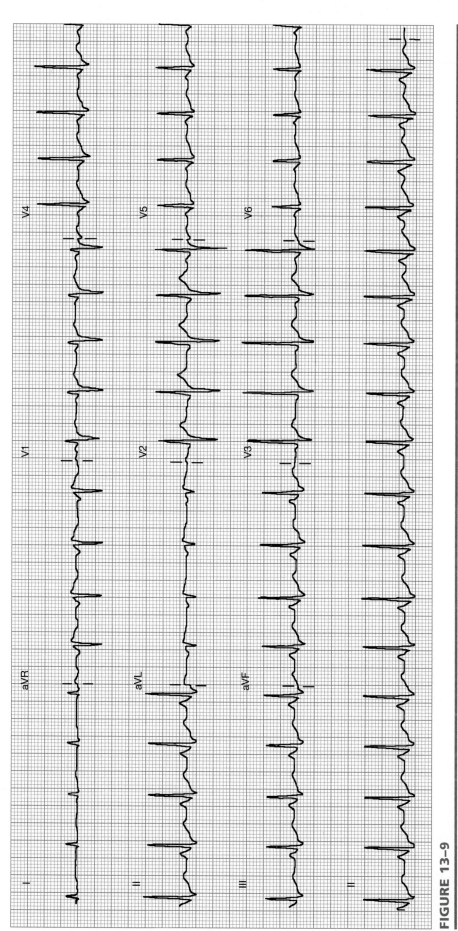

**FIGURE 13–9**

Mr. Cameron's resting EKG.

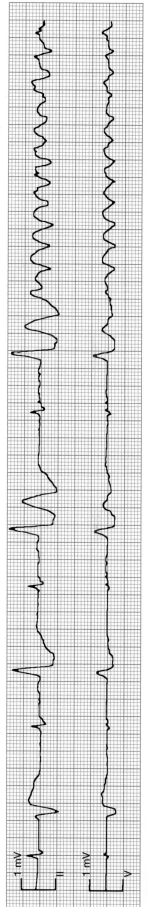

**FIGURE 13–10**

Mr. Cameron's rhythm when he loses consciousness.

# Appendix

## Answers

### CHAPTER ONE
### Practice Quiz

1. The function of the heart is to **pump enough blood to meet the body's metabolic needs.**
2. The three layers of the heart are the **endocardium, myocardium, and epicardium.**
3. The four chambers of the heart are the **right atrium, left atrium, right ventricle,** and **left ventricle.**
4. The four heart valves are the **tricuspid, mitral, pulmonic,** and **aortic valves.**
5. The purpose of the heart valves is to **prevent backflow of blood.**
6. The five great vessels are the **aorta, pulmonary artery, pulmonary veins, superior vena cava,** and **inferior vena cava.**
7. The phases of diastole are **rapid filling, diastasis,** and **atrial kick.**
8. The phases of systole are **isovolumetric contraction, ventricular ejection, protodiastole,** and **iovolumetric relaxation.**
9. The two divisions of the autonomic nervous system are the **sympathetic** and **parasympathetic nervous systems.**
10. The two main coronary arteries are the **left main coronary artery and the right coronary artery.**

2. Here are the following structures numbered 1 to 14 in order of blood flow through the heart:
   - 1 superior and inferior vena cava
   - 3 tricuspid valve
   - 10 mitral valve
   - 12 aortic valve
   - 5 pulmonic valve
   - 14 body
   - 13 aorta
   - 6 pulmonary artery
   - 7 lungs
   - 8 pulmonary veins
   - 2 right atrium
   - 9 left atrium
   - 4 right ventricle
   - 11 left ventricle

3. If the chordae tendineae of the tricuspid and mitral valves "snapped" loose, the valves would lose their ability to remain closed during systole, allowing blood to flow backward into the atria.

## Critical Thinking Exercises

1.

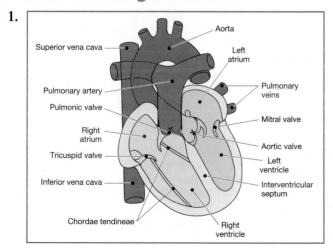

## CHAPTER TWO
# Waves and Complexes Identification Practice

1.
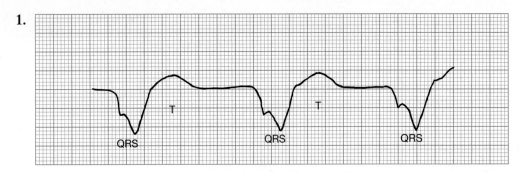

2.
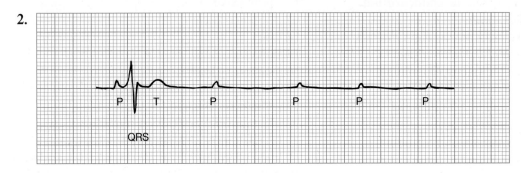

3.
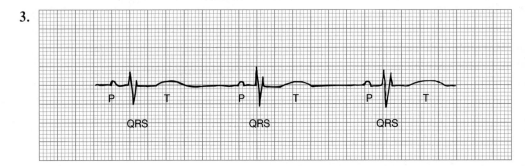

4.
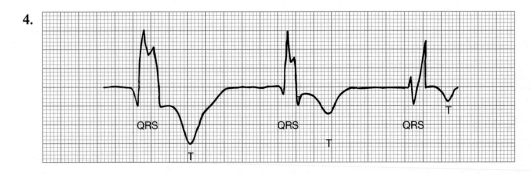

5.
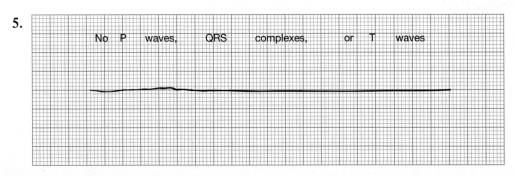

## QRS Nomenclature Practice
## "Name the waves"

1. R.
2. QS. This cannot be called a Q or an S because there is no R wave to precede or follow, so the QRS complex that is completely negative is called QS.
3. QR.
4. RS.
5. QRS.
6. RSR'

## "Draw the QRS complexes"

1.
2.
3.
4.
5.
6.

## Intervals Practice

1. PR 0.12, QRS 0.08, QT 0.24.
2. PR 0.12, QRS 0.14, QT 0.32.
3. PR 0.24, QRS 0.08, QT 0.28.

## Intervals Practice on normal-size EKG paper

Note: For the intervals, it is acceptable if your answer is within 0.02 secs of displayed answer.

1. PR 0.20, QRS 0.08, QT 0.36.
2. PR 0.22, QRS 0.08, QT 0.32.
3. PR 0.08, QRS 0.12, QT 0.36.
4. PR 0.10, QRS 0.08, QT 0.32.
5. PR 0.16, QRS 0.06, QT 0.36.
6. PR 0.16, QRS 0.08, QT 0.30.
7. PR 0.16, QRS 0.08, QT 0.30.
8. PR 0.14, QRS 0.09, QT 0.38.
9. PR 0.16, QRS 0.10, QT 0.37.
10. PR 0.14, QRS 0.08, QT 0.30.

## Practice Quiz

1. Cardiac cells at rest are electrically **negative.**
2. Depolarization and repolarization are **electrical events.**
3. Phase 4. **The cardiac cell is at rest.**
   Phase 0. **Depolarization occurs when sodium rushes into the cell.**
   Phase 1. **Early repolarization. Calcium is released.**
   Phase 2. **The plateau phase of early repolarization. Calcium is released.**
   Phase 3. **Rapid repolarization. Sodium rushes out of the cell.**
4. The P wave represents **atrial depolarization.**
   The QRS complex represents **ventricular depolarization.**
   The T wave represents **ventricular repolarization.**
5. **No impulse can result in depolarization during the absolute refractory period.**
6. The four characteristics of heart cells are **automaticity, conductivity, excitability,** and **contractility.**
7. The inherent rates of the pacemaker cells are **sinus node—60 to 100, AV junction—40 to 60, ventricle—20 to 40.**
8. The structures of the cardiac conduction pathway are **sinus node, interatrial tracts, atrium, internodal tracts, AV node, bundle of His, bundle branches, Purkinje fibers,** and **ventricle.**
9. **Escape occurs when the prevailing pacemaker slows or fails and a lower pacemaker takes over as the pacemaker at a slower rate than before.**
10. **Usurpation occurs when a lower pacemaker becomes "hyper" and fires at an accelerated rate, stealing control away from the predominant pacemaker and providing a faster heart rate than before.**

## Critical Thinking Exercises

1. If the sinus node is firing at a rate of 65 and the AV junction kicks in at a rate of 70, **the AV junction will usurp the sinus node and become the heart's pacemaker.** The sinus node would be inhibited and would stop firing out impulses as long as the AV junction is faster. Remember, the fastest pacemaker at any given time is the one in control.
2. If your patient's PR interval last night was 0.16 seconds and this morning it is 0.22, **the AV node is becoming incapable of transmitting impulses at its normal rate, causing the PR interval to prolong.**
3. The heart's pumping ability can fail, but its electrical conduction ability remains **intact if there is a heart attack or other condition that damages the myocardium but leaves the conduction system unaffected.** The conduction system would send out its impulses as usual, but the damaged myocardium would be unable to respond by pumping.

4.

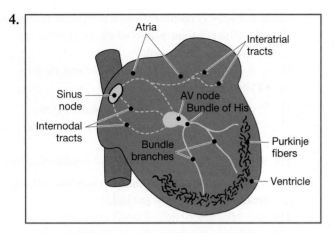

## CHAPTER THREE
## Practice Quiz

1. Electrocardiography **is the recording of the heart's electrical impulses by electrodes placed on the arms, legs, and chest**.
2. The three bipolar leads are **Leads I, II,** and **III. Lead I connects the right and left arms. Lead II connects the right arm and left leg. Lead III connects the left arm and left leg.**
3. The three augmented leads are as follows:

    aVR    **Positive pole is on the right arm.**
    aVL    **Positive pole is on the left arm.**
    aVF    **Positive pole is on the left leg.**

4. The six leads comprising the hexiaxial diagram are **Leads I, II, III, aVR, aVL,** and **aVF.**
5. The precordial leads see the heart from the **horizontal plane.**
6. The precordial leads and their locations are as follows:

    $V_1$    **4th ICS, RSB**
    $V_2$    **4th ICS, LSB**
    $V_3$    **Between $V_2$ and $V_4$**
    $V_4$    **5th ICS, MCL**
    $V_5$    **5th ICS, AAL**
    $V_6$    **5th ICS, MAL**

7. The two leads most commonly used for continuous monitoring are **Leads II** and $V_1/MCL_1$.
8. An impulse traveling toward a positive electrode writes a **positive** complex on the EKG.
9. The aVR should have a **negative** QRS complex.
10. The QRS complexes in the precordial leads start out primarily **negative.**

## Critical Thinking Exercises

1. If Lead I + Lead III do not equal Lead II, it could imply that **the electrodes were placed on the incorrect limbs.**
2. If the QRS complex in Lead III is isoelectric, **the heart's current is traveling perpendicular to that lead.**
3. If your patient has a heart rhythm in which the current starts in the left ventricle and travels upward toward the sinus node, the frontal leads would look like the following: **Lead I's QRS would be negative, Lead II would be negative, Lead III would be negative, aVR would be positive, aVL would be negative, and aVF would be negative.** You'll note this is the exact opposite of how the frontal leads normally look. This is because the current would be traveling away from all the positive electrodes except aVR's. Recall that aVR's positive electrode sits on the right arm and would be watching this current come straight toward it, resulting in a positive QRS in aVR.

## CHAPTER FOUR
## Artifact Troubleshooting Practice

1. The artifact is in Leads **I, III,** and **aVL.** Corrective action is to check for and reattach or reconnect loose or disconnected electrodes or lead wires on the **left arm.** If an electrode patch is loose or missing, put on a new patch. *Never put a used patch back on. It will not stick well enough to ensure good impulse transmission.* How do we know the problem is on the left arm? Refer to Figure 4-6. What is the common limb shared by all these leads? Lead I connects right arm and left arm; III connects left arm and left leg; aVL involves left arm only. The common limb is the left arm. Direct corrective efforts there.
2. The artifact is in Leads **II, III,** and **aVF.** Corrective action is to check the **left leg** for loose or disconnected electrodes or lead wires and to reattach/reconnect them as necessary. What is the common limb? Lead II connects right arm and left leg; III connects left arm and left leg; aVF involves left leg only. The common limb is the left leg.
3. The artifact is in Leads **I, II,** and **aVR.** Corrective action is to check the **right arm** for loose or

disconnected electrodes or lead wires and to reattach/reconnect them as necessary. What is the common limb? Lead I connects right arm and left arm; II connects right arm and left leg; III involves right arm only. The common limb is the right arm.

## Practice Quiz

1. The function of the EKG machine is **to print out a representation of the electrical signals generated by the heart.**
2. Normal chart speed for running a 12-lead EKG is **25** millimeters per second.
3. The gain **adjusts the height of the waves and complexes.**
4. If the technician changes any of the settings (the chart speed or the gain) when doing an EKG, **he or she should document this on the EKG.**
5. Macroshock **is a high-voltage electrical shock that results from inadequate grounding of electrical equipment.**
6. Microshock is **a lower voltage shock that involves a conduit directly into the patient, such as a pacemaker.**
7. Artifact is **unwanted interference or jitter on the EKG tracing.**
8. The four kinds of artifact are **somatic tremors, baseline sway, 60-cycle interference,** and **broken recording.**
9. If there is artifact in I, aVR, and II, troubleshooting efforts should be directed toward the **right arm.**
10. Ways to determine if a rhythm is real or artifact include any of the following three: **Observe the rhythm in another lead such as V₁. Check to see if the rhythm meets the normal criteria. Check the monitor wires and patches. See if the patient has any muscle tremors that could cause artifact. Check the patient's vital signs for evidence of decreased cardiac output.**

## Critical Thinking Exercises

1. If your patient, who is on telemetry monitoring, is noted to have two electrodes that have fallen off—the right arm and left leg, **you would expect to see artifact in any leads that use either or both of those limbs: Lead I, Lead II, Lead III, aVR, and aVF.**

2. You would know that your patient is having artifact and not a life-threatening arrhythmia by **assessing the patient for signs of decreased cardiac output, checking the rhythm in another lead, checking the electrode patches and wires to see if any are loose or detached, and assessing for any muscle tremors or twitches that could mimic artifact.**

## CHAPTER FIVE
## Practice Strips: Regularity of Rhythms

1. **Irregular.** The R-R intervals are all over the place, with no hint of regularity.
2. **Regular.** The R-R intervals are all about 56 little blocks.
3. **Regular but interrupted.** This is the strip shown earlier as an example of regular but interrupted rhythms. Look back if you don't recognize it.
4. **Regular but interrupted.** The R-R intervals are all 28 to 29 blocks except for the long pause that interrupts this otherwise regular rhythm.
5. **Regular but interrupted.** Again, the R-R intervals are regular before and after the premature beat (and the expected short pause after it).

## Practice Strips: Calculating Heart Rate

1. This is a regular rhythm, so choose any two consecutive QRS complexes and calculate the heart rate there. There are 15 little blocks between QRSs. Divide 1,500 by 15 for the little block method. The heart rate is **100.**
2. Another regular rhythm. The heart rate is **75.**
3. This is a regular rhythm interrupted by a premature beat. We therefore ignore the premature beat for the purposes of heart rate calculation. The heart rate is **107,** as there are 14 little blocks between QRS complexes.
4. Although at first glance this rhythm appears regular, closer examination reveals that the R-R intervals vary from 9-1/2 to 12-1/2 little blocks apart. Because it is an irregular rhythm, we need the heart rate range along with the mean rate. The range is **about 120 to 155, with a mean rate of 140.**
5. This is a regular rhythm interrupted by a pause, so we calculate the range and the mean rate. There are 35 little blocks during the pause, and 20 little

blocks between the regular QRS complexes. The heart rate range is therefore **43 to 75, with a mean rate of 70.**

6. This is an irregular rhythm. The **mean heart rate is 80 and the range is 56 to 107.** The first two QRS complexes are the farthest apart on the strip and thus represent the slowest heart rate (56). The 6th and 7th QRS complexes are the closest together and represent the fastest heart rate on the strip (107).

7. Here the rhythm is regular. Heart rate is **50.**

8. The QRS complexes are *huge* on this strip, but the rhythm is regular. Heart rate is **75.**

9. The rhythm is irregular. Heart rate **range is 52 to 81, with a mean rate of 70.**

10. The rhythm is regular. Heart rate is **130.**

## Practice Quiz

1. The three methods for calculating heart rate are the **6-second strip method,** the **little block method,** and the **memory method.**

2. The least accurate method of calculating heart rate is the **6-second strip method.**

3. When using the little block method, count the number of little blocks between QRS complexes and divide into **1,500.**

4. The memory method is **300–150–100–75–60–50–43–37–33–30.**

5. With regular rhythms interrupted by premature beats, the heart rate is calculated by **ignoring the premature beat and calculating the heart rate on an uninterrupted portion of the strip.**

6. The three types of regularity are **regular, regular but interrupted,** and **irregular.**

7. A rhythm with R-R intervals that vary throughout the strip is an **irregular** rhythm.

8. A rhythm that is regular except for premature beats or pauses is a **regular but interrupted** rhythm.

9. A rhythm in which the R-R intervals vary by only one or two little blocks is a **regular** rhythm.

10. R-R interval is defined as **the distance between two consecutive QRS complexes.**

## Critical Thinking Exercises

1. A rhythm whose R-R intervals are 23, 24, 23, 23, 12, 24, 23, 24, 23, 23 would be considered **regular but interrupted (by a premature beat). The heart rate would be 65 (1,500 divided by 23).** On a rhythm that's regular but interrupted by a premature beat, ignore the premature beat (the R-R interval of 12) and the short pause that normally follows it (R-R of 24) and just find an uninterrupted part of the strip. Most R-R intervals are 23, so calculate the heart rate based on this.

2. A rhythm with R-R intervals of 12, 17, 22, 45, 10, and 18 would be considered **irregular. Heart rate would be mean rate of 70 and a range of 33 to 150.** How did we come up with the mean rate? To get the first R-R of 12 requires two QRS complexes. Then each R-R is one more QRS for a total of 7 on the strip. So the mean rate is 70. Then for the heart rate range, find the two QRS complexes the farthest apart (R-R of 45) and the two closest together (R-R of 10) and divide each set into 1,500. Slowest heart rate is 33; fastest is 150.

3. A rhythm with R-R intervals of 22, 23, 22, 22, 23, 22, 22, 22 would be considered **regular. Heart rate is 68 (R-R of 22 divided into 1,500).**

## CHAPTER SIX
## Practice Quiz

1. A heart rate that is greater than 100 is said to be a **tachycardia.**

2. A heart rate less than 60 is a **bradycardia.**

3. **Is.** A sudden drop in heart rate from a tachycardia of 125 to a normal heart rate of 65 is indeed cause for concern, as it may cause the cardiac output (the amount of blood pumped out by the heart each minute) to drop. This could cause the patient to have symptoms such as low blood pressure, dizziness, cold clammy skin, or other problems.

4. Arrhythmia means **abnormal heart rhythm.**

5. The five steps to rhythm interpretation are
   ■ Evaluate the QRS complexes.
   ■ Assess rhythm regularity.
   ■ Calculate the heart rate.
   ■ Assess P waves.
   ■ Assess PR interval and QRS intervals.

## CHAPTER SEVEN
## Practice Strips: Sinus Rhythms

Note: For the intervals, it is acceptable if your answer is within 0.02 secs of displayed answer.

1. **QRS complexes:** present, all shaped the same. **Regularity:** regular. **Heart rate:** 56. **P waves:** upright, matching, one per QRS; P-P interval regular. **PR:** 0.18. **QRS:** 0.12 (wider than normal). **Interpretation:** sinus bradycardia with wide QRS.

2. **QRS complexes:** present, all shaped the same. **Regularity:** regular. **Heart rate:** 125. **P waves:** upright, matching, one per QRS; P-P interval regular. **PR:** 0.14. **QRS:** 0.08. **Interpretation:** sinus tachycardia.

3. **QRS complexes:** present, all shaped the same. **Regularity:** regular. **Heart rate:** 115. **P waves:** upright, matching, one per QRS; P-P interval regular. **PR:** 0.12. **QRS:** 0.10. **Interpretation:** sinus tachycardia.

4. **QRS complexes:** present, all shaped the same. **Regularity:** regular. **Heart rate:** 45. **P waves:** upright, matching, one per QRS; P-P interval regular. **PR:** 0.16. **QRS:** 0.14 (wider than normal). **Interpretation:** sinus bradycardia.

5. **QRS complexes:** present, all shaped the same. **Regularity:** regular but interrupted (by a pause). **Heart rate:** 21 to 54, with a mean rate of 40. **P waves:** upright, matching, one per QRS; P-P interval irregular due to the pause. **PR:** 0.18. **QRS:** 0.10. **Interpretation:** sinus bradycardia with a 3.08-second sinus arrest.

6. **QRS complexes:** present, all shaped the same. **Regularity:** regular (R-R intervals vary by only two small blocks). **Heart rate:** about 68. **P waves:** upright, matching, one per QRS; P-P interval regular. **PR:** 0.16. **QRS:** 0.08. **Interpretation:** sinus rhythm.

7. **QRS complexes:** present, all shaped the same. **Regularity:** regular. **Heart rate:** about 130. **P waves:** upright, matching, one per QRS. The heart rate is so fast that the T waves and P waves merge together. Do you see the notch at the top of the T wave? That's the P wave popping out. P-P interval regular. **PR:** cannot measure. **QRS:** 0.08. **Interpretation:** sinus tachycardia.

8. **QRS complexes:** present, all shaped the same. **Regularity:** regular. **Heart rate:** 88. **P waves:** biphasic (counts as upright), matching, one per QRS; P-P interval regular. **PR:** 0.12. **QRS:** 0.10. **Interpretation:** sinus rhythm.

9. **QRS complexes:** present, all shaped the same. **Regularity:** irregular; the R-R intervals vary from 25 to 29 small blocks. **Heart rate:** 52 to 60, with a mean rate of 60. **P waves:** upright, matching, one per QRS; P-P interval irregular. **PR:** 0.16. **QRS:** 0.06. **Interpretation:** sinus arrhythmia.

10. **QRS complexes:** present, all shaped the same. **Regularity:** regular. **Heart rate:** about 47. **P waves:** upright, matching, one preceding each QRS; P-P interval regular. **PR:** 0.16. **QRS:** 0.08. **Interpretation:** sinus bradycardia.

11. **QRS complexes:** present, all shaped the same within each lead. **Regularity:** regular. **Heart rate:** 75. **P waves:** upright in Lead I and inverted in $V_1$ (you'll recall this is OK for this lead), matching, one per QRS; P-P interval regular. **PR:** 0.10 (unusually short). **QRS:** 0.10. **Interpretation:** sinus rhythm.

12. **QRS complexes:** present, all shaped the same within each lead. **Regularity:** irregular. **Heart rate:** 43 to 63, with a mean rate of 60. **P waves:** upright, matching, one per QRS. P-P interval irregular. **PR:** 0.16. **QRS:** 0.12. **Interpretation:** sinus arrhythmia.

13. **QRS complexes:** present, all shaped the same within each lead. **Regularity:** regular. **Heart rate:** 83. **P waves:** upright, matching, one per QRS; P-P interval regular. **PR:** 0.14. **QRS:** 0.14. **Interpretation:** sinus rhythm.

14. **QRS complexes:** present, all shaped the same within each lead. **Regularity:** regular. **Heart rate:** 71. **P waves:** upright, matching, one per QRS; P-P interval regular. **PR:** 0.16. **QRS:** 0.76. **Interpretation:** sinus rhythm.

15. **QRS complexes:** present, all shaped the same within each lead. **Regularity:** regular. **Heart rate:** 125. **P waves:** upright, matching, one preceding each QRS; P-P interval regular. **PR:** 0.12. **QRS:** 0.08. **Interpretation:** sinus tachycardia.

16. **QRS complexes:** present, all shaped the same within each lead. **Regularity:** regular. **Heart rate:** 136. **P waves:** upright, matching, one per QRS; P-P interval regular. **PR:** 0.12. **QRS:** 0.08. **Interpretation:** sinus tachycardia.

17. **QRS complexes:** present, all shaped the same within each lead. **Regularity:** regular. **Heart rate:** 42. **P waves:** upright, matching, one per QRS; P-P interval regular. **PR:** 0.16. **QRS:** 0.08. **Interpretation:** sinus bradycardia. Thank goodness this is a double-lead strip because if we had only the top strip, we'd be hard pressed to interpret it.

18. **QRS complexes:** present, all shaped the same within each lead. **Regularity:** regular. **Heart rate:** 79. **P waves:** upright, matching, one per QRS; P-P interval regular. **PR:** 0.20. **QRS:** 0.10. **Interpretation:** sinus rhythm.

19. **QRS complexes:** present, all shaped the same within each lead. **Regularity:** regular. **Heart rate:** 115. **P waves:** upright, matching, one per QRS; P-P interval regular. **PR:** 0.14. **QRS:** 0.06. **Interpretation:** sinus tachycardia.

20. **QRS complexes:** present, all shaped the same within each lead. **Regularity:** regular. **Heart**

rate: 115. **P waves:** upright, matching, one per QRS; P-P interval regular. **PR:** 0.16. **QRS:** 0.12. **Interpretation:** sinus tachycardia.

21. **QRS complexes:** present, all shaped the same within each lead. **Regularity:** irregular. **Heart rate:** 48 to 71, mean rate 60. **P waves:** upright, matching, one per QRS; P-P interval irregular. **PR:** 0.16–0.18. **QRS:** 0.06. **Interpretation:** sinus arrhythmia.

22. **QRS complexes:** present, all shaped the same within each lead. **Regularity:** regular. **Heart rate:** 54. **P waves:** upright, matching, one per QRS; P-P interval regular. **PR:** 0.12. **QRS:** 0.12. **Interpretation:** sinus bradycardia.

23. **QRS complexes:** present, all shaped the same within each lead. **Regularity:** regular. **Heart rate:** 137. **P waves:** upright, matching, one per QRS; P-P regular. **PR:** 0.12. **QRS:** 0.06. **Interpretation:** sinus tachycardia.

24. **QRS complexes:** present, all shaped the same within each lead. **Regularity:** regular. **Heart rate:** 88. **P waves:** upright, matching, one per QRS; P-P regular. **PR:** 0.16. **QRS:** 0.08. **Interpretation:** sinus rhythm.

25. **QRS complexes:** present, all shaped the same within each lead. **Regularity:** regular. **Heart rate:** 60. **P waves:** upright, matching, one per QRS; P-P regular. **PR:** 0.18. **QRS:** 0.08. **Interpretation:** sinus rhythm.

## Practice Quiz

1. **False.** Most rhythms from the sinus node are regular rhythms.
2. The only difference in interpretation between sinus rhythm, sinus bradycardia, and sinus tachycardia is the **heart rate.**
3. Sinus arrhythmia is typically caused by the **breathing pattern.**
4. A sinus exit block differs from a sinus arrest in that **in a sinus exit block, the pause is a multiple of the previous R-R intervals. In sinus arrest, the pause is not a multiple.**
5. **False.** Atropine is inappropriate for sinus tachycardia, as it would speed up the already fast heart rate even more.
6. An individual with a fever of 103°F would be expected to be in **sinus tachycardia.**
7. A regular rhythm from the sinus node with heart rate of 155 is called **sinus tachycardia.**
8. **True.** That is the most basic criterion for sinus rhythms.

9. **Atropine causes the heart rate to increase.**
10. **False.** Atropine is indicated for sinus bradycardia with symptoms. Remember, athletes very often have sinus bradycardia and tolerate it well.

## Critical Thinking Exercises

1. The rhythm is **sinus rhythm.** Note the matching upright P waves and the heart rate between 60 and 100.
2. The rhythm is **sinus tachycardia,** rate 115.
3. The change in heart rate is most likely caused by **Mr. Cavernum's increasing temperature.** Recall that the heart rate speeds up about 10 beats per minute for every one degree increase in temp. Since his temp has climbed just over two degrees, his heart rate has increased by about 20 beats per minute.
4. **Acetaminophen** is the medication Mr. Cavernum needs. It will lower his body temperature and that will decrease his heart rate. Atropine is indicated for bradycardias, not tachycardias. Beta-blockers would indeed lower the heart rate, but because it is likely the heart rate is related to the fever, acetaminophen or ibuprofen is the best choice.
5. The rhythm is **sinus arrhythmia.** Note the irregularity. The first two QRS complexes are 37 little blocks apart. The last two are 41 blocks apart—enough to say this rhythm is irregular and is, therefore, sinus arrhythmia.
6. As long as Mr. Cavernum is tolerating the rhythm without ill effects, **he requires no emergency treatment.** If he did show signs of decreased cardiac output, however, he'd probably need atropine to speed up his heart rate. Although his heart rate is slow (between 37 and 40), it is not necessarily in need of treatment.
7. **Past history of sleep apnea** is a possible cause of sinus arrhythmia.

## CHAPTER EIGHT
## Practice Strips: Atrial Rhythms

Note: For the intervals, it is acceptable if your answer is within 0.02 secs of displayed answer.

1. **QRS complexes:** present, all shaped the same. **Regularity:** regular. **Heart rate:** 150. **P waves:** none visible. **PR:** not applicable. **QRS:** 0.08. **Interpretation:** SVT.
2. **QRS complexes:** present, all shaped the same. **Regularity:** regular but interrupted (by a premature

beat). Remember it's normal to have a short pause after a premature beat. **Heart rate:** 56. **P waves:** upright and matching, except for the fourth P wave, which is premature and shaped differently. (There is a tiny notch on the downstroke of the premature P wave.) P-P interval is irregular because of the premature beat. **PR:** 0.12. **QRS:** 0.08. **Interpretation:** sinus bradycardia with a PAC.

3. **QRS complexes:** present, all shaped the same. **Regularity:** regular. **Heart rate:** atrial rate 375; ventricular rate 79. **P waves:** none present; flutter waves present instead. **PR:** not applicable. **QRS:** 0.10. **Interpretation:** atrial flutter with 5:1 and 6:1 conduction.

4. **QRS complexes:** present, all shaped the same. **Regularity:** irregular. **Heart rate:** 88 to 137, with a mean rate of 110. **P waves:** none present; wavy baseline present instead. **PR:** not applicable. **QRS:** 0.08. **Interpretation:** atrial fibrillation.

5. **QRS complexes:** present, all shaped the same. **Regularity:** regular but interrupted (by a pause). **Heart rate:** atrial rate 300; ventricular rate 98 to 158, with a mean rate of 150. **P waves:** none present; flutter waves present instead. **PR:** not applicable. **QRS:** 0.08. **Interpretation:** atrial flutter with 2:1 and 4:1 conduction.

6. **QRS complexes:** present, all shaped the same. **Regularity:** irregular. **Heart rate:** 100 to 125, with a mean rate of 110. **P waves:** at least three different shapes; P-P interval irregular. **PR:** varies. **QRS:** 0.08. **Interpretation:** multifocal atrial tachycardia.

7. **QRS complexes:** present, all shaped the same. **Regularity:** regular but interrupted (by a pause). **Heart rate:** 43 to 83. **P waves:** upright and matching, one before each beat. See the T wave of the last beat before the pause? It's a bit taller than the other Ts. There is a P hiding inside it, distorting its normal shape. That P in the T is premature, so that makes it a PAC. **PR:** 0.16. **QRS:** 0.10. **Interpretation:** sinus rhythm with a nonconducted PAC.

8. **QRS complexes:** present, all shaped the same. **Regularity:** irregular. **Heart rate:** 52 to 75, with a mean rate of 70. **P waves:** none present; wavy baseline present instead. **PR:** not applicable. **QRS:** 0.10. **Interpretation:** atrial fibrillation.

9. **QRS complexes:** present, all shaped the same. **Regularity:** regular but interrupted (by a premature beat). **Heart rate:** 100. **P waves:** upright, all matching except for the premature P wave preceding the sixth QRS complex. There is one P wave preceding each QRS complex; P-P interval irregular. **PR:** 0.16. **QRS:** 0.08. **Interpretation:** sinus rhythm with a PAC.

10. **QRS complexes:** present, all shaped the same. **Regularity:** regular. **Heart rate:** about 150. **P waves:** Is that a tall pointy P wave distorting the T waves? Maybe. But it's also a possibility that those are flutter waves between the QRS complexes. We just can't be sure. **PR:** not applicable. **QRS:** 0.08. **Interpretation:** SVT.

11. **QRS complexes:** present, all shaped the same. **Regularity:** irregular. **Heart rate:** 22 to 75, mean rate 40. **P waves:** none noted; wavy baseline present instead. **PR:** not applicable. **QRS:** 0.08. **Interpretation:** atrial fibrillation.

12. **QRS complexes:** present, all shaped the same. **Regularity:** regular. **Heart rate:** 187. **P waves:** not seen. The wave between the QRS complexes may just be a T wave without a P wave. **PR:** not applicable. **QRS:** 0.06. **Interpretation:** SVT.

13. **QRS complexes:** present, all shaped the same. **Regularity:** regular but interrupted (by a premature beat). **Heart rate:** 75. **P waves:** biphasic, all matching except for the premature P wave preceding the fifth QRS. There is one P wave preceding each QRS; P-P interval irregular. **PR:** 0.14. **QRS:** 0.08. **Interpretation:** sinus rhythm with a PAC.

14. **QRS complexes:** present, all shaped the same. **Regularity:** irregular. **Heart rate:** 16 to 44, mean rate 30. **P waves:** none noted; wavy baseline present instead. **PR:** not applicable. **QRS:** 0.08. **Interpretation:** atrial fibrillation.

15. **QRS complexes:** present, all shaped the same. **Regularity:** regular. **Heart rate:** about 136. **P waves:** Is that a pointy P wave distorting the T waves in the top strip? Maybe—can't be sure. There are no hints of a P wave in the bottom strip. **PR:** not applicable. **QRS:** 0.10. **Interpretation:** SVT. This may indeed be a sinus tachycardia with the P wave hidden in the T wave of the preceding beat, but we can't be sure.

16. **QRS complexes:** present, all shaped the same. **Regularity:** regular. **Heart rate:** 150. **P waves:** No P waves—those are flutter waves between the QRS complexes. See the asterisks under the flutter waves toward the end of the strip on the bottom lead? **PR:** not applicable. **QRS:** 0.08. **Interpretation:** atrial flutter with 2:1 conduction. There are two flutter waves to each QRS.

17. **QRS complexes:** present, all shaped the same. **Regularity:** irregular. **Heart rate:** 136 to 231, mean rate 170. **P waves:** at least three different

shapes; P-P interval irregular. **PR:** varies. **QRS:** 0.06. **Interpretation:** multifocal atrial tachycardia.

18. **QRS complexes:** present, all shaped the same. **Regularity:** irregular. **Heart rate:** 88 to 150, mean rate 120. **P waves:** none noted; wavy baseline present instead. **PR:** not applicable. **QRS:** 0.08. **Interpretation:** atrial fibrillation.

19. **QRS complexes:** present, all shaped the same. **Regularity:** regular but interrupted (by a pause). **Heart rate:** 26 to 65, mean rate 50. **P waves:** none seen. On the top strip is a very fine wavy baseline. The bottom strip has flutter waves. **PR:** not applicable. **QRS:** 0.08. **Interpretation:** This one is up for grabs. It could be either atrial fibrillation or atrial flutter (top strip looks like fib, bottom strip like flutter). It would help to have more leads to examine. Statistically, it's more likely that this is atrial flutter rather than fibrillation because atrial fib tends to be much more irregular. On this rhythm, the QRS complexes are regular except for the pause.

20. **QRS complexes:** present, all shaped the same. **Regularity:** regular but interrupted (by premature beats). Remember that premature beats are followed by a short pause; that does not make the rhythm irregular. The fourth, seventh, and tenth beats are premature. **Heart rate:** 83. **P waves:** upright, matching except for the P waves on the premature beats; P-P interval irregular. **PR:** 0.14 on the sinus beats, 0.06 on the premature beats. **QRS:** 0.14. **Interpretation:** sinus rhythm with PACs.

21. **QRS complexes:** present, all shaped the same. **Regularity:** regular but interrupted (by a pause). **Heart rate:** 50 to 75, mean rate 70. **P waves:** none; flutter waves present instead. **PR:** not applicable. **QRS:** 0.08. **Interpretation:** atrial flutter with 4:1 and 6:1 conduction.

22. **QRS complexes:** present, all shaped the same. **Regularity:** irregular. **Heart rate:** 40 to 115, mean rate 80. **P waves:** none; fibrillatory waves present instead. **PR:** not applicable. **QRS:** 0.08–0.10. **Interpretation:** atrial fibrillation.

23. **QRS complexes:** present, shape varies; some are smaller than others. **Regularity:** irregular. **Heart rate:** 167 to 250, mean rate 210. **P waves:** none; fibrillatory waves present instead. **PR:** not applicable. **QRS:** 0.14. **Interpretation:** atrial fibrillation.

24. **QRS complexes:** present, shape varies. **Regularity:** regular but interrupted (by premature beats). **Heart rate:** 94. **P waves:** upright, shape varies. **PR:** 0.10–0.12. **QRS:** 0.12. **Interpretation:** sinus rhythm with two PACs. See the dots?

Beneath them are PACs. Notice those beats pop in early and their P wave is shaped differently from the sinus beats that surround them. The QRS shapes vary a bit also—not sure of the significance there.

25. **QRS complexes:** present, all shaped the same. **Regularity:** irregular. **Heart rate:** 45 to 94, mean rate 70. **P waves:** none; fibrillatory waves present instead. **PR:** not applicable. **QRS:** 0.10–0.12. **Interpretation:** atrial fibrillation with a wide QRS. Note the bottom half of the strip is not a rhythm—it's a printout of the patient's oxygen saturation wave as read through a sensor on the finger. So ignore this part of the strip when analyzing the rhythm.

## Practice Quiz

1. The complication of atrial fibrillation that can be prevented by the use of anticoagulants is **blood clots.**
2. The rhythm that is the same as wandering atrial pacemaker except for the heart rate is **multifocal atrial tachycardia.**
3. The rhythm that produces V-shaped waves between QRS complexes is **atrial flutter.**
4. Atrial rhythms take **the normal conduction pathway to the ventricles after depolarizing the atria.**
5. All rhythms that originate in a pacemaker other than the sinus node are called **ectopic rhythms.**
6. Treatment for atrial fibrillation is dependent **on its duration—specifically whether or not the atrial fibrillation has lasted longer than 48 hours.**
7. **False.** Some PACs are nonconducted.
8. The classic cause of multifocal atrial tachycardia is **chronic lung disease.**
9. The test that can determine the presence of atrial blood clots in an emergency is **transesophageal echocardiogram.**
10. If the rhythm is regular, heart rate is 130 or greater, and P waves cannot be identified, the rhythm is called **SVT.**

## Critical Thinking Exercises

1. The rhythm is **atrial fibrillation.** Heart rate varies from a **low of 71 to a high of 166. Mean rate is 110.** Note the rhythm is very irregular with a wavy baseline and no P waves between QRS complexes.
2. Mr. Baldo is relatively asymptomatic, with stable vital signs. He does feel intermittent

palpitations but this is not unusual. **This is NOT an emergency.**

3. **Coumadin** (or **Heparin**), an anticoagulant, is not needed in this situation, because the duration of atrial fibrillation is less than 48 hours.

4. Appropriate treatment could include **beta-blockers, calcium channel blockers, amiodarone,** or **digitalis. Electrical cardioversion** could also be performed, but this is usually reserved for emergencies or for patients in whom medications have not been successful.

5. This rhythm strip catches Mr. Baldo converting from **atrial fibrillation to sinus rhythm.**

6. The rhythm on discharge is **sinus rhythm.**

## CHAPTER NINE
## Practice Strips: Junctional Rhythms

Note: For the intervals, it is acceptable if your answer is within 0.02 secs of displayed answer.

1. **QRS complexes:** present, all shaped the same. **Regularity:** regular. **Heart rate:** 94. **P waves:** none visible. **PR:** not applicable. **QRS:** 0.08. **Interpretation:** accelerated junctional rhythm.

2. **QRS complexes:** present, all shaped the same. **Regularity:** regular but interrupted. **Heart rate:** 100. **P waves:** matching and upright on all except the sixth beat. That beat has no visible P wave at all. P-P interval is regular except for that sixth beat, which is premature. **PR:** 0.14. **QRS:** 0.08. **Interpretation:** sinus rhythm with a PJC.

3. **QRS complexes:** present, all shaped the same. **Regularity:** regular. **Heart rate:** 48. **P waves:** none visible. **PR:** not applicable. **QRS:** 0.08. **Interpretation:** junctional rhythm.

4. **QRS complexes:** present, all shaped the same. **Regularity:** regular but interrupted. **Heart rate:** 47. **P waves:** matching upright Ps present except on the third beat, which has an inverted P wave preceding the QRS. **PR:** 0.16 on the beats with upright Ps; 0.06 on the third beat. **QRS:** 0.08. **Interpretation:** sinus bradycardia with a PJC. Remember, it is normal for the R-R cycle immediately following a premature beat to be a little longer than usual. Consider this when determining the regularity.

5. **QRS complexes:** present, all shaped the same. **Regularity:** regular. **Heart rate:** 28. **P waves:** inverted following the QRS complexes. **PR:** not applicable. **QRS:** 0.08. **Interpretation:** junctional bradycardia.

6. **QRS complexes:** present, all shaped the same. **Regularity:** regular. **Heart rate:** 75. **P waves:** none visible. **PR:** not applicable. **QRS:** 0.08. **Interpretation:** accelerated junctional rhythm.

7. **QRS complexes:** present, all shaped the same. **Regularity:** regular. **Heart rate:** 72. **P waves:** none visible. **PR:** not applicable. **QRS:** 0.10. **Interpretation:** accelerated junctional rhythm.

8. **QRS complexes:** present, all shaped the same. **Regularity:** regular. **Heart rate:** 38. **P waves:** none visible. **PR:** not applicable. **QRS:** 0.10. **Interpretation:** junctional bradycardia.

9. **QRS complexes:** present, all shaped the same. **Regularity:** regular. **Heart rate:** 100. **P waves:** inverted preceding each QRS. **PR:** 0.10–0.12. **QRS:** 0.08. **Interpretation:** accelerated junctional rhythm.

10. **QRS complexes:** present, all shaped the same. **Regularity:** regular. **Heart rate:** 150. **P waves:** none visible. **PR:** not applicable. **QRS:** 0.08. **Interpretation:** SVT. Although this could indeed be a junctional tachycardia, it is best to call it SVT because P waves cannot be seen. Had there been an inverted P wave present, we'd have known for sure the rhythm was junctional in origin. Without those P waves, we can't be sure the rhythm is junctional. It could be atrial or even sinus in origin (with the P waves hidden inside the T waves).

11. **QRS complexes:** present, all shaped the same. **Regularity:** regular. **Heart rate:** 60. **P waves:** none visible. **PR:** not applicable. **QRS:** 0.08. **Interpretation:** junctional rhythm.

12. **QRS complexes:** present, all shaped the same. **Regularity:** regular. **Heart rate:** 26. **P waves:** none visible. **PR:** not applicable. **QRS:** 0.06–0.08. **Interpretation:** junctional bradycardia. This is an extremely slow junctional bradycardia. This patient is probably either in cardiac arrest or soon will be.

13. **QRS complexes:** present, all shaped the same. **Regularity:** regular. **Heart rate:** 115 to 125. **P waves:** none visible. **PR:** not applicable. **QRS:** 0.08. **Interpretation:** junctional tachycardia.

14. **QRS complexes:** present, all shaped the same. **Regularity:** regular but interrupted (by a premature beat). The third beat is early. **Heart rate:** 48. **P waves:** upright and matching on all but the premature beat. That beat has no P wave. **PR:** 0.16. **QRS:** 0.10. **Interpretation:** sinus bradycardia with one PJC.

15. **QRS complexes:** present, all shaped the same. **Regularity:** regular. **Heart rate:** 88. **P waves:** none visible. **PR:** not applicable. **QRS:** 0.08. **Interpretation:** accelerated junctional rhythm.

## Practice Quiz

1. The three possible locations for the P waves in junctional rhythms are **before the QRS complex, after the QRS complex,** and **hidden inside the QRS complex.**
2. The P wave is inverted in junctional rhythms because **the impulse travels in a backward direction to reach the atria.**
3. A junctional rhythm with a heart rate greater than 100 is **junctional tachycardia.**
4. **False.** PJCs do not imply that a lethal arrhythmia is imminent.
5. A junctional rhythm with a heart rate less than 40 is **junctional bradycardia.**
6. Treatment for junctional bradycardia could consist of the following: **atropine, epinephrine or dopamine infusion if the patient is symptomatic, oxygen, discontinuing or decreasing the dosage of any medications that could slow the heart rate down, and a pacemaker.**
7. PJCs cause the regularity to be **regular but interrupted.**
8. Junctional bradycardia is usually the result of **escape.**
9. Junctional tachycardia is best called SVT if the P waves are **hidden inside the QRS.**
10. Junctional tachycardia is the result of **usurpation.**

## Critical Thinking Exercises

1. The medication used to speed up the heart rate is **atropine.** That's what Mrs. Dubos would have been given.
2. The rhythm is **junctional bradycardia with a heart rate of 37.**
3. **The ER nurse was incorrect** in her assertion that the rhythm was sinus bradycardia. Recall all rhythms from the sinus node have matching upright P waves. Because this rhythm has no P waves at all, it cannot be sinus. Additionally, the heart rate is slower than the ER nurse reported.
4. The treatment in the ER would have been **atropine** and/or a **pacemaker,** which would have been appropriate for any slow rhythm that produced symptoms. So even though the nurse identified the rhythm incorrectly, the treatment was still correct.
5. Mrs. Dubos **complained of chest pain and shortness of breath, both of which can imply decreased cardiac output.** If the heart rate is too slow, the myocardium is deprived of oxygen and chest pain can result. Shortness of breath is a result of the slow heart rate's inability to transport

adequate oxygen throughout the body. The low blood pressure, rapid respiratory rate, and the dazed and confused demeanor are also signs of decreased cardiac output.

## CHAPTER TEN
## Practice Strips: Ventricular Rhythms

Note: For the intervals, it is acceptable if your answer is within 0.02 secs of displayed answer.

1. **QRS complexes:** present, both shaped the same—very wide and bizarre. **Regularity:** cannot tell as only two QRS complexes are shown. **Heart rate:** 14. **P waves:** not present. **PR:** not applicable. **QRS:** 0.38. **Interpretation:** agonal rhythm.
2. **QRS complexes:** present, varying in shapes and sizes. **Regularity:** irregular. **Heart rate:** 375 to 500. **P waves:** absent. **PR:** not applicable. **QRS:** varies—some QRS intervals are not measurable; others are 0.12. **Interpretation:** torsades de pointes.
3. **QRS complexes:** present, all but the third QRS shaped the same. The third QRS is wider. **Regularity:** regular but interrupted (by a premature beat). **Heart rate:** 115. **P waves:** matching and upright on all beats except the third, which has no P wave. **PR:** 0.12 on the sinus beats. **QRS:** 0.10 on the sinus beats; 0.16 on the premature beat. **Interpretation:** sinus tachycardia with one PVC.
4. **QRS complexes:** present, wide, all shaped the same; spike noted preceding each QRS complex. **Regularity:** regular. **Heart rate:** 40. **P waves:** none noted. **PR:** not applicable. **QRS:** 0.16. **Interpretation:** ventricular pacing.
5. **QRS complexes:** absent. **Regularity:** not applicable. **Heart rate:** zero. **P waves:** upright, matching, atrial rate 26. **PR:** not applicable. **QRS:** not applicable. **Interpretation:** P wave asystole.
6. **QRS complexes:** absent; wavy baseline present instead. **Regularity:** not applicable. **Heart rate:** not measurable. **P waves:** absent. **PR:** not applicable. **QRS:** not applicable. **Interpretation:** ventricular fibrillation.
7. **QRS complexes:** present, two different shapes—some narrow, others wide and bizarre. **Regularity:** regular but interrupted (by a run of premature beats). **Heart rate:** 107 while in the narrow-QRS rhythm; 187 when in the wide-QRS rhythm. **P waves:** upright and matching on the narrow beats; none noted on the wide beats. **PR:** 0.12 on the narrow beats; not applicable on the wide beats. **QRS:** 0.06 on the narrow beats; 0.12 on the wide

beats. **Interpretation:** sinus tachycardia with an 11-beat run of ventricular tachycardia.

8. **QRS complexes:** present, all shaped the same—extremely wide and bizarre. **Regularity:** regular. **Heart rate:** 28. **P waves:** absent. **PR:** not applicable. **QRS:** 0.28. **Interpretation:** idioventricular rhythm.

9. **QRS complexes:** present, every third beat wider than the rest. **Regularity:** regular but interrupted (by premature beats). **Heart rate:** 94. **P waves:** matching and upright on all narrow beats. P waves are noted in the T waves of the wide beats. **PR:** 0.16. **QRS:** 0.06 on the narrow beats; 0.14 on the wide beats. **Interpretation:** sinus rhythm with PVCs in trigeminy.

10. **QRS complexes:** present, all shaped the same—wide QRS complexes. **Regularity:** irregular. **Heart rate:** 16 to 47, with a mean rate of 30. **P waves:** none noted. **PR:** not applicable. **QRS:** 0.28. **Interpretation:** agonal rhythm. Although in places this rate exceeds 20, the very irregular nature of it points to agonal rhythm rather than idioventricular rhythm.

11. **QRS complexes:** none seen—just a coarse zigzag baseline. **Regularity:** not applicable. **Heart rate:** not measurable. **P waves:** absent. **PR:** not applicable. **QRS:** not applicable. **Interpretation:** ventricular fibrillation. (But there could be an argument for torsades de pointes. The rhythm does appear to oscillate toward the middle. It would be helpful to have a longer strip for a better look at the rhythm.)

12. **QRS complexes:** present, all but two shaped the same. Two are wider than the others. **Regularity:** regular but interrupted (by premature beats). **Heart rate:** 88. **P waves:** upright and matching on the narrow-QRS beats; no P wave preceding the wide-QRS beats. **PR:** 0.20. **QRS:** 0.06 on the narrow-QRS beats; 0.16 on the wide-QRS beats. **Interpretation:** sinus rhythm with two PVCs.

13. **QRS complexes:** present, all shaped the same—very wide with a preceding spike. **Regularity:** regular. **Heart rate:** 115. **P waves:** one present—noted on the downstroke of the second T wave on the strip. **PR:** not applicable. **QRS:** 0.16. **Interpretation:** ventricular pacing.

14. **QRS complexes:** present, all shaped the same—very wide and bizarre. **Regularity:** regular. **Heart rate:** 136. **P waves:** not present. **PR:** not applicable. **QRS:** 0.28. **Interpretation:** ventricular tachycardia. Note the unusually wide QRS complexes—this is often a sign that the patient's blood potassium level is extremely high, a condition seen most often in renal failure.

15. **QRS complexes:** only one present—very wide and bizarre. **Regularity:** not applicable as only one QRS complex is shown. **Heart rate:** zero after that one beat. **P waves:** not present. **PR:** not applicable. **QRS:** 0.20. **Interpretation:** agonal rhythm, then asystole.

16. **QRS complexes:** only one present. **Regularity:** not applicable as only one QRS complex is shown. **Heart rate:** zero after that one beat. **P waves:** upright, matching, one preceding the QRS complex and then continuing on; P-P interval irregular. **PR:** 0.24 on the one beat with a QRS. **QRS:** 0.08. **Interpretation:** one beat, then P wave asystole.

17. **QRS complexes:** present, all shaped the same—very wide and bizarre. **Regularity:** regular. **Heart rate:** 150. **P waves:** not present. **PR:** not applicable. **QRS:** 0.20. If you measured a bit wider than that, rest assured it is often difficult to measure QRS complexes when they merge into the T wave so well—hard to tell where the QRS ends and the T wave begins. **Interpretation:** ventricular tachycardia.

18. **QRS complexes:** present, all shaped the same—wide and preceded by a spike. **Regularity:** regular. **Heart rate:** 68. **P waves:** upright, matching; one preceding each QRS spike; P-P interval regular. **PR:** 0.20. **QRS:** 0.12. **Interpretation:** ventricular pacing.

19. **QRS complexes:** present, all but two shaped the same—two are wide and bizarre. **Regularity:** regular but interrupted (by premature beats). **Heart rate:** 94. **P waves:** upright and matching preceding the narrow-QRS beats; none preceding the wide-QRS beats. **PR:** 0.16. **QRS:** 0.06 on the narrow beats; 0.12 on the wide beats. **Interpretation:** sinus rhythm with two PVCs.

20. **QRS complexes:** very wide and bizarre. **Regularity:** not applicable as only one QRS complex is shown. **Heart rate:** zero after that one beat. **P waves:** not present. **PR:** not applicable. **QRS:** 0.16. **Interpretation:** agonal rhythm.

21. **QRS complexes:** very wide and bizarre. **Regularity:** regular. **Heart rate:** 20. **P waves:** not present. **PR:** not applicable. **QRS:** 0.20. **Interpretation:** idioventricular rhythm.

22. **QRS complexes:** none present; baseline looks like static. **Regularity:** not applicable. **Heart rate:** not measureable. **P waves:** not present. **PR:** not applicable. **QRS:** not applicable. **Interpretation:** coarse ventricular fibrillation.

23. **QRS complexes:** present, uniform shape. **Regularity:** regular. **Heart rate:** 75. **P waves:** present; pacemaker spike preceding P waves. **PR:** 0.28 (called the *AV interval* here—measure from the pacer spike to the QRS). **QRS:** 0.08. **Interpretation:** atrial pacing.

24. **QRS complexes:** present—very wide and bizarre. **Regularity:** regular. **Heart rate:** 107. **P waves:** not present. **PR:** not applicable. **QRS:** 0.20. **Interpretation:** ventricular tachycardia.

25. **QRS complexes:** present—very wide and bizarre, uniform shape. **Regularity:** regular. **Heart rate:** 88. **P waves:** not present. **PR:** not applicable. **QRS:** 0.16. **Interpretation:** accelerated idioventricular rhythm.

## Practice Quiz

1. The three main causes of PVCs are **heart disease, hypokalemia,** and **hypoxia.**

2. The rhythm that has no QRS complexes, but instead has a wavy, static-looking baseline is **ventricular fibrillation.**

3. Appropriate treatment for PVCs interrupting a sinus bradycardia with a heart rate of 32 would be **atropine** or **epinephrine** to increase the heart rate. Do not give amiodarone or lidocaine!

4. *Torsades de pointes* is a French term meaning **twisting of the points.**

5. Asystole differs from P wave asystole in that **asystole is flat line** and **P wave asystole still has P waves.**

6. For a patient with a ventricular rhythm with a heart rate of 39 and no pulse, the treatment would be **CPR, epinephrine, and oxygen.**

7. **False.** Asystole is *not* treated with electric shock to the heart. Electric shock's goal is to recoordinate the heart's electrical activity. In asystole, there is no electrical activity to coordinate.

8. The treatment of choice for ventricular fibrillation is **defibrillation.**

9. **True.** Pacemakers can pace the atrium, the ventricle, or both.

10. **False.** Antiarrhythmics should *not* be used to treat agonal rhythm. Those medications would suppress the only pacemaker this person has left—the ventricle—and would likely be fatal. Try atropine or epinephrine instead to speed up the heart rate. A pacemaker is usually not indicated for agonal rhythm, because it is likely that this is a terminal event, but it can be used at the physician's discretion.

## Critical Thinking Exercises

1. The rhythm is **sinus rhythm with PVCs in trigeminy and quadrigeminy.**

2. **No, this rhythm does not require emergency treatment.** The patient is stable.

3. Three causes of PVCs **are hypoxia, hypokalemia, and MI.**

4. **This is ventricular fibrillation.**

5. **Yes, this is an emergency.** Patients in V-fib have no pulse and no breathing.

6. **Mr. Winston needs immediate defibrillation. Medications such as amiodarone or lidocaine can also be given to make defibrillation more successful, but they will not convert this lethal rhythm back to normal on their own. The treatment for V-fib is to defib!**

## CHAPTER ELEVEN
## Practice Strips: AV Blocks

Note: For the intervals, it is acceptable if your answer is within 0.02 secs of displayed answer.

1. **QRS complexes:** present, all shaped the same. **Regularity:** regular but interrupted (by a pause). **Heart rate:** 31 to 68, with a mean rate of 50. **P waves:** biphasic, matching; more than one per QRS at times; P-P interval is regular; atrial rate is 62. **PR:** varies. **QRS:** 0.08. **Interpretation:** Wenckebach. Look at the P directly preceding the second QRS complex. The PR interval there is 0.24. The PR preceding the last QRS on the strip is 0.28. The PR interval prolongs and there are blocked P waves. The rhythm starts out as 2:1 AV block and then becomes an obvious Wenckebach. The 2:1 AV block here is, therefore, also Wenckebach.

2. **QRS complexes:** present, all shaped the same. **Regularity:** regular. **Heart rate:** 88. **P waves:** upright, matching; one to each QRS complex; atrial rate is 88; P-P interval is regular. **PR:** 0.24. **QRS:** 0.10. **Interpretation:** sinus rhythm with first-degree AV block.

3. **QRS complexes:** present, all shaped the same. **Regularity:** regular. **Heart rate:** 83. **P waves:** upright, matching; one to each QRS; P-P interval is regular; atrial rate is 83. **PR:** 0.24. **QRS:** 0.10. **Interpretation:** sinus rhythm with first-degree AV block.

4. **QRS complexes:** present, all shaped the same. **Regularity:** regular. **Heart rate:** 33. **P waves:** upright, matching; three to each QRS; P-P interval

is regular; atrial rate is 100. **PR:** 0.16. **QRS:** 0.08. **Interpretation:** Mobitz II second-degree AV block. The block here is probably at the AV node, as evidenced by the narrow QRS. This is a kind of **high-grade AV block,** a block in which more than half the P waves are not conducted.

5. **QRS complexes:** present, all shaped the same. **Regularity:** regular. **Heart rate:** 30. **P waves:** upright, matching; more than one per QRS; P-P interval is regular; atrial rate is 75. **PR:** varies. **QRS:** 0.08. **Interpretation:** third-degree AV block and a junctional escape rhythm. We know the junction is the pacemaker controlling the ventricles because the QRS interval is <0.12.

6. **QRS complexes:** present, all shaped the same. **Regularity:** regular. **Heart rate:** 37. **P waves:** upright, matching; two per QRS; P-P interval is regular; atrial rate is 75. **PR:** 0.36. **QRS:** 0.08. **Interpretation:** 2:1 AV block (probably Wenckebach, because the QRS is narrow and there is a prolonged PR interval).

7. **QRS complexes:** present, all shaped the same. **Regularity:** irregular. **Heart rate:** 37 to 68. **P waves:** upright, matching; one to each QRS except for the fifth QRS, which has two P waves preceding it; P-P interval is regular; atrial rate is 60. **PR:** varies—prolongs progressively. **QRS:** 0.08. **Interpretation:** Wenckebach.

8. **QRS complexes:** present, all shaped the same. **Regularity:** irregular. **Heart rate:** 25 to 75, with a mean rate of 40. **P waves:** matching, upright; one for the first two QRS complexes, then three per QRS; P-P interval is regular; atrial rate is 75. **PR:** 0.16. **QRS:** 0.16. **Interpretation:** Mobitz II second-degree AV block.

9. **QRS complexes:** present, all shaped the same. **Regularity:** regular but interrupted (by a pause). **Heart rate:** 42 to 60, with a mean rate of 50. **P waves:** matching, upright; one preceding each QRS except the fourth QRS, which has two P waves preceding it (there's a P in the T wave of the third beat); P-P interval is *irregular;* atrial rate is 60 to 125. **PR:** 0.16. **QRS:** 0.10. **Interpretation:** sinus rhythm with a nonconducted PAC. Did you think this was an AV block? It's easy to mistake a nonconducted PAC for an AV block. How do you tell the difference? AV blocks have regular P-P intervals. Here the P-P is *not regular,* is it? One P is premature. That makes it a PAC. And because there is no QRS following it, that makes it a nonconducted PAC.

10. **QRS complexes:** present, all shaped the same. **Regularity:** regular but interrupted (by pauses).

**Heart rate:** 42 to 68, with a mean rate of 50. **P waves:** upright, matching; more than one per QRS at times; P-P interval is regular; atrial rate is 75. **PR:** varies. **QRS:** 0.08. **Interpretation:** Wenckebach.

11. **QRS complexes:** present, all shaped the same within each lead. **Regularity:** regular but interrupted (by a pause). **Heart rate:** 48 to 79, with a mean rate of 70. **P waves:** upright, matching; more than one per QRS at times; P-P interval is regular; atrial rate is 88. **PR:** varies. **QRS:** 0.12. **Interpretation:** Wenckebach. Look at the P wave directly preceding the first QRS complex. The PR interval there is 0.22. The PR preceding the sixth QRS (the last QRS before the pause) is 0.32. The PR interval prolongs until a P wave is blocked. This is typical of Wenckebach.

12. **QRS complexes:** present, all shaped the same within each lead. **Regularity:** regular. **Heart rate:** 68. **P waves:** upright, matching; one per QRS; P-P interval is regular. **PR:** 0.24. **QRS:** 0.08. **Interpretation:** sinus rhythm with first-degree AV block.

13. **QRS complexes:** present, all shaped the same within each lead. **Regularity:** regular but interrupted (by a pause). **Heart rate:** 38 to 68, with a mean rate of 60. **P waves:** upright, matching; more than one per QRS at times; P-P interval is regular; atrial rate is 75. **PR:** varies. **QRS:** 0.08. **Interpretation:** Wenckebach. Look at the first PR interval on the strip—it is 0.24. The PR preceding the fourth QRS is 0.36. The PR interval prolongs and there is a blocked P wave—classic Wenckebach.

14. **QRS complexes:** present, all shaped the same within each lead. **Regularity:** regular. **Heart rate:** 38. **P waves:** upright in top strip, biphasic in bottom, matching; two P waves per QRS (except first QRS has only one because the start of the strip cut off the other P wave); P-P interval is regular; atrial rate is 79. **PR:** 0.28. **QRS:** 0.12. **Interpretation:** 2:1 AV block.

15. **QRS complexes:** present, all shaped the same within each lead. **Regularity:** irregular. **Heart rate:** 30 to 37, with a mean rate of 40. **P waves:** biphasic, matching; one per QRS; P-P interval is irregular. **PR:** 0.28. **QRS:** 0.13. **Interpretation:** sinus arrhythmia with first degree AV block.

16. **QRS complexes:** present, all shaped the same within each lead. **Regularity:** regular. **Heart rate:** 37. **P waves:** upright, matching; two per QRS; P-P interval is regular; atrial rate is 75. **PR:** varies. **QRS:** 0.09. **Interpretation:** third-degree

AV block. This is not 2:1 AV block because the PR intervals are not constant here, as they should be for 2:1 AV block. Notice the first PR interval on the strip is 0.20 and the last one is 0.06, with the P wave "crawling up onto" the QRS complex.

17. **QRS complexes:** present, all shaped the same within each lead. **Regularity:** regular. **Heart rate:** 41. **P waves:** upright in top strip, biphasic in bottom; matching; more than one per QRS; P-P interval is regular; atrial rate is 79. **PR:** varies. **QRS:** 0.08. **Interpretation:** third-degree AV block with junctional escape rhythm.

18. **QRS complexes:** present, all shaped the same within each lead. **Regularity:** regular but interrupted (by a pause). **Heart rate:** 37 to 75, with a mean rate of 60. **P waves:** upright, matching; more than one per QRS at times; P-P interval is regular; atrial rate is 75. **PR:** varies. **QRS:** 0.10. **Interpretation:** Wenckebach. Note the first PR interval on the strip is shorter than the second and third, then there is a blocked P wave. After the pause, the PR is short again, but lengthens by the next beat.

19. **QRS complexes:** present, all shaped the same within each lead. **Regularity:** regular but interrupted (by a premature beat). **Heart rate:** 81. **P waves:** upright, all but the fifth matching (the fifth is a premature P wave of a different shape); P-P interval is irregular. **PR:** 0.28. **QRS:** 0.08. **Interpretation:** sinus rhythm with a PAC (the fifth QRS is premature) and first-degree AV block.

20. **QRS complexes:** present, all shaped the same within each lead. **Regularity:** regular but interrupted (by a pause). **Heart rate:** 36 to 75, with a mean rate of 60. **P waves:** upright, matching; more than one per QRS at times; P-P interval is regular; atrial rate is 75. **PR:** varies. **QRS:** 0.10. **Interpretation:** Wenckebach. The PR intervals prolong until a P wave is blocked.

21. **QRS complexes:** present, all shaped the same within each lead. **Regularity:** regular. **Heart rate:** 42. **P waves:** upright, matching; two per QRS; P-P interval is regular; atrial rate is 83. **PR:** 0.24. **QRS:** 0.08. **Interpretation:** 2:1 AV block. Note there are two P waves to each QRS—right after the T wave and right before the QRS.

22. **QRS complexes:** present, all shaped the same within each lead. **Regularity:** regular. **Heart rate:** 60. **P waves:** upright, matching; one per QRS; P-P interval is regular; atrial rate is 60. **PR:** 0.32. **QRS:** 0.08–0.10. **Interpretation:** sinus rhythm with first-degree AV block.

23. **QRS complexes:** present, all shaped the same within each lead. **Regularity:** regular. **Heart rate:** 25. **P waves:** upright, matching; more than one per QRS; P-P interval is regular; atrial rate is 60. **PR:** varies. **QRS:** 0.16. **Interpretation:** third-degree AV block with a ventricular escape rhythm.

24. **QRS complexes:** present, all shaped the same within each lead. **Regularity:** regular. **Heart rate:** 68. **P waves:** upright, matching; one per QRS; P-P interval is regular; atrial rate is 68. **PR:** 0.26. **QRS:** 0.16. **Interpretation:** sinus rhythm with first-degree AV block.

25. **QRS complexes:** present, all shaped the same within each lead. **Regularity:** regular. **Heart rate:** 45. **P waves:** upright, matching; more than one per QRS; P-P interval is regular; atrial rate is about 68. **PR:** varies. **QRS:** 0.12. **Interpretation:** third-degree AV block. The QRS interval is right at 0.12 seconds, so it could be either a junctional or a ventricular escape pacemaker providing the QRS. With a heart rate of 45, it's probably the junction.

## Practice Quiz

1. The two typical locations for the block in AV blocks are the **AV node** and the **bundle branches.**
2. **False.** First-degree AV block causes no symptoms and does not require pacemaker insertion.
3. Wenckebach is another name for **Mobitz I second-degree AV block.**
4. AV dissociation is a hallmark of **third-degree AV block.**
5. **False.** Atropine has no effect on blocks at the bundle branches.
6. The AV block that merely results in a prolonged PR interval is **first-degree AV block.**
7. Atropine's mode of action is **to speed up the sinus node's rate of firing and to accelerate conduction through the AV node.**
8. The most dangerous type of AV block is **third-degree AV block.**
9. The least dangerous type of AV block is **first-degree AV block.**
10. **False.** First-degree AV blocks do not require atropine or epinephrine.

## Critical Thinking Exercises

1. The rhythm is **sinus rhythm with first-degree AV block** (PR interval 0.24), heart rate 68.
2. **No, this is not an emergency.** First-degree AV block does not cause symptoms, and the underlying rhythm is sinus, which is normal.

3. The rhythm has changed to **Wenckebach.**
4. Both **digoxin** and **beta-blockers** can cause decreased conduction through the AV node, resulting in AV blocks. Insulin is not a likely cause of this rhythm.
5. Treatment should include **withholding digoxin until her level returns to normal, teaching her not to take extra medication without approval from her physician, and perhaps giving atropine if her heart rate slows enough to cause her symptoms.** The "funny" spell in the physician's office could have reflected a slower heart rate, which might have been missed by the time the second rhythm strip was obtained. Atropine should be close by in case Ms. Watson needs it.

## CHAPTER TWELVE
## Rhythms for Practice

Note: For the intervals, it is acceptable if your answer is within 0.02 secs of displayed answer.

1. **QRS complexes:** present, all shaped the same. **Regularity:** regular. **Heart rate:** 68. **P waves:** matching, upright; one preceding each QRS; P-P interval regular. **PR interval:** 0.42. **QRS interval:** 0.16. **Interpretation:** sinus rhythm with first-degree AV block and a wide QRS.
2. **QRS complexes:** present, all shaped the same. **Regularity:** regular. **Heart rate:** 37. **P waves:** none seen. **PR interval:** not applicable. **QRS interval:** 0.12. **Interpretation:** junctional bradycardia with wide QRS.
3. **QRS complexes:** present, all shaped the same. **Regularity:** regular. **Heart rate:** 71. **P waves:** matching, upright; one preceding each QRS; P-P interval regular. **PR interval:** 0.24. **QRS interval:** 0.12. **Interpretation:** sinus rhythm with first-degree AV block and wide QRS.
4. **QRS complexes:** present, all shaped the same. **Regularity:** regular. **Heart rate:** 125. **P waves:** an occasional dissociated P can be seen. **PR interval:** cannot measure. **QRS interval:** 0.22. **Interpretation:** ventricular tachycardia.
5. **QRS complexes:** present, all shaped the same. **Regularity:** irregular. **Heart rate:** 65 to 94, with a mean rate of 80. **P waves:** none present; wavy, undulating baseline is present. **PR interval:** not applicable. **QRS interval:** 0.06. **Interpretation:** atrial fibrillation.
6. **QRS complexes:** Present, all shaped the same, low voltage. **Regularity:** regular. **Heart rate:** 125. **P waves:** matching, upright; one preceding each QRS, low voltage; P-P interval regular. **PR interval:** 0.16. **QRS interval:** 0.06. **Interpretation:** sinus tachycardia.
7. **QRS complexes:** present, all shaped the same. **Regularity:** regular. **Heart rate:** 32. **P waves:** upright, matching, some nonconducted; P-P interval regular; atrial rate 125. **PR interval:** varies. **QRS interval:** 0.13. **Interpretation:** third-degree AV block and a ventricular escape rhythm.
8. **QRS complexes:** present, all shaped the same. **Regularity:** regular. **Heart rate:** 150. **P waves:** none present; regular sawtooth-shaped waves between QRS complexes present instead, two to each QRS; atrial rate about 300. **PR interval:** not applicable. **QRS interval:** 0.06. **Interpretation:** atrial flutter with 2:1 conduction. Did you think it was something else? Look at the tail end of the QRS complex. See how it looks rounded at the bottom? That rounded part looks a lot like the other rounded wave that follows it, doesn't it? Those are both flutter waves. You'll notice these flutter waves march out—they're all the same distance from one another. Always be very suspicious when the heart rate is 150—it may be atrial flutter with 2:1 conduction.
9. **QRS complexes:** present, all shaped the same. **Regularity:** regular but interrupted (by two pauses). **Heart rate:** 44 to 75, with a mean rate of 60. **P waves:** upright; one preceding each QRS; shape varies slightly, but not enough to be significant. Don't get too hyper about the P wave shapes. Slight variability can be caused by fine baseline artifact. Different P wave shapes will be much more obvious. If you have to agonize over whether the P waves are shaped the same or are different, they're probably not different enough to be significant in terms of rhythm interpretation. **PR interval:** 0.20–0.22. **QRS interval:** 0.08. **Interpretation:** sinus rhythm with two sinus pauses. Why is this not a sinus arrhythmia? Sinus arrhythmia is cyclic, with slow periods, then faster periods. And it's irregular. Here the rhythm is regular, with an R-R interval of about 20 small blocks, except during the pauses. Sinus arrhythmia would be more irregular across the strip. Pay close attention to the regularity and it should lead the way.
10. **QRS complexes:** present, all shaped the same. They look different, you say? Hold on—the explanation is coming soon. **Regularity:** irregular. **Heart rate:** 100 to 150, with a mean rate of 120. **P waves:** upright and matching on the first four beats, then changes to flutter waves after that. **PR interval:** 0.16 on the first four beats, not applicable

after that. **QRS interval:** 0.08. **Interpretation:** sinus tachycardia converting after four beats to atrial flutter with variable conduction. The QRS complexes in atrial flutter here are distorted by the flutter waves. That's why they look different.

11. **QRS complexes:** present, all shaped the same. **Regularity:** regular. **Heart rate:** 44. **P waves:** upright, matching, some nonconducted; P-P interval regular; atrial rate 150. **PR interval:** varies. **QRS interval:** 0.14. **Interpretation:** third-degree AV block and a ventricular escape rhythm.

12. **QRS complexes:** present, all shaped the same. **Regularity:** regular. **Heart rate:** 125. **P waves:** upright, matching; one preceding each QRS; P-P interval regular. **PR interval:** 0.16. **QRS interval:** 0.06. **Interpretation:** sinus tachycardia.

13. **QRS complexes:** present, all but three shaped the same. Three beats are wide and bizarre in shape. **Regularity:** regular but interrupted (by premature beats). **Heart rate:** 125. **P waves:** upright and matching on the narrow beats, absent on the wide beats. **PR interval:** 0.12. **QRS interval:** 0.08 on the narrow beats, 0.16 on the wide beats. **Interpretation:** sinus tachycardia with unifocal PVCs in quadrigeminy (every fourth beat is a PVC).

14. **QRS complexes:** present, all shaped the same. **Regularity:** regular. **Heart rate:** 137. **P waves:** none seen. **PR interval:** not applicable. **QRS interval:** 0.10. **Interpretation:** SVT.

15. **QRS complex:** present, all shaped the same, very low voltage. **Regularity:** regular. **Heart rate:** about 135. **P waves:** not discernible. **PR interval:** cannot measure. **QRS interval:** 0.08. **Interpretation:** SVT.

16. **QRS complex:** present, all shaped the same. **Regularity:** irregular. **Heart rate:** 56 to 71, with a mean rate of 70. **P waves:** upright, matching; one preceding each QRS; P-P interval irregular. **PR interval:** 0.12. **QRS interval:** 0.10. **Interpretation:** sinus arrhythmia. Note the longest R-R interval is between the last two QRS complexes on the strip, ending with the barely there QRS at the very end. That R-R interval is 27 small blocks. The shortest R-R is between the third and fourth QRS complexes. That R-R is 21 small blocks. Because the rhythm is irregular, the longest R-R exceeds the shortest by four or more small blocks, and this is definitely sinus in origin, it's a sinus arrhythmia. If you thought there was a sinus pause here, remember that sinus pause usually interrupts an otherwise regular rhythm. This rhythm is irregular.

17. **QRS complexes:** present, all shaped the same. **Regularity:** slightly irregular. R-R intervals vary from 22 to 25 small blocks. **Heart rate:** 60 to 68, with a mean rate of 60. **P waves:** upright, matching; one preceding each QRS. **PR interval:** 0.12. **QRS interval:** 0.10. **Interpretation:** sinus rhythm versus sinus arrhythmia. This one is a bit odd. It's really not irregular enough to call it a sinus arrhythmia, because the longest R-R interval does not exceed the shortest by four or more small blocks. On the other hand, it's a bit irregular for the typical sinus rhythm. Because we're in a gray area here, it's OK to call it one versus the other. It would be nice to have a longer rhythm strip to evaluate. If, on the longer strip, the rhythm is an obvious sinus rhythm or an obvious sinus arrhythmia, then this little stretch of the total rhythm is probably also that same rhythm.

18. **QRS complexes:** present, all shaped the same. **Regularity:** regular. **Heart rate:** 75. **P waves:** none seen. **PR interval:** not applicable. **QRS interval:** around 0.20 to 0.28. This is a guesstimate, because it's hard to tell where the QRS ends and the ST segment begins. **Interpretation:** accelerated idioventricular rhythm.

19. **QRS complexes:** present, all shaped the same. **Regularity:** regular. **Heart rate:** 167. **P waves:** occasionally seen hidden in the T waves. Note the T waves between the first and second and eleventh and twelfth QRS complexes. Those T waves reveal the hidden P waves. **PR interval:** cannot measure, as we cannot see the beginning of the P wave. **QRS interval:** 0.08. **Interpretation:** atrial tachycardia or SVT. It's probably more correct to call it atrial tachycardia, because the P waves are evident in places, but it's acceptable to say SVT.

20. **QRS complexes:** present, all shaped the same. **Regularity:** regular but interrupted (by premature beats). Remember it's normal to have a short pause following each premature beat. That's why this is not an irregular rhythm. **Heart rate:** about 85. Where did that heart rate come from? The first two beats on the strip are sinus beats with a rate of 85. From then on, every other beat is a PAC, so the heart rate cannot be determined accurately there. **P waves:** upright, two different shapes; almost every other P wave is premature and of a different shape. **PR interval:** 0.12 on the sinus beats, 0.16 on the premature beats. **QRS interval:** 0.08. **Interpretation:** sinus rhythm with frequent PACs, most of it in bigeminy.

21. **QRS complexes:** none present; wavy, static-looking baseline present instead. **Regularity:** not

applicable. **Heart rate:** cannot measure, has no QRS complexes. **P waves:** none. **PR interval:** not applicable. **QRS interval:** not applicable. **Interpretation:** ventricular fibrillation.

22. **QRS complexes:** present, two different shapes. Some QRS complexes are narrow; others are wide. **Regularity:** regular but interrupted (by premature beats). **Heart rate:** 94. **P waves:** upright and matching preceding the narrow QRS complexes and seen in the T wave following the premature beats. **PR interval:** 0.18 on the narrow beats; not calculated on the premature beats, as the P is retrograde. **QRS interval:** 0.08 on the narrow beats, 0.14 on the wide beats. **Interpretation:** sinus rhythm with unifocal PVCs in trigeminy.

23. **QRS complexes:** present, all shaped the same. **Regularity:** irregular. **Heart rate:** 48 to 81, with a mean rate of 60. **P waves:** upright, matching, some nonconducted; P-P interval regular. **PR interval:** varies. **QRS interval:** 0.11. **Interpretation:** Wenckebach. Note how the PR interval gradually prolongs, and then a beat is dropped.

24. **QRS complexes:** present, all shaped the same. **Regularity:** regular. **Heart rate:** 79. **P waves:** none present; regular sawtooth-shaped waves present instead. **PR interval:** not applicable. **QRS interval:** 0.08. **Interpretation:** atrial flutter with 4:1 conduction.

25. **QRS complexes:** present, all but one having the same shape. One is very wide compared to the others. **Regularity:** regular but interrupted (by a premature beat). **Heart rate:** 107. **P waves:** upright and matching on the narrow beats, absent on the wide beat. **PR interval:** 0.12–0.14. **QRS interval:** 0.08 on the narrow beats, 0.16 on the wide beat. **Interpretation:** sinus tachycardia with one PVC.

26. **QRS complexes:** none. **Regularity:** not applicable, as there are no QRS complexes. **Heart rate:** zero. **P waves:** none. **PR interval:** not applicable. **QRS interval:** not applicable. **Interpretation:** asystole.

27. **QRS complexes:** present, all shaped the same. **Regularity:** regular. **Heart rate:** 50. **P waves:** upright, matching; P-P interval regular; one P wave is hidden inside the last QRS; atrial rate 88. **PR interval:** varies. **QRS interval:** 0.14. **Interpretation:** third-degree AV block and a ventricular escape rhythm.

28. **QRS complexes:** present, all shaped the same. **Regularity:** regular. **Heart rate:** 79. **P waves:** matching, upright; one preceding each QRS; P-P interval regular. **PR interval:** 0.28. **QRS interval:** 0.08. **Interpretation:** sinus rhythm with first-degree AV block.

29. **QRS complexes:** present, all shaped the same. **Regularity:** regular. **Heart rate:** 68. **P waves:** none present; regular sawtooth-shaped waves present instead. **PR interval:** not applicable. **QRS interval:** about 0.10. The end of the QRS is distorted by a flutter wave, making the QRS look artificially wide. **Interpretation:** atrial flutter with 4:1 conduction. Two of the flutter waves are hidden inside the QRS and T waves. So how can we tell the flutter waves are even there if we can't see them? We can definitely see two obvious flutter waves between the QRS complexes. Because we know that flutter waves are regular, we simply note the distance between the two flutter waves we see together, and then march out where the rest of them should be.

30. **QRS complexes:** present, most shaped the same. An occasional QRS is missing the notch on the downstroke. **Regularity:** regular. **Heart rate:** 187. **P waves:** an occasional dissociated P wave is seen. **PR interval:** not applicable. **QRS interval:** 0.14. **Interpretation:** ventricular tachycardia.

31. **QRS complexes:** present, all shaped the same. **Regularity:** irregular. **Heart rate:** 50 to 63, with a mean rate of 60. You'll notice the mean heart rate is not a mathematical average of the high and low. It is merely a head count of the number of QRS complexes—and the mean is a multiple of 10. So if there are more QRS complexes closely spaced than there are narrowly spaced, the mean could actually be higher than the high heart rate. **P waves:** all upright, but there are at least three different shapes; P-P interval irregular. **PR interval:** 0.24–0.28. **QRS interval:** 0.10. **Interpretation:** wandering atrial pacemaker.

32. **QRS complexes:** present, all shaped the same. **Regularity:** regular but interrupted (by a premature beat). **Heart rate:** 71. **P waves:** none present; regular sawtooth-shaped waves present instead. **PR interval:** not applicable. **QRS interval:** 0.10. **Interpretation:** atrial flutter with 2:1 and 4:1 conduction. The one episode of the 2:1 conduction is responsible for the interruption of this otherwise regular 4:1 conduction. This beat that comes in early because of the conduction ratio change is not, per se, a premature beat in the way that PVCs are, but nevertheless it does arrive earlier than expected, given the surrounding R-R intervals. For this reason the regularity is called *regular but interrupted* rather than irregular. All R-R intervals except this short one are about the same.

33. **QRS complexes:** present, all shaped the same. **Regularity:** regular but interrupted (by pauses).

**Heart rate:** 62 to 107, with a mean rate of 90.
**P waves:** upright, matching; some nonconducted, others hidden inside T waves; P-P interval regular; atrial rate about 115. **PR interval:** varies. **QRS interval:** 0.08. **Interpretation:** Wenckebach.

34. **QRS complexes:** present, all shaped the same. **Regularity:** regular but interrupted (by premature beats). **Heart rate:** 79. **P waves:** biphasic except for the two that are inside the T wave. There are two different shapes of P waves; P-P interval varies. **PR interval:** 0.18 on the normal beats, approximately 0.22 on the premature beats. **QRS interval:** 0.08. **Interpretation:** sinus rhythm with two PACs.

35. **QRS complexes:** present, all shaped the same, one shorter than the rest. **Regularity:** regular but interrupted (by a pause). **Heart rate:** 19 to 54, with a mean rate of 50. **P waves:** upright, matching; none present on the beat ending the pause; P-P interval irregular. **PR interval:** 0.16–0.18. **QRS interval:** 0.09. **Interpretation:** sinus bradycardia with a 3.28-second sinus arrest ending with a junctional escape beat. Whenever there is a pause, the length of it must be recorded. If there is a sinus arrest, the beat ending the pause may be an escape beat from a lower pacemaker. Whichever pacemaker takes over should also be recorded.

36. **QRS complexes:** present, all shaped the same. **Regularity:** regular; the R-R intervals vary only by two small blocks. **Heart rate:** about 50. **P waves:** upright and matching; one preceding each QRS; P-P interval regular. **PR interval:** 0.20. **QRS interval:** 0.08. **Interpretation:** sinus bradycardia. A PR interval of 0.20 is still normal. There's no first-degree AV block.

37. **QRS complexes:** present, all shaped the same. **Regularity:** regular. **Heart rate:** 61. **P waves:** inverted inside ST segment following the QRS complexes. **PR interval:** not applicable. **QRS interval:** 0.12. **Interpretation:** accelerated junctional rhythm with a wide QRS.

38. **QRS complexes:** present, all shaped the same. **Regularity:** regular. **Heart rate:** 88. **P waves:** upright and matching; one preceding each QRS; P-P interval regular. **PR interval:** 0.24. **QRS interval:** 0.10. **Interpretation:** sinus rhythm with first-degree AV block.

39. **QRS complexes:** present, all shaped the same. **Regularity:** regular. The R-R intervals vary by only two small blocks. **Heart rate:** about 36. **P waves:** upright and matching; one preceding each QRS; P-P interval regular. **PR interval:** 0.16. **QRS interval:** 0.12. **Interpretation:** sinus bradycardia

with a wide QRS; there's a prominent U wave following the T waves.

40. **QRS complexes:** present, all shaped the same. **Regularity:** regular. **Heart rate:** 60. **P waves:** upright, notched, and matching; one preceding each QRS; P-P interval regular. **PR interval:** 0.16. **QRS interval:** 0.08. **Interpretation:** sinus rhythm.

41. **QRS complexes:** present, all shaped the same. **Regularity:** irregular. The R-R intervals vary from 11 to 15 small blocks. **Heart rate:** 100 to 137, with a mean rate of 120. **P waves:** none seen. **PR interval:** not applicable. **QRS interval:** 0.20. **Interpretation:** ventricular tachycardia. Remember V-tach is usually regular but can be irregular at times.

42. **QRS complexes:** present, all shaped the same. **Regularity:** irregular. **Heart rate:** 39 to 88, with a mean rate of 60. **P waves:** none present; wavy, undulating baseline present instead. **PR interval:** not applicable. **QRS interval:** 0.06. **Interpretation:** atrial fibrillation.

43. **QRS complexes:** present, all shaped the same. **Regularity:** regular. **Heart rate:** 115. **P waves:** upright and matching; one preceding each QRS; P-P interval regular. **PR interval:** 0.12. **QRS interval:** 0.10. **Interpretation:** sinus tachycardia.

44. **QRS complexes:** present, all shaped the same. **Regularity:** irregular. **Heart rate:** 83 to 167, with a mean rate of 140. **P waves:** none present; wavy, undulating baseline present instead. **PR interval:** not applicable. **QRS interval:** 0.04. **Interpretation:** atrial fibrillation.

45. **QRS complexes:** present, all shaped the same. **Regularity:** regular. **Heart rate:** about 52. **P waves:** upright, matching; one preceding each QRS. **PR interval:** 0.18. **QRS interval:** 0.13. **Interpretation:** sinus bradycardia with a wide QRS.

46. **QRS complexes:** present, all shaped the same. **Regularity:** regular. **Heart rate:** 28. **P waves:** upright, matching; some nonconducted; P-P interval regular; atrial rate 83. **PR interval:** 0.16. **QRS interval:** 0.06. **Interpretation:** Mobitz II second-degree AV block.

47. **QRS complexes:** present, all but one shaped the same. **Regularity:** regular. **Heart rate:** 26. **P waves:** matching, upright, some nonconducted; P-P interval regular; atrial rate 75. **PR interval:** varies. **QRS interval:** 0.04–0.08. **Interpretation:** third-degree AV block and a junctional escape rhythm. This heart rate is extremely slow for the junction. Remember, it normally escapes at a rate of 40 to 60. This patient not only has an AV block, but also

a sick AV node in terms of its pacemaking ability. Also of concern is the ventricle as a pacemaker. It normally escapes at a rate of 20 to 40. Where is it? Why didn't it kick in as the pacemaker at a faster rate than we have here? This rhythm indicates a very sick heart.

48. **QRS complexes:** present, all shaped the same. **Regularity:** regular. The R-R intervals vary by only two small blocks. **Heart rate:** 88. **P waves:** biphasic, matching; one preceding each QRS; P-P interval regular. **PR interval:** 0.12. **QRS interval:** 0.10. **Interpretation:** sinus rhythm.

49. **QRS complexes:** present, both shaped the same, although one is shorter than the other. **Regularity:** cannot assess as only two QRS complexes are present (at least three QRS complexes are needed to determine regularity). **Heart rate:** about 11. **P waves:** none present; wavy, undulating baseline present instead. **PR interval:** not applicable. **QRS interval:** 0.12. **Interpretation:** atrial fibrillation with a wide QRS. This could also be called atrial fib-flutter, as it does look quite fluttery in places. It is best not to call this an outright atrial flutter, though, as the waves dampen out in the middle of the strip, causing the waves to look different throughout the strip. This is a drastic representation of how slow the heart rate can go with atrial fibrillation. This is a 5.6-second pause, erroneously labeled on the strip as 5.52 seconds. This patient was lucky to be asleep and had no problems. A pause this long could easily have caused symptoms of decreased cardiac output.

50. **QRS complexes:** present, all shaped the same. **Regularity:** slightly irregular. The R-R intervals vary by three small blocks. **Heart rate:** 30 to 32. **P waves:** upright, three different shapes; one preceding each QRS; P-P interval slightly irregular. **PR interval:** 0.16–0.20. **QRS interval:** 0.10. **Interpretation:** wandering atrial pacemaker.

51. **QRS complexes:** present, all shaped the same. **Regularity:** regular. **Heart rate:** 94. **P waves:** matching, biphasic; two to each QRS; atrial rate 187. **PR interval:** 0.06. **QRS interval:** 0.08. **Interpretation:** atrial tachycardia with 2:1 block. One P wave is easy to see between the QRS complexes. The other is right *on* the QRS, distorting the shape of the QRS and the P a little. It wouldn't be correct to call this atrial flutter, because there is an obvious flat baseline between the P waves. You'll recall atrial flutter has no flat isoelectric line— flutter waves all zigzag one after the other.

52. **QRS complexes:** present, all shaped the same. **Regularity:** regular. **Heart rate:** 68. **P waves:** negative; one preceding each QRS; P-P interval regular. **PR interval:** 0.24. **QRS interval:** 0.20. **Interpretation:** sinus rhythm with first-degree AV block and a wide QRS. Although the lead is not recorded on this strip, it's probably $V_1$. Sinus rhythms can have a negative P wave in $V_1$. This is a very sick heart. The AV node is sick, as evidenced by the first-degree block, but also the bundle branches are sick, as evidenced by the width of the QRS complexes. Many cardiologists believe that to some extent a patient's ventricular function can be predicted by the QRS interval. This patient was predicted to have a low-functioning heart, and that was borne out by further studies.

53. **QRS complexes:** present, all shaped the same. **Regularity:** regular. **Heart rate:** about 103. **P waves:** upright, matching; one preceding each QRS. **PR interval:** 0.16. **QRS interval:** 0.08. **Interpretation:** sinus tachycardia.

54. **QRS complexes:** present, all shaped the same. **Regularity:** irregular. **Heart rate:** 29 to 83, with a mean rate of 50. **P waves:** none present; *very* low-voltage wavy, undulating baseline present instead. **PR interval:** not applicable. **QRS interval:** 0.08. **Interpretation:** atrial fibrillation. This is an example of what's sometimes called *straight-line* atrial fibrillation. There is barely a bobble of the baseline between QRS complexes. The most obvious feature that suggests atrial fibrillation is the irregularity of the rhythm. Then you notice the fine fibrillatory waves. This patient has probably been in atrial fibrillation for years.

55. **QRS complexes:** present, all shaped the same. **Regularity:** irregular. **Heart rate:** 37 to 52, with a mean rate of 30. Here the mean rate is so low because the strip starts in the middle of a 2.6-second pause. With only three QRS complexes on the strip, the mean cannot possibly be higher than 30. **P waves:** none present. Regular sawtooth-shaped waves present instead. **PR interval:** not applicable. **QRS interval:** 0.08. **Interpretation:** atrial flutter with variable conduction.

56. **QRS complexes:** present, all shaped the same. **Regularity:** regular. **Heart rate:** 94. **P waves:** upright, matching; one preceding each QRS. **PR interval:** 0.16. **QRS interval:** 0.14. **Interpretation:** sinus rhythm with wide QRS.

57. **QRS complexes:** present, all shaped the same. **Regularity:** irregular. **Heart rate:** about 19 to 23, with a mean rate of 30. **P waves:** none present. **PR interval:** not applicable. **QRS interval:** 0.28. **Interpretation:** agonal rhythm. Although the heart rate is a little fast for agonal rhythm, it must be

called this because it is so irregular. Idioventricular rhythm is usually more regular.

58. **QRS complexes:** present, all shaped the same. **Regularity:** regular. R-R intervals vary by only one small block. **Heart rate:** 60. **P waves:** upright, matching; one preceding each QRS; P-P interval regular. **PR interval:** 0.12. **QRS interval:** 0.10. **Interpretation:** sinus rhythm.

59. **QRS complexes:** none present; wavy, static-looking baseline present instead. **Regularity:** not applicable. **Heart rate:** cannot measure. **P waves:** none present. **PR interval:** not applicable. **QRS interval:** not applicable. **Interpretation:** ventricular fibrillation.

60. **QRS complexes:** present, all shaped the same. **Regularity:** irregular. The R-R intervals vary by four small blocks. **Heart rate:** about 37 to 40, with a mean rate of 40. **P waves:** upright, matching; one preceding each QRS; P-P interval slightly irregular. **PR interval:** 0.13. **QRS interval:** 0.09. **Interpretation:** sinus arrhythmia.

61. **QRS complexes:** present, all but one having the same shape. One is much wider than the others. **Regularity:** regular but interrupted (by a premature beat). **Heart rate:** 115. **P waves:** upright, matching; one preceding all QRS complexes except the wide one. **PR interval:** 0.14. **QRS interval:** 0.06 on the narrow beats, 0.14 on the wide beat. **Interpretation:** sinus tachycardia with a PVC.

62. **QRS complexes:** none present. **Regularity:** cannot determine because there are no QRS complexes. **Heart rate:** zero. **P waves:** upright and matching; P-P interval irregular. **PR interval:** not applicable. **QRS interval:** not applicable. **Interpretation:** P wave asystole.

63. **QRS complexes:** present, all shaped the same. **Regularity:** regular. **Heart rate:** about 110. **P waves:** upright, matching; one preceding each QRS; P-P interval regular. **PR interval:** 0.16. **QRS interval:** 0.08. **Interpretation:** sinus tachycardia.

64. **QRS complexes:** present, all but one shaped the same. One is wider than the others. **Regularity:** regular but interrupted (by a premature beat). **Heart rate:** 62. **P waves:** upright, matching; one preceding all QRS complexes except the premature one. There is a P wave in the premature beat's ST segment. **PR interval:** 0.20. **QRS interval:** 0.10 on the narrow beats, 0.18 on the wide beat. **Interpretation:** sinus rhythm with a PVC.

65. **QRS complexes:** present, all shaped the same. **Regularity:** irregular. **Heart rate:** 68 to 125, with a mean rate of 100. **P waves:** upright, matching, some nonconducted; P-P interval regular; atrial rate 115. **PR interval:** varies. **QRS interval:** 0.10. **Interpretation:** Wenckebach.

66. **QRS complexes:** present, all shaped the same. **Regularity:** regular. **Heart rate:** 65. **P waves:** upright, matching; one preceding each QRS; P-P interval regular. **PR interval:** 0.22. **QRS interval:** 0.10. **Interpretation:** sinus rhythm with first-degree AV block.

67. **QRS complexes:** present, all shaped the same. **Regularity:** irregular. **Heart rate:** 62 to 137, with a mean rate of 110. **P waves:** none present; wavy, undulating baseline present instead. **PR interval:** not applicable. **QRS interval:** 0.08. **Interpretation:** atrial fib-flutter. Although this may indeed be a true atrial flutter, the flutter waves are not as obvious at the beginning of the strip as they are later on, so it's possible this may be a combination of fib and flutter.

68. **QRS complexes:** present, all shaped the same. **Regularity:** regular. **Heart rate:** 44. **P waves:** upright, matching, some nonconducted; P-P interval regular; atrial rate 137. **PR interval:** 0.28–0.40. **QRS interval:** 0.14. **Interpretation:** third-degree AV block and ventricular escape rhythm. There are three P waves to each QRS. If you counted only two, look again. Note the distance between two consecutive P waves. March out where the rest of them are. There's more here than first meets the eye. Always march out the P waves!

69. **QRS complexes:** present, all shaped the same. **Regularity:** regular. **Heart rate:** 71. **P waves:** upright, matching; one preceding each QRS; P-P interval regular. **PR interval:** 0.28. **QRS interval:** 0.10. **Interpretation:** sinus rhythm with first-degree AV block.

70. **QRS complexes:** present, all shaped the same. **Regularity:** irregular. **Heart rate:** 60 to 94, with a mean rate of 70. **P waves:** none present; wavy, undulating baseline present instead. **PR interval:** not applicable. **QRS interval:** 0.10. **Interpretation:** atrial fibrillation.

71. **QRS complexes:** present, all shaped the same. **Regularity:** regular. **Heart rate:** 56. **P waves:** upright, matching; one preceding each QRS; P-P interval regular. **PR interval:** 0.14. **QRS interval:** 0.10. **Interpretation:** sinus bradycardia.

72. **QRS complexes:** present, all shaped the same. **Regularity:** regular. **Heart rate:** 79. **P waves:** none present; regular, sawtooth-shaped waves present instead. Also note the pacemaker spike preceding each QRS. **PR interval:** not applicable.

**QRS interval:** 0.12. **Interpretation:** ventricular pacing with underlying atrial flutter.

73. **QRS complexes:** present, all shaped the same. **Regularity:** regular. **Heart rate:** 94. **P waves:** upright, matching; one preceding each QRS; P-P interval regular. **PR interval:** 0.12. **QRS interval:** 0.08. **Interpretation:** sinus rhythm. Baseline sway artifact is present.

74. **QRS complexes:** present, all shaped the same. **Regularity:** irregular. **Heart rate:** 75 to 107, with a mean rate of 90. **P waves:** none present; regular sawtooth-shaped waves present instead. **PR interval:** not applicable. **QRS interval:** 0.08. **Interpretation:** atrial flutter with variable conduction.

75. **QRS complexes:** present, all shaped the same. **Regularity:** irregular. **Heart rate:** 37 to 62, with a mean rate of 60. **P waves:** upright, matching; one preceding each QRS complex; P-P interval irregular. **PR interval:** 0.12. **QRS interval:** 0.10. **Interpretation:** sinus arrhythmia. If you count out the R-R intervals, you'll note they grow steadily longer throughout the strip.

76. **QRS complexes:** present, all shaped the same. **Regularity:** regular. **Heart rate:** 79. **P waves:** upright, matching; one preceding each QRS complex; P-P interval regular. **PR interval:** 0.14. **QRS interval:** 0.08. **Interpretation:** sinus rhythm.

77. **QRS complexes:** present, all shaped the same. **Regularity:** regular. **Heart rate:** 27. **P waves:** none present. **PR interval:** not applicable. **QRS interval:** 0.08. **Interpretation:** junctional bradycardia.

78. **QRS complexes:** present, all shaped the same. **Regularity:** regular. **Heart rate:** 45. **P waves:** upright, matching; one preceding each QRS; P-P interval regular. **PR interval:** 0.20. **QRS interval:** 0.08. **Interpretation:** sinus bradycardia. Note also a prominent U wave.

79. **QRS complexes:** present, all shaped the same. **Regularity:** regular. **Heart rate:** 115. **P waves:** upright, matching; one preceding each QRS; P-P interval regular. **PR interval:** 0.12. **QRS interval:** 0.06. **Interpretation:** sinus tachycardia.

80. **QRS complexes:** present, all shaped the same. **Regularity:** regular. **Heart rate:** 107. **P waves:** biphasic, matching; one preceding each QRS; P-P interval regular. **PR interval:** 0.14. **QRS interval:** 0.10. **Interpretation:** sinus tachycardia.

81. **QRS complexes:** present, all shaped the same. **Regularity:** irregular. **Heart rate:** 137 to 167, with a mean rate of 150. **P waves:** none seen. **PR interval:** not applicable. **QRS interval:** 0.08.

**Interpretation:** atrial fibrillation. If you thought it was ventricular tachycardia, look again. The QRS complexes are not wide enough to be ventricular. Because it's irregular, it can't be called SVT. Although there are no obvious fibrillatory waves, it's prudent to call this atrial fibrillation because of its irregularity and lack of P waves.

82. **QRS complexes:** present, all shaped the same. **Regularity:** regular. **Heart rate:** 60. **P waves:** upright, matching; one preceding each QRS; P-P interval regular. **PR interval:** 0.12. **QRS interval:** 0.10. **Interpretation:** sinus rhythm.

83. **QRS complexes:** present, all shaped the same. **Regularity:** irregular. **Heart rate:** 88 to 115, with a mean rate of 110. **P waves:** none present; regular sawtooth-shaped waves present instead. **PR interval:** not applicable. **QRS interval:** 0.08. **Interpretation:** atrial flutter with variable conduction.

84. **QRS complexes:** present, all shaped the same. **Regularity:** irregular. **Heart rate:** 79 to 137, with a mean rate of 110. **P waves:** none present; wavy, undulating baseline present instead. **PR interval:** not applicable. **QRS interval:** 0.10. **Interpretation:** atrial fibrillation.

85. **QRS complexes:** present, all shaped the same. **Regularity:** regular. **Heart rate:** 88. **P waves:** upright, matching; one preceding each QRS; P-P interval regular. **PR interval:** 0.22. **QRS interval:** 0.12. **Interpretation:** sinus rhythm with first-degree AV block and wide QRS.

86. **QRS complexes:** present, all shaped the same. **Regularity:** regular. **Heart rate:** 60. **P waves:** none present; regular sawtooth-shaped waves present instead. **PR interval:** not applicable. **QRS interval:** 0.10. **Interpretation:** atrial flutter with variable conduction. Many of the flutter waves are lost inside the big inverted T wave.

87. **QRS complexes:** present, all shaped the same. **Regularity:** regular. **Heart rate:** 59. **P waves:** upright, matching; two to each QRS. The T wave has a double hump—do you see it? The first hump is the first P wave. The second P is right in front of the QRS. P-P interval is regular; atrial rate 115. **PR interval:** 0.24. **QRS interval:** 0.08. **Interpretation:** 2:1 AV block, probably Wenckebach.

88. **QRS complexes:** present, all shaped the same. **Regularity:** irregular. **Heart rate:** 33 to 137, with a mean rate of 50. **P waves:** none present; wavy, undulating baseline present instead. **PR interval:** not applicable. **QRS interval:** 0.08. **Interpretation:** atrial fibrillation.

89. **QRS complexes:** present, all shaped the same. **Regularity:** regular. **Heart rate:** 115. **P waves:** upright, matching; one preceding each QRS; P-P interval regular. **PR interval:** 0.16. **QRS interval:** 0.12. **Interpretation:** sinus tachycardia with wide QRS.

90. **QRS complexes:** present, all shaped the same. **Regularity:** regular. **Heart rate:** 75. **P waves:** upright, matching; one preceding each QRS; P-P interval regular. **PR interval:** 0.12. **QRS interval:** 0.06. **Interpretation:** sinus rhythm.

91. **QRS complexes:** present, sawtooth-shaped. **Regularity:** irregular. **Heart rate:** 187 to 300, with a mean rate of 230. **P waves:** none seen. **PR interval:** not applicable. **QRS interval:** cannot measure, as we cannot tell where QRS ends and T wave begins. **Interpretation:** ventricular tachycardia.

92. **QRS complexes:** present. **Regularity:** regular but interrupted (by premature beats). **Heart rate:** about 85. **P waves:** inverted, matching; one preceding all the narrow QRS complexes. **PR interval:** 0.16. **Interpretation:** sinus rhythm with a unifocal ventricular couplet and a PVC. Wait a minute. The P wave here is negative. Why is this not a junctional rhythm? This is $V_1$—see the notation at the top of the strip? Recall the P wave can be normally inverted in $V_1$. So that doesn't necessarily imply a junctional pacemaker. Also, a junctional rhythm would have had a shorter PR interval, less than 0.12 seconds.

93. **QRS complexes:** present, all shaped the same. **Regularity:** irregular. **Heart rate:** 29, then slower. **P waves:** none present. **PR interval:** not applicable. **QRS interval:** 0.24–0.28. **Interpretation:** agonal rhythm.

94. **QRS complexes:** present, different shapes. **Regularity:** irregular. **Heart rate:** >300 in places. **P waves:** none seen. **PR interval:** not applicable. **QRS interval:** cannot measure, as we cannot tell where QRS ends and T wave begins. **Interpretation:** torsades de pointes. Remember torsades is identified more by its classic shape than by any other criteria.

95. **QRS complexes:** present, all shaped the same. **Regularity:** regular. **Heart rate:** 43. **P waves:** inverted following each QRS complex in the ST segment. **PR interval:** not applicable. **QRS interval:** 0.08. **Interpretation:** junctional rhythm.

96. **QRS complexes:** only one present—at the beginning of the strip. Then a wavy, static-looking baseline is seen. **Regularity:** not applicable. **Heart rate:** zero after that first beat. **P waves:** none present. **PR interval:** not applicable.

**QRS interval:** 0.28 on the only QRS complex on the strip. **Interpretation:** one ventricular beat, then ventricular fibrillation.

97. **QRS complexes:** none present; wavy, static-looking baseline present instead. **Regularity:** not applicable. **Heart rate:** cannot measure. **P waves:** none present. **PR interval:** not applicable. **QRS interval:** not applicable. **Interpretation:** ventricular fibrillation.

98. **QRS complexes:** none present. **Regularity:** not applicable, as there are no QRS complexes. **Heart rate:** zero. **P waves:** biphasic, matching; P-P interval regular. **PR interval:** not applicable. **QRS interval:** not applicable. **Interpretation:** P wave asystole.

99. **QRS complexes:** present, all shaped the same. **Regularity:** irregular. **Heart rate:** 100 to 167, with a mean rate of 130. **P waves:** none present; wavy, undulating baseline present instead. **PR interval:** not applicable. **QRS interval:** 0.12. **Interpretation:** atrial fibrillation with wide QRS.

100. **QRS complexes:** present, all shaped the same. **Regularity:** regular. **Heart rate:** 60. **P waves:** none present. **PR interval:** not applicable. **QRS interval:** 0.16–0.22. **Interpretation:** accelerated idioventricular rhythm.

101. **QRS complexes:** present, all shaped the same. **Regularity:** regular but interrupted (by a premature beat). **Heart rate:** 68. **P waves:** upright and matching except for the last beat, which has a tiny inverted P wave. One P wave precedes each QRS; P-P interval is irregular. **PR interval:** 0.14 on all but the last beat. The PR interval of the last beat is 0.12. **QRS interval:** 0.12. **Interpretation:** sinus rhythm with a PJC and wide QRS.

102. **QRS complexes:** present, all shaped the same. **Regularity:** regular but interrupted (by a premature beat and also a pause). **Heart rate:** 39 to 100, with a mean rate of 70. **P waves:** upright and matching on all but the third beat, which has a tiny upright P wave at the end of the preceding T wave. There is also a tiny upright P wave just before the downstroke of the third T wave (inside the pause). P-P interval is irregular. **PR interval:** 0.18 on the normal beats, 0.22 on the premature beat. **QRS interval:** 0.06. **Interpretation:** sinus rhythm with a PAC and a nonconducted PAC. The third beat is the PAC. The P wave at the downstroke of the third beat's T wave is the nonconducted PAC. If you called this an AV block of some kind, remember that in AV blocks, the P-P interval is regular. Here we have two premature P waves.

103. **QRS complexes:** present, all shaped the same. **Regularity:** irregular. **Heart rate:** 28 to 38, with a mean rate of 40. Again, keep in mind that the mean rate is not a mathematical average of the high and low heart rates and can at times be a number slightly higher than the high heart rate calculated using the other method. **P waves:** none present; wavy, undulating baseline present instead. **PR interval:** not applicable. **QRS interval:** 0.08. **Interpretation:** atrial fibrillation.

104. **QRS complexes:** present, all shaped the same. **Regularity:** regular but interrupted (by a premature beat). **Heart rate:** 100. **P waves:** biphasic and matching on all but the third beat, which is premature and has a different shape P wave. **PR interval:** 0.14 on the normal beats, 0.12 on the premature beat. **QRS interval:** 0.06. **Interpretation:** sinus rhythm with a PAC.

105. **QRS complexes:** present, all shaped the same. **Regularity:** regular but interrupted (by premature beats and pauses). **Heart rate:** 38 to 125, with a mean rate of 80. **P waves:** upright and matching on all but the P wave following the second QRS and also the P wave preceding the sixth QRS. Those P waves have a different shape. P-P interval is irregular. **PR interval:** 0.14 on the normal beats, 0.12 on the sixth beat. **QRS interval:** 0.08. **Interpretation:** sinus rhythm with a PAC (the sixth beat) and a nonconducted PAC (the premature P after the second QRS).

106. **QRS complexes:** present, all but one shaped the same. One is wider and taller than the others. **Regularity:** regular but interrupted (by a premature beat). **Heart rate:** 125. **P waves:** upright and matching on all but the wide QRS beat, which has no P wave. **PR interval:** 0.16. **QRS interval:** 0.08 on the normal beats, 0.14 on the premature beat. **Interpretation:** sinus tachycardia with a PVC.

107. **QRS complexes:** present, all shaped the same. **Regularity:** regular. **Heart rate:** about 130. **P waves:** upright, matching; one preceding each QRS; P-P interval regular. **PR interval:** 0.14. **QRS interval:** 0.08. **Interpretation:** sinus tachycardia.

108. **QRS complexes:** present, all shaped the same. **Regularity:** irregular. **Heart rate:** 68 to 125, with a mean rate of 90. **P waves:** at least three different shapes; P-P interval irregular. **PR interval:** varies. **QRS interval:** 0.10. **Interpretation:** wandering atrial pacemaker.

109. **QRS complexes:** present, all shaped the same. **Regularity:** regular. **Heart rate:** 38. **P waves:** upright and matching directly preceding the QRS. There is an extra premature P wave at the end of each T wave. That P has a different shape— it's pointy. **PR interval:** 0.20. **QRS interval:** 0.08. **Interpretation:** sinus bradycardia with bigeminal nonconducted PACs. This strip looks like sinus bradycardia, doesn't it? But do you see the premature P wave now that it's been pointed out? Always be suspicious of T waves with humps on their downslopes. That hump might just be a P wave.

110. **QRS complexes:** present, all shaped the same. **Regularity:** irregular. **Heart rate:** 29 to 60, with a mean rate of 40. **P waves:** none present; wavy, undulating baseline present instead. **PR interval:** not applicable. **QRS interval:** 0.08. **Interpretation:** atrial fibrillation.

111. **QRS complexes:** present, most but not all shaped the same. **Regularity:** irregular. **Heart rate:** 167 to 250, with a mean rate of 200. **P waves:** none present; wavy, undulating baseline present instead. **PR interval:** not applicable. **QRS interval:** 0.06– 0.08. **Interpretation:** atrial fibrillation. If you were tempted to call this SVT, remember that SVT is a regular rhythm. This strip is not regular.

112. **QRS complexes:** present, all shaped the same. **Regularity:** regular. **Heart rate:** 62. **P waves:** none seen. **PR interval:** not applicable. **QRS interval:** 0.20. **Interpretation:** accelerated idioventricular rhythm.

113. **QRS complexes:** present, all shaped the same, although some are deeper than others. **Regularity:** regular but interrupted (by a run of premature beats). **Heart rate:** 88 when in sinus tachycardia, about 187 when in atrial tachycardia. **P waves:** upright and matching on all but the very rapid beats, whose P waves are inside the preceding T wave. **PR interval:** 0.20 on the normal beats, unable to measure on the rapid beats, as the P is inside the T wave. **QRS interval:** 0.08. **Interpretation:** sinus tachycardia with a 10-beat run of PAT. We know this is PAT, as we can see the PAC (the fourth beat) that initiates it.

114. **QRS complexes:** present, all shaped the same. **Regularity:** irregular. **Heart rate:** 150 to 250, with a mean rate of 190. **P waves:** none present; wavy, undulating baseline present instead. **PR interval:** not applicable. **QRS interval:** 0.06. **Interpretation:** atrial fibrillation.

115. **QRS complexes:** present, all shaped the same. **Regularity:** irregular. **Heart rate:** 150 to 250, with a mean rate of 190. **P waves:** none present; wavy, undulating baseline present instead. **PR interval:** not applicable. **QRS interval:** 0.06. **Interpretation:** atrial fibrillation.

116. **QRS complexes:** present, all shaped the same. **Regularity:** regular but interrupted (by a pause). **Heart rate:** 37 to 72, with a mean heart rate of 70. **P waves:** upright and matching except for the premature P wave inside the fourth T wave. **PR interval:** 0.24. **QRS interval:** 0.08. **Interpretation:** sinus rhythm with a nonconducted PAC.

117. **QRS complexes:** present, all shaped the same. **Regularity:** regular. **Heart rate:** 71. **P waves:** tiny inverted P waves present preceding the QRS complexes. **PR interval:** about 0.06. **QRS interval:** 0.10. **Interpretation:** accelerated junctional rhythm.

118. **QRS complexes:** present, all shaped the same. **Regularity:** regular but interrupted (by pauses). **Heart rate:** 48 to 88, with a mean rate of 80. **P waves:** upright and matching except for the premature P waves inside the third and sixth T waves. **PR interval:** 0.18. **QRS interval:** 0.08. **Interpretation:** sinus rhythm with two nonconducted PACs.

119. **QRS complexes:** present, all shaped the same. **Regularity:** regular. **Heart rate:** 29. **P waves:** none present. **PR interval:** not applicable. **QRS interval:** 0.28. **Interpretation:** idioventricular rhythm.

120. **QRS complexes:** present, all shaped the same. **Regularity:** regular but interrupted (by a pause). **Heart rate:** 32 to 58, with a mean rate of 50. **P waves:** upright, matching; sometimes more than one per QRS; atrial rate 60. **PR interval:** varies. **QRS interval:** 0.10. **Interpretation:** Wenckebach. See how the PR interval gradually prolongs until a P wave is blocked (not followed by a QRS)?

121. **QRS complexes:** present, all shaped the same. **Regularity:** regular. **Heart rate:** 45. **P waves:** upright, matching, some nonconducted; atrial rate 137. **PR interval:** varies. **QRS interval:** 0.16. **Interpretation:** third-degree AV block and a ventricular escape rhythm. Did you think this was Mobitz II second-degree AV block? The differentiating factor here is the changing PR intervals. Mobitz II has constant PR intervals. Did you think it was Wenckebach? Wenckebach does not have regular R-R intervals. So it could only be third-degree AV block.

122. **QRS complexes:** present, all shaped the same. **Regularity:** irregular. **Heart rate:** 60 to 83, with a mean rate of 80. **P waves:** upright, matching; one per QRS; P-P interval irregular. **PR interval:** 0.14. **QRS interval:** 0.08. **Interpretation:** sinus arrhythmia.

123. **QRS complexes:** present, all shaped the same. **Regularity:** regular. **Heart rate:** 83. **P waves:** none noted. **PR interval:** not applicable. **QRS interval:** 0.16. **Interpretation:** accelerated idioventricular rhythm.

124. **QRS complexes:** present, all shaped the same. **Regularity:** regular. **Heart rate:** 125. **P waves:** none seen. **PR interval:** not applicable. **QRS interval:** 0.20. **Interpretation:** ventricular tachycardia.

125. **QRS complexes:** present, all shaped the same. **Regularity:** regular. **Heart rate:** 58. **P waves:** none seen. There's a U wave immediately following the T waves—don't confuse those with P waves. **PR interval:** not applicable. **QRS interval:** 0.10. **Interpretation:** junctional rhythm.

126. **QRS complexes:** present, all shaped the same. **Regularity:** irregular. **Heart rate:** 42 to 47, with a mean rate of 50. Recall the mean is not a mathematical average of the high and low heart rates—it's merely a count of the number of QRS complexes on the six-second strip—and it can at times be a bit higher than the high heart rate calculated using the other method. **P waves:** at least three different shapes; one preceding each QRS. **PR interval:** varies. **QRS interval:** 0.10. **Interpretation:** wandering atrial pacemaker.

127. **QRS complexes:** present, all shaped the same. **Regularity:** irregular. **Heart rate:** 100 to 150, with a mean rate of 130. **P waves:** none noted; wavy, undulating baseline present instead. **PR interval:** not applicable. **QRS interval:** 0.06. **Interpretation:** atrial fibrillation.

128. **QRS complexes:** present, all shaped the same. **Regularity:** irregular. **Heart rate:** 85 to 137, with a mean rate of 100. **P waves:** none present; sawtooth-shaped waves present between QRS complexes. **PR interval:** not applicable. **QRS interval:** 0.10. **Interpretation:** atrial flutter with variable conduction.

129. **QRS complexes:** present with differing shapes, if indeed those are real QRS complexes and not just spiked fibrillatory waves. **Regularity:** irregular. **Heart rate:** around 300 to 375, but difficult to count as QRS shapes change. **P waves:** none seen. **PR interval:** not applicable. **QRS interval:** cannot measure at times. **Interpretation:** torsades de pointes versus ventricular fibrillation. This is a judgment call, as this rhythm might well be ventricular fibrillation. You will find that torsades and V-fib can be easily mistaken for each other.

130. **QRS complexes:** present, all shaped the same. **Regularity:** regular. **Heart rate:** 79. **P waves:** upright, matching; one preceding each QRS; P-P interval regular. **PR interval:** 0.14. **QRS interval:** 0.12. **Interpretation:** sinus rhythm.

131. **QRS complexes:** present, all shaped the same. **Regularity:** regular. **Heart rate:** 51. **P waves:** none seen. **PR interval:** not applicable. **QRS interval:** 0.10. **Interpretation:** junctional rhythm.

132. **QRS complexes:** present, all shaped the same. **Regularity:** regular but interrupted (by premature beats). **Heart rate:** 65. **P waves:** upright, all except the third and fourth P waves matching. The third and fourth P waves are premature and shaped a bit differently. P-P interval is irregular. **PR interval:** 0.16–0.20. **QRS interval:** 0.06. **Interpretation:** sinus rhythm with two PACs (the third and fourth beats).

133. **QRS complexes:** present, all shaped the same. **Regularity:** irregular. **Heart rate:** 71 to 110, with a mean rate of 90. **P waves:** none present; wavy, undulating baseline present instead. **PR interval:** not applicable. **QRS interval:** 0.08. **Interpretation:** atrial fibrillation. In places it looks pretty fluttery, doesn't it? You might have been tempted to call this atrial flutter. The problem is that the fluttery pattern is not consistent. Its waves could never be marched out, as they dampen out so much in places. It's safer to call this atrial fibrillation (or fib-flutter).

134. **QRS complexes:** present, all shaped the same. **Regularity:** regular. **Heart rate:** 60. **P waves:** none noted. **PR interval:** not applicable. **QRS interval:** 0.20. **Interpretation:** accelerated idioventricular rhythm.

135. **QRS complexes:** present, all shaped the same, although two are distorted by artifact. **Regularity:** regular. **Heart rate:** 137. **P waves:** none seen. **PR interval:** not applicable. **QRS interval:** 0.18. **Interpretation:** ventricular tachycardia.

136. **QRS complexes:** present, all shaped the same. **Regularity:** regular. **Heart rate:** 60. **P waves:** none seen; wavy, undulating baseline present instead. **PR interval:** not applicable. **QRS interval:** 0.10. **Interpretation:** atrial fibrillation. Although normally atrial fibrillation is an irregular rhythm, you can see that it may look regular at times. This is not common, but you should be aware it does happen sometimes, typically in individuals who've been in atrial fibrillation for years.

137. **QRS complexes:** present, all shaped the same. **Regularity:** regular. **Heart rate:** 137. **P waves:** upright, matching; one preceding each QRS; P-P interval regular. **PR interval:** 0.16. **QRS interval:** 0.08. **Interpretation:** sinus tachycardia.

138. **QRS complexes:** present, all shaped the same. **Regularity:** regular. **Heart rate:** 42. **P waves:** upright, matching (some a little distorted by artifact); one preceding each QRS; P-P interval regular. **PR interval:** 0.16. **QRS interval:** 0.10. **Interpretation:** sinus bradycardia.

139. **QRS complexes:** present, all shaped the same. **Regularity:** regular. **Heart rate:** 60. **P waves:** upright, matching; one preceding each QRS; P-P interval regular. **PR interval:** 0.14. **QRS interval:** 0.08. **Interpretation:** sinus rhythm.

140. **QRS complexes:** present, all shaped the same. **Regularity:** irregular. **Heart rate:** 71 to 107, with a mean rate of 90. **P waves:** none present; sawtooth-shaped waves present instead. **PR interval:** not applicable. **QRS interval:** 0.06. **Interpretation:** atrial flutter with variable conduction.

141. **QRS complexes:** present, all shaped the same. **Regularity:** regular. **Heart rate:** about 73. **P waves:** none noted; sawtooth-shaped waves present instead. **PR interval:** not applicable. **QRS interval:** 0.12, although difficult to measure as QRS is distorted by flutter waves. **Interpretation:** atrial flutter with variable conduction and a possible wide QRS.

142. **QRS complexes:** cannot distinguish. **Regularity:** cannot tell. **Heart rate:** cannot tell. **P waves:** cannot distinguish. **PR interval:** not applicable. **QRS interval:** not applicable. **Interpretation:** unknown rhythm with artifact. Why is this strip even in here if you can't possibly tell what it is? Because it's important for you to know *not to even try to interpret a rhythm this obscured by artifact.* There is no way to tell what the underlying rhythm is here. Check the patient's monitor lead wires and electrode patches or change the lead the patient is being monitored in to get a better tracing, and try again with a clearer strip.

143. **QRS complexes:** present, all shaped the same. **Regularity:** regular. **Heart rate:** about 130. **P waves:** upright, matching; one preceding each QRS; P-P interval regular. **PR interval:** 0.16. **QRS interval:** 0.06. **Interpretation:** sinus tachycardia.

144. **QRS complexes:** present, all shaped the same. **Regularity:** regular. **Heart rate:** 83. **P waves:** upright, matching; one preceding each QRS; P-P interval regular. **PR interval:** 0.10. **QRS interval:** 0.08. **Interpretation:** sinus rhythm with short PR interval.

145. **QRS complexes:** present, all shaped the same. **Regularity:** regular. **Heart rate:** 88. **P waves:** upright, matching; one preceding each QRS; P-P interval regular. **PR interval:** 0.12. **QRS interval:** 0.12. **Interpretation:** sinus rhythm with wide QRS.

146. **QRS complexes:** present, all shaped the same. **Regularity:** regular. **Heart rate:** 60. **P waves:** upright, matching; one preceding each QRS; P-P interval regular. **PR interval:** 0.16. **QRS interval:** 0.08. **Interpretation:** sinus rhythm.

147. **QRS complexes:** present, all shaped the same. **Regularity:** regular. **Heart rate:** 68. **P waves:** upright, matching; one preceding each QRS; P-P interval regular. **PR interval:** 0.18. **QRS interval:** 0.14. **Interpretation:** sinus rhythm with wide QRS.

148. **QRS complexes:** present, all shaped the same. **Regularity:** regular. **Heart rate:** about 57. **P waves:** upright, matching; one preceding each QRS; P-P interval regular. **PR interval:** 0.16. **QRS interval:** 0.08. **Interpretation:** sinus bradycardia.

149. **QRS complexes:** present, all shaped the same. **Regularity:** irregular. **Heart rate:** 56 to 83, with a mean rate of 70. **P waves:** none noted; wavy, undulating baseline present instead. **PR interval:** not applicable. **QRS interval:** 0.10. **Interpretation:** atrial fibrillation.

150. **QRS complexes:** present, all shaped the same. **Regularity:** regular. **Heart rate:** 43. **P waves:** upright, matching; one preceding each QRS; P-P interval regular. **PR interval:** 0.16. **QRS interval:** 0.08. **Interpretation:** sinus bradycardia.

151. **QRS complexes:** present, all shaped the same. **Regularity:** regular. **Heart rate:** 83. **P waves:** upright, matching; one preceding each QRS; P-P interval regular. **PR interval:** 0.14. **QRS interval:** 0.10. **Interpretation:** sinus rhythm.

152. **QRS complexes:** present, all shaped the same. **Regularity:** regular. **Heart rate:** about 35. **P waves:** upright, matching; one preceding each QRS; P-P interval regular. **PR interval:** 0.16. **QRS interval:** 0.10. **Interpretation:** sinus bradycardia.

153. **QRS complexes:** present, most but not all shaped the same. Some have an S wave, but others do not. **Regularity:** irregular. **Heart rate:** 150 to 250, with a mean rate of 190. **P waves:** none noted; wavy, undulating baseline present instead. **PR interval:** not applicable. **QRS interval:** 0.06 to 0.08. **Interpretation:** atrial fibrillation.

154. **QRS complexes:** present, all shaped the same. **Regularity:** regular. **Heart rate:** 62. **P waves:** upright, matching; one preceding each QRS; P-P interval regular. **PR interval:** 0.20. **QRS interval:** 0.08. **Interpretation:** sinus rhythm.

155. **QRS complexes:** present, all shaped the same. **Regularity:** regular. **Heart rate:** 115. **P waves:** upright, matching; one preceding each QRS; P-P interval regular. **PR interval:** 0.12. **QRS interval:** 0.10. **Interpretation:** sinus tachycardia.

156. **QRS complexes:** present, all shaped the same. **Regularity:** irregular. **Heart rate:** 107 to 167, with a mean rate of 140. **P waves:** none seen; wavy, undulating baseline present instead. **PR interval:** not applicable. **QRS interval:** 0.08. **Interpretation:** atrial fibrillation.

157. **QRS complexes:** one present; wavy, static-looking baseline present instead. **Regularity:** not applicable. **Heart rate:** cannot determine, as there is only one QRS complexes. **P waves:** none seen. **PR interval:** not applicable. **QRS interval:** not applicable. **Interpretation:** ventricular fibrillation.

158. **QRS complexes:** present, all shaped the same. **Regularity:** irregular. **Heart rate:** 36 to 42, with a mean rate of 40. **P waves:** upright, matching; one preceding each QRS; P-P interval irregular. **PR interval:** 0.16. **QRS interval:** 0.10. **Interpretation:** sinus arrhythmia.

159. **QRS complexes:** present, all shaped the same. **Regularity:** regular but interrupted (by pauses). **Heart rate:** 75 to 125, with a mean rate of 110. **P waves:** upright, many hidden in T waves. Some P waves are nonconducted. P-P interval is regular; atrial rate 137. **PR interval:** varies. **QRS interval:** 0.06. **Interpretation:** Wenckebach. This is not an obvious Wenckebach, is it? See the pause between the third and fourth QRS complexes? Note the P wave preceding the fourth QRS. Now back up to the T wave of the third beat. See how deformed the T wave's shape is? That's because there's a P wave inside it. Note the P-P interval between those two P waves and you can march out where the rest of the P waves are. You'll find the P-P intervals are all regular and the PR intervals gradually prolong until a beat is dropped.

160. **QRS complexes:** present, all shaped the same. **Regularity:** irregular. **Heart rate:** 75 to 107, with a mean rate of 100. **P waves:** none noted; wavy, undulating baseline present instead. **PR interval:** not applicable. **QRS interval:** 0.10. **Interpretation:** atrial fibrillation.

161. **QRS complexes:** present, all shaped the same. **Regularity:** regular. **Heart rate:** about 130. **P waves:** none seen. **PR interval:** not applicable. **QRS interval:** 0.08. **Interpretation:** SVT.

162. **QRS complexes:** cannot be sure if there are QRS complexes of varying shapes or if it is just a static-looking baseline without QRS complexes. **Regularity:** irregular. **Heart rate:** 250 to 300, with a mean rate of about 280. **P waves:** none seen. **PR interval:** not applicable. **QRS interval:** 0.12 or greater. **Interpretation:** either torsades de pointes or ventricular fibrillation. It oscillates like torsades but looks more uncoordinated, like V-fib. The treatment for these is similar, thankfully, so calling it either torsades or V-fib would still get appropriate treatment for the patient.

163. **QRS complexes:** present, all shaped the same. **Regularity:** irregular. **Heart rate:** 60 to 107, with a mean rate of 90. **P waves:** none seen; wavy, undulating baseline present instead. **PR interval:** not applicable. **QRS interval:** 0.06. **Interpretation:** atrial fibrillation.

164. **QRS complexes:** present, all shaped the same. **Regularity:** regular. **Heart rate:** about 80. **P waves:** none seen; wavy, undulating baseline present instead. **PR interval:** not applicable. **QRS interval:** 0.10. **Interpretation:** atrial fibrillation. This is another example of a regular spell of atrial fibrillation.

165. **QRS complexes:** present, all but one shaped the same. One is shorter than the rest. **Regularity:** irregular. **Heart rate:** 45 to 65, with a mean rate of 50. **P waves:** none noted; wavy, undulating baseline present instead. **PR interval:** not applicable. **QRS interval:** 0.08. **Interpretation:** atrial fibrillation.

166. **QRS complexes:** present, all shaped the same. **Regularity:** regular. **Heart rate:** 75. **P waves:** upright, matching; one preceding each QRS; P-P interval regular. **PR interval:** 0.16. **QRS interval:** 0.14. **Interpretation:** sinus rhythm with wide QRS.

167. **QRS complexes:** present, all shaped the same. **Regularity:** irregular. **Heart rate:** 88 to 187, with a mean rate of 120. **P waves:** present, at least three different shapes; P-P interval irregular. **PR interval:** varies. **QRS interval:** 0.08. **Interpretation:** multifocal atrial tachycardia.

168. **QRS complexes:** present, all shaped the same. **Regularity:** regular. **Heart rate:** around 90. **P waves:** upright, matching; one preceding each QRS; P-P interval regular. **PR interval:** 0.14. **QRS interval:** 0.08. **Interpretation:** sinus rhythm.

169. **QRS complexes:** present, all shaped the same. **Regularity:** irregular. **Heart rate:** 83 to 137, with a mean rate of 110. **P waves:** none noted; sawtooth-shaped waves present instead. **PR interval:** not applicable. **QRS interval:** 0.08. **Interpretation:** atrial flutter with variable conduction.

170. **QRS complexes:** present, all shaped the same. **Regularity:** regular. **Heart rate:** 150. **P waves:** upright, matching; one preceding each QRS; P-P interval regular. **PR interval:** 0.10. **QRS interval:** 0.10. **Interpretation:** sinus tachycardia with short PR interval.

171. **QRS complexes:** present, all shaped the same. **Regularity:** regular. **Heart rate:** 45. **P waves:** upright, matching, two preceding each QRS; P-P interval regular; atrial rate 88. **PR interval:** 0.36. **QRS interval:** 0.08. **Interpretation:** 2:1 AV block.

172. **QRS complexes:** present, all shaped the same. **Regularity:** regular but interrupted (by pauses). **Heart rate:** 44 to 83, with a mean rate of 60. **P waves:** upright, matching, some nonconducted; P-P interval regular; atrial rate 88. **PR interval:** 0.36. **QRS interval:** 0.08. **Interpretation:** Mobitz II second-degree AV block.

173. **QRS complexes:** present, all shaped the same. **Regularity:** regular. **Heart rate:** 137. **P waves:** none seen. **PR interval:** not applicable. **QRS interval:** 0.06. **Interpretation:** SVT.

174. **QRS complexes:** only one mammoth QRS on the strip. Believe it or not, that huge wave at the beginning of the strip is a QRS and T wave. **Regularity:** cannot determine. **Heart rate:** cannot determine. **P waves:** none seen. **PR interval:** not applicable. **QRS interval:** about 0.60, but that's a guesstimate. **Interpretation:** agonal rhythm. It is unusual for an agonal rhythm's QRS complexes to be this wide. It's likely this patient has an *extremely elevated* potassium level in his or her bloodstream, which can cause the QRS to widen out more than usual.

175. **QRS complexes:** none seen. **Regularity:** not applicable. **Heart rate:** zero. **P waves:** none seen. **PR interval:** not applicable. **QRS interval:** not applicable. **Interpretation:** asystole.

176. **QRS complexes:** present, differing shapes. **Regularity:** irregular. **Heart rate:** about 375. **P waves:** none seen. **PR interval:** not applicable. **QRS interval:** 0.12 or greater. **Interpretation:** torsades de pointes.

177. **QRS complexes:** none; wavy, static-looking baseline present instead. **Regularity:** not applicable. **Heart rate:** cannot measure. **P waves:** none seen. **PR interval:** not applicable. **QRS interval:** not applicable. **Interpretation:** ventricular fibrillation.

178. **QRS complexes:** none; wavy, static-looking baseline present instead. **Regularity:** not applicable. **Heart rate:** cannot measure. **P waves:** none seen. **PR interval:** not applicable. **QRS interval:** not applicable. **Interpretation:** ventricular fibrillation.

179. **QRS complexes:** present, all shaped the same. **Regularity:** regular. **Heart rate:** just a hair over 100. **P waves:** upright, matching; one preceding each QRS; P-P interval regular. **PR interval:** 0.22. **QRS interval:** 0.10. **Interpretation:** sinus tachycardia with a first-degree AV block.

180. **QRS complexes:** present, all shaped the same. **Regularity:** irregular. **Heart rate:** 80 to 167, with a mean rate of 110. **P waves:** present, at least three different shapes. **PR interval:** not applicable. **QRS interval:** 0.06. **Interpretation:** multifocal atrial tachycardia. If you thought it was atrial fibrillation, remember that *atrial fibrillation has no P waves.* There are obvious P waves on this strip.

181. **QRS complexes:** present, all shaped the same. **Regularity:** regular. **Heart rate:** 68. **P waves:** none seen. **PR interval:** not applicable. **QRS interval:** 0.18. **Interpretation:** accelerated idioventricular rhythm.

182. **QRS complexes:** present, all shaped the same. **Regularity:** regular. **Heart rate:** 125. **P waves:** upright, matching; one preceding each QRS; P-P interval regular. **PR interval:** 0.16. **QRS interval:** 0.06. **Interpretation:** sinus tachycardia.

183. **QRS complexes:** present, all shaped the same. **Regularity:** regular. **Heart rate:** 56. **P waves:** upright, matching; one preceding each QRS; P-P interval regular; P waves are small. **PR interval:** 0.16. **QRS interval:** 0.16. **Interpretation:** sinus bradycardia with wide QRS. Look again at this strip if you thought this was atrial fibrillation. There are obvious, although tiny, P waves. And if you thought this was a ventricular rhythm of some kind because of the QRS width, note the matching upright P waves. Ventricular rhythms don't have that. Remember—the width of the QRS does not determine whether a rhythm can be sinus. The P waves are the key criterion.

184. **QRS complexes:** present, all shaped the same. **Regularity:** regular. **Heart rate:** 83. **P waves:** upright, matching; one preceding each QRS; P-P interval regular. **PR interval:** 0.13. **QRS interval:** 0.10. **Interpretation:** sinus rhythm. Did you think this was a 2:1 AV block? The T wave does look like the P wave, doesn't it? Remember, AV blocks have regular P-P intervals. If this T wave were hiding a P wave, the P-P intervals would not be regular. So it's not an AV block.

185. **QRS complexes:** present, all shaped the same. **Regularity:** regular. **Heart rate:** 167. **P waves:** upright, matching; one preceding each QRS; P-P interval regular. **PR interval:** 0.12. **QRS interval:** 0.06. **Interpretation:** atrial tachycardia. Remember, the sinus node does not usually fire at rates above 160 in supine resting adults. Because this rate is above 160, we must call it atrial tachycardia.

186. **QRS complexes:** present, all shaped the same. **Regularity:** irregular. **Heart rate:** 20 to 75, with a mean rate of 50. **P waves:** none seen; very fine wavy, undulating baseline present instead. **PR interval:** not applicable. **QRS interval:** 0.08. **Interpretation:** atrial fibrillation.

187. **QRS complexes:** present, all shaped the same. **Regularity:** irregular. **Heart rate:** 28 to 62, with a mean rate of 50. **P waves:** none seen; wavy, undulating baseline present instead. **PR interval:** not applicable. **QRS interval:** 0.10. **Interpretation:** atrial fibrillation.

188. **QRS complexes:** present, all shaped the same. **Regularity:** irregular. **Heart rate:** 60 to 79, with a mean rate of 70. **P waves:** upright, matching; one preceding each QRS; P-P interval regular. **PR interval:** 0.18. **QRS interval:** 0.08. **Interpretation:** sinus arrhythmia.

189. **QRS complexes:** present, all shaped the same. **Regularity:** regular. **Heart rate:** 60. **P waves:** upright, matching (the ones that can be seen); one preceding each QRS; P-P interval regular, as far as can be seen. **PR interval:** 0.18. **QRS interval:** 0.08. **Interpretation:** sinus rhythm partially obscured by artifact. Unlike some strips with artifact, this strip has measurable waves and complexes. Because we can pick out the QRS complexes throughout the strip, we can deduce that the P waves continue as well during the artifact spells. Even so, it would be better not to mount a strip like this in the patient's chart, because one cannot be entirely sure what is happening during the periods of artifact.

190. **QRS complexes:** present, all shaped the same. **Regularity:** regular but interrupted (by pauses). **Heart rate:** 75 to 125. **P waves:** upright, some hidden in T waves, some nonconducted; P-P interval regular; atrial rate 137. **PR interval:** varies. **QRS interval:** 0.06. **Interpretation:** Wenckebach.

191. **QRS complexes:** present, all but two shaped the same (two are taller and wider). **Regularity:** regular but interrupted (by premature beats). **Heart rate:** 88. **P waves:** upright and matching on the narrow beats, none on the wide beats; P-P regular. **PR interval:** 0.24. **QRS interval:** 0.08 on the narrow beats, 0.14 on the wide beats. **Interpretation:** sinus rhythm with PVCs and a first-degree AV block.

192. **QRS complexes:** present, all shaped the same. **Regularity:** regular. **Heart rate:** 88. **P waves:** notched, matching; one preceding each QRS; P-P interval regular. **PR interval:** 0.20. **QRS interval:** 0.08. **Interpretation:** sinus rhythm.

193. **QRS complexes:** present, all shaped the same. **Regularity:** regular. **Heart rate:** 71. **P waves:** upright, matching; one preceding each QRS; P-P interval regular. **PR interval:** 0.22. **QRS interval:** 0.08. **Interpretation:** sinus rhythm with a first-degree AV block.

194. **QRS complexes:** present, all shaped the same. **Regularity:** regular. **Heart rate:** 36. **P waves:** upright, matching; one preceding each QRS; P-P interval regular. **PR interval:** 0.16. **QRS interval:** 0.10. **Interpretation:** sinus bradycardia.

195. **QRS complexes:** only one seen on the strip. **Regularity:** cannot determine. **Heart rate:** cannot determine from just one QRS complex. **P waves:** cannot distinguish due to artifact. **PR interval:** not applicable. **QRS interval:** cannot measure, as it's distorted by artifact. **Interpretation:** probably agonal rhythm obscured by CPR artifact. This strip looks a lot like the example of CPR artifact in Chapter 3, doesn't it? In order to know for sure what this rhythm is, CPR would need to be stopped briefly to allow a strip without artifact to be analyzed.

196. **QRS complexes:** none present; wavy, static-looking baseline present instead. **Regularity:** not applicable. **Heart rate:** not applicable. **P waves:** none seen. **PR interval:** not applicable. **QRS interval:** not applicable. **Interpretation:** ventricular fibrillation.

197. **QRS complexes:** present, all shaped the same. **Regularity:** regular but interrupted (by a premature beat). **Heart rate:** 75. **P waves:** upright and matching except for the premature P wave on the seventh beat; P-P interval irregular because of this premature beat. **PR interval:** 0.16. **QRS interval:** 0.10. **Interpretation:** sinus rhythm with a PAC.

198. **QRS complexes:** present, all shaped the same. **Regularity:** regular but interrupted (by a premature beat). **Heart rate:** about 77. **P waves:** tiny, biphasic, and matching except for the third beat, which is premature. The P-P interval is irregular because of this premature beat. **PR interval:** 0.14–0.16. **QRS interval:** 0.06. **Interpretation:** sinus rhythm with a PAC. This premature beat is not a PJC because the PR interval of that beat is greater than 0.12.

199. **QRS complexes:** present, two different shapes. **Regularity:** regular but interrupted (by premature beats). **Heart rate:** 115. **P waves:** upright and matching on the narrow beats, none on the wide beats. **PR interval:** 0.14. **QRS interval:** 0.08 on the narrow beats, 0.16 on the wide beats. **Interpretation:** sinus tachycardia with two PVCs.

200. **QRS complexes:** present, all shaped the same. **Regularity:** irregular. **Heart rate:** 79 to 125, with an atrial rate of 100. **P waves:** none present, sawtooth-shaped waves present instead. **PR interval:** not applicable. **QRS interval:** 0.08. **Interpretation:** atrial flutter with variable conduction.

201. **QRS complexes:** present, all shaped the same within each lead. **Regularity:** regular. **Heart rate:** 38. **P waves:** upright in Lead II, biphasic in $V_1$, matching within each lead. **PR interval:** 0.26. **QRS interval:** 0.10. **Interpretation:** sinus bradycardia with first-degree AV block.

202. **QRS complexes:** present, all shaped the same. **Regularity:** regular. **Heart rate:** 65. **P waves:** upright, matching. **PR interval:** 0.10. **QRS interval:** 0.10. **Interpretation:** sinus rhythm.

203. **QRS complexes:** present, all shaped the same within each lead. **Regularity:** regular. **Heart rate:** 150. **P waves:** none noted. **PR interval:** not applicable. **QRS interval:** 0.06. **Interpretation:** SVT.

204. **QRS complexes:** absent. **Regularity:** not applicable. **Heart rate:** zero. **P waves:** none present. **PR interval:** not applicable. **QRS interval:** not applicable. **Interpretation:** asystole.

205. **QRS complexes:** present, all shaped the same within each lead. **Regularity:** regular. **Heart rate:** 65. **P waves:** upright in Lead II, biphasic in $V_1$, matching within each lead. **PR interval:** 0.20. **QRS interval:** 0.10. **Interpretation:** sinus rhythm.

206. **QRS complexes:** present, all shaped the same within each lead. **Regularity:** irregular. **Heart rate:** 41 to 68, with a mean rate of 50. **P waves:** upright in Lead II, biphasic in $V_1$, matching within each lead. P-P interval is regular; atrial rate 79. **PR interval:** varies. **QRS interval:** 0.14. **Interpretation:** Wenckebach with wide QRS.

207. **QRS complexes:** present, all shaped the same within each lead. **Regularity:** regular but

interrupted (by a pause). **Heart rate:** 36 to 79, with a mean rate of 50. **P waves:** upright, matching; P-P interval regular; atrial rate 75. **PR interval:** varies. **QRS interval:** 0.10. **Interpretation:** Wenckebach.

208. **QRS complexes:** present, all shaped the same within each lead. **Regularity:** regular but interrupted (by a premature beat). The fifth QRS complex is premature. **Heart rate:** 75. **P waves:** upright in Lead II, biphasic in $V_1$, matching within each lead except for the fifth P wave, which is shaped differently and is premature. **PR interval:** 0.12. **QRS interval:** 08. **Interpretation:** sinus rhythm with PAC.

209. **QRS complexes:** present, all shaped the same within each lead. **Regularity:** regular. **Heart rate:** 38. **P waves:** upright in Lead II, biphasic in $V_1$, matching within each lead. P-P interval is regular; atrial rate 79. **PR interval:** 0.28. **QRS interval:** 0.14. **Interpretation:** 2:1 AV block with wide QRS.

210. **QRS complexes:** present, all shaped the same within each lead. **Regularity:** regular. **Heart rate:** 102. **P waves:** matching, inverted following the QRS in both leads. **PR interval:** not applicable. **QRS interval:** 0.08. **Interpretation:** junctional tachycardia. See the blips following the QRS complexes? Those are the inverted P waves.

211. **QRS complexes:** present, all shaped the same within each lead. **Regularity:** regular. **Heart rate:** 71. **P waves:** cannot see in Lead II, inverted in $V_1$. **PR interval:** 0.11. **QRS interval:** 0.06. **Interpretation:** accelerated junctional rhythm.

212. **QRS complexes:** present, all shaped the same. **Regularity:** irregular. **Heart rate:** 71 to 125, with a mean rate of 90. **P waves:** none noted; wavy baseline present between QRS complexes. **PR interval:** not applicable. **QRS interval:** 0.10 **Interpretation:** atrial fibrillation.

213. **QRS complexes:** present, all shaped the same. **Regularity:** regular. **Heart rate:** 65. **P waves:** matching, upright. **PR interval:** 0.20. **QRS interval:** 0.12. **Interpretation:** sinus rhythm with borderline first-degree AV block and wide QRS.

214. **QRS complexes:** present, all shaped the same. **Regularity:** regular but interrupted (by premature beats). **Heart rate:** 88. **P waves:** matching on all but the second, fourth, and sixth beats—those P waves are shaped differently. **PR interval:** 0.13. **QRS interval:** 0.14. **Interpretation:** sinus rhythm with three PACs and wide QRS.

215. **QRS complexes:** present, all shaped the same. **Regularity:** regular but interrupted (by a run of rapid beats). **Heart rate:** 68, then 150.

**P waves:** upright and matching on the first four beats, then shaped differently during the tachycardia. **PR interval:** 0.16. **QRS interval:** 0.10. **Interpretation:** sinus rhythm, then atrial tachycardia (the fifth beat is a PAC, which starts off a run of PACs—this run of PACs is called atrial tachycardia).

216. **QRS complexes:** present, all shaped the same. **Regularity:** regular. **Heart rate:** 83. **P waves:** upright, matching; one preceding each QRS. **PR interval:** 0.16. **QRS interval:** 0.08. **Interpretation:** sinus rhythm.

217. **QRS complexes:** present, all shaped the same within each lead. **Regularity:** regular. **Heart rate:** 94. **P waves:** cannot see in Lead I, inverted preceding the QRS in Lead II. **PR interval:** 0.08. **QRS interval:** 0.06. **Interpretation:** accelerated junctional rhythm.

218. **QRS complexes:** present, all different shapes. **Regularity:** irregular. **Heart rate:** up to 500. **P waves:** none seen. **PR interval:** not applicable. **QRS interval:** 0.04–0.08 (hard to measure). **Interpretation:** torsades de pointes. Note the characteristic oscillating (bigger-smaller-bigger) pattern.

219. **QRS complexes:** None present—chaotic, wavy baseline noted instead. **Regularity:** not applicable as there are no QRS complexes. **Heart rate:** cannot measure. **P waves:** none. **PR interval:** not applicable. **QRS interval:** not applicable. **Interpretation:** ventricular fibrillation. Note the sudden wild change in baseline on the strip along with the notation of a shock delivered to the heart. This was an attempt to defibrillate the heart. Note that the V-fib continues even after the shock.

220. **QRS complexes:** present, all shaped the same within each lead. **Regularity:** regular. **Heart rate:** 187. **P waves:** an occasional dissociated P wave is noted. See the blip following the 5th, 8th, 10th, 12th, and 14th QRS complexes? Those are P waves. **PR interval:** not applicable. **QRS interval:** 0.14. **Interpretation:** ventricular tachycardia.

221. **QRS complexes:** present, all shaped the same within each lead. **Regularity:** irregular. **Heart rate:** from less than 30 to 62, with a mean rate of 40. **P waves:** none seen; wavy baseline noted between QRS complexes. **PR interval:** not applicable. **QRS interval:** 0.06. **Interpretation:** atrial fibrillation.

222. **QRS complexes:** present, all shaped the same within each lead. **Regularity:** regular. **Heart rate:** 88. **P waves:** matching and upright in both

leads. **PR interval:** 0.18. **QRS interval:** 0.10. **Interpretation:** sinus rhythm.

223. **QRS complexes:** present, all shaped the same within each lead. **Regularity:** regular. **Heart rate:** 75. **P waves:** matching, upright in both leads. **PR interval:** 0.16. **QRS interval:** 0.12. **Interpretation:** sinus rhythm with wide QRS.

224. **QRS complexes:** present, all shaped the same within each lead. **Regularity:** irregular. **Heart rate:** 68 to 94, with a mean rate of 80. **P waves:** none present; wavy baseline noted between QRS complexes. **PR interval:** not applicable. **QRS interval:** 0.09. **Interpretation:** atrial fibrillation.

225. **QRS complexes:** present, all shaped the same within each lead. **Regularity:** regular. **Heart rate:** 68. **P waves:** matching, upright in both leads. **PR interval:** 0.14. **QRS interval:** 0.06. **Interpretation:** sinus rhythm.

226. **QRS complexes:** present, all shaped the same within each lead. **Regularity:** regular. **Heart rate:** 62. **P waves:** matching, right in both leads. **PR interval:** 0.12. **QRS interval:** 0.10. **Interpretation:** sinus rhythm.

227. **QRS complexes:** present, all shaped the same within each lead. **Regularity:** regular but interrupted (by a premature beat). **Heart rate:** 75. **P waves:** matching, upright in both leads. **PR interval:** 0.22. **QRS interval:** 0.08. **Interpretation:** sinus rhythm with first-degree AV block.

228. **QRS complexes:** present, all shaped the same within each lead. **Regularity:** regular. **Heart rate:** 83. **P waves:** matching, upright in both leads. **PR interval:** 0.12. **QRS interval:** 0.08. **Interpretation:** sinus rhythm.

229. **QRS complexes:** present, all shaped the same. **Regularity:** regular. **Heart rate:** 62. **P waves:** matching, M-shaped. **PR interval:** 0.20. **QRS interval:** 0.10. **Interpretation:** sinus rhythm.

230. **QRS complexes:** present, all shaped the same within each lead. **Regularity:** regular. **Heart rate:** 88. **P waves:** none seen. **PR interval:** not applicable. **QRS interval:** 0.08. **Interpretation:** accelerated junctional rhythm.

231. **QRS complexes:** none noted. **Regularity:** not applicable. **Heart rate:** zero. **P waves:** none. **PR interval:** not applicable. **QRS interval:** not applicable. **Interpretation:** asystole.

232. **QRS complexes:** present, all shaped the same within each lead. **Regularity:** regular. **Heart rate:** 107. **P waves:** matching, inverted following the QRS in both leads. **PR interval:** not applicable. **QRS interval:** 0.08. **Interpretation:** junctional

tachycardia. See the blips following the QRS complexes? Those are the inverted P waves.

233. **QRS complexes:** present, all shaped the same within each lead. **Regularity:** regular. **Heart rate:** 100. **P waves:** matching, upright in both leads. **PR interval:** 0.20. **QRS interval:** 0.08. **Interpretation:** sinus rhythm.

234. **QRS complexes:** present, all shaped the same within each lead. **Regularity:** regular. **Heart rate:** 137. **P waves:** none seen. **PR interval:** not applicable. **QRS interval:** hard to measure, but probably about 0.20. **Interpretation:** ventricular tachycardia.

235. **QRS complexes:** present, all shaped the same. **Regularity:** regular. **Heart rate:** 150. **P waves:** matching, upright. **PR interval:** 0.12. **QRS interval:** 0.08. **Interpretation:** sinus tachycardia.

236. **QRS complexes:** present, all shaped the same within each lead. **Regularity:** regular. **Heart rate:** 43. **P waves:** upright and matching in Lead II, biphasic and matching in $V_1$. **PR interval:** 0.26. **QRS interval:** 0.10. **Interpretation:** sinus bradycardia with first-degree AV block.

237. **QRS complexes:** present, all shaped the same. **Regularity:** irregular. **Heart rate:** 45 to 54, with a mean rate of 50. **P waves:** matching, upright. **PR interval:** 0.18. **QRS interval:** 0.10. **Interpretation:** sinus bradycardia.

238. **QRS complexes:** present, all shaped the same within each lead. **Regularity:** irregular. **Heart rate:** 35 to 60, with mean rate of 50. **P waves:** upright and matching in both leads. The fourth QRS has a P wave at the top of its T wave. P-P interval is regular; atrial rate 60. **PR interval:** 0.24. **QRS interval:** 0.08. **Interpretation:** Mobitz II second-degree AV block.

239. **QRS complexes:** present, all shaped the same within each lead. **Regularity:** irregular. **Heart rate:** 54 to 68, with a mean rate of 60. **P waves:** matching, upright in both leads. **PR interval:** 0.16. **QRS interval:** 0.08. **Interpretation:** sinus arrhythmia.

240. **QRS complexes:** present, all shaped the same within each lead. **Regularity:** irregular. **Heart rate:** 100 to 150, with a mean rate of 140. **P waves:** none noted. **PR interval:** not applicable. **QRS interval:** 0.12. **Interpretation:** ventricular tachycardia.

241. **QRS complexes:** present, all shaped the same within each lead. **Regularity:** regular. **Heart rate:** 107. **P waves:** matching, inverted preceding the QRS. **PR interval:** 0.09. **QRS interval:** 0.08. **Interpretation:** junctional tachycardia.

242. **QRS complexes:** present, all shaped the same within each lead. **Regularity:** regular. **Heart rate:** 137. **P waves:** none noted. **PR interval:** not applicable. **QRS interval:** 0.10. **Interpretation:** SVT.

243. **QRS complexes:** present, all shaped the same within each lead. **Regularity:** irregular. **Heart rate:** 86 to 150, with a mean rate of 120. **P waves:** none seen; wavy baseline noted between QRS complexes. **PR interval:** not applicable. **QRS interval:** 0.08. **Interpretation:** atrial fibrillation.

244. **QRS complexes:** present, all shaped the same. **Regularity:** regular. **Heart rate:** 102. **P waves:** none noted; sawtooth-shaped waves noted between QRS complexes. **PR interval:** not applicable. **QRS interval:** 0.08. **Interpretation:** atrial flutter.

245. **QRS complexes:** present, all shaped the same. **Regularity:** regular. **Heart rate:** 79. **P waves:** matching, upright in Lead II, cannot see Ps in $V_1$. **PR interval:** 0.14. **QRS interval:** 0.12. **Interpretation:** sinus rhythm with wide QRS.

246. **QRS complexes:** present, all shaped the same within each lead except for beat number 3, which is a different shape. **Regularity:** regular but interrupted (by a premature beat). **Heart rate:** 50. **P waves:** matching, upright in Lead II, biphasic in $V_1$. The third QRS has no P wave. **PR interval:** 0.14. **QRS interval:** 0.08. **Interpretation:** sinus bradycardia with a PJC. The PJC beat has a wide QRS.

247. **QRS complexes:** present, all shaped the same within each lead. **Regularity:** regular. **Heart rate:** 107. **P waves:** matching, upright in both leads. **PR interval:** 0.14. **QRS interval:** 0.08. **Interpretation:** sinus tachycardia.

248. **QRS complexes:** present, all but the sixth shaped the same. The sixth QRS is wider. **Regularity:** regular but interrupted (by a premature beat). **Heart rate:** 71. **P waves:** upright and matching in both leads. **PR interval:** 0.14. **QRS interval:** 0.08. **Interpretation:** sinus rhythm with PVC.

249. **QRS complexes:** only one present; then chaotic, spiked, wavy baseline. **Regularity:** not applicable. **Heart rate:** unable to calculate, as only one QRS. **P waves:** none noted. **PR interval:** not applicable **QRS interval:** 0.06 on the one QRS. **Interpretation:** one sinus beat, then V-fib.

250. **QRS complexes:** present, the first two and the last one shaped the same. In between is a run of differently shaped beats. **Regularity:** irregular. **Heart rate:** 94 for the first two beats, then 187 on the run of beats. **P waves:** matching and upright on the first two and the last one beat; no Ps on the other beats. **PR interval:** 0.16. **QRS interval:** 0.10 on the narrow beats, 0.12 on the other beats. **Interpretation:** sinus rhythm with a run of V-tach.

# CHAPTER THIRTEEN
## Stress Test Assessment Practice

1. **Continue.** The EKG shows sinus tachycardia, which is expected. There are no ST segment changes that warrant stopping the test.

2. **Terminate.** The heart rate before the test was 70 and now varies from about 33 to 58. Note the P wave shapes vary also. The heart rate during a stress test should increase, not decrease. This decreased heart rate could signal decreased cardiac reserve.

3. **Terminate.** This is third-degree AV block, an ominous development during a stress test. The heart rate should speed up during the test.

4. **Terminate.** There is marked ST segment elevation in Leads II, III, aVF, and $V_5$ to $V_6$. This is an indication of an MI in progress. Note the reciprocal ST depression in I, aVL, and $V_2$ to $V_4$.

5. **Continue.** Sinus tachycardia is expected during a stress test. As long as the patient is tolerating the rhythm, the test may continue.

6. **False positive.** The stress test is positive for CAD—note the >1.5 mm ST segment depression in I, aVL, and $V_5$ to $V_6$. But the angiogram is negative, and that's the gold standard for diagnosing CAD. The stress test result is, therefore, a false positive.

7. **False negative.** The stress test is negative—no ST depression—but the angiogram is positive.

8. **False positive.** The stress test is positive—striking ST depression in $V_1$ to $V_6$—but the angiogram is negative.

9. **True positive.** Both stress test and angiogram are positive. Note the ST depression in $V_1$ to $V_6$.

10. **True negative.** Both stress test and angiogram are negative.

## Practice Quiz

1. The type of monitor worn for 24 hours to uncover any arrhythmias or ST segment changes that might be causing the patient's symptoms is the **Holter monitor.**

2. Indications for stress testing are the following (choose any three): **to determine the presence or absence of CAD, for post-CABG and post-PTCA evaluation, for diagnosis and treatment of exercise-induced arrhythmias, as follow-up to cardiac rehab, and to evaluate individuals with a family history of heart disease.**

3. Bayes's theorem says that **the validity of a test result depends not only on the test accuracy, but also on the probability that the patient in question would have the disease.**

4. ST segment elevation of 5 mm is **indicative of a positive stress test.** ST elevation that high indicates an infarction beginning.

5. **True.** Patients on beta-blockers and nitrates might be advised to avoid taking these medications for a period of time before the stress test.

6. Target heart rate is **220 minus the patient's age.**

7. Event monitoring differs from Holter monitoring in that **event monitoring can be worn or used over a prolonged period,** whereas Holter monitoring is typically used for only 24 hours. Also, Holter monitoring involves continuous recording of the rhythm, whereas **event monitoring records only abnormalities or rhythms it's programmed to record or that are present when activated by the patient.**

8. The most commonly used protocol for treadmill stress testing is the **Bruce protocol.**

9. The protocol used most often for post-MI patients just before or following hospital discharge is the **Naughton protocol.**

10. A MET is a **metabolic equivalent, a measurement of oxygen consumption, with which 1 MET is the resting oxygen consumption of a seated adult.**

## Critical Thinking Exercises

1. Of only slight concern on this EKG is the sinus tachycardia that is present at rest. Mr. Cameron is overweight and a smoker and is probably nervous about the test, so it is not surprising that his heart rate is a little elevated.

2. Mr. Cameron is overweight and a smoker, so his getting short of breath early on is not of too much concern.

3. The test should continue as these changes are normal and expected.

4. The rhythm is a bradycardia with bigeminal PVCs, then ventricular fibrillation.

5. The appropriate course of action is to get Mr. Cameron off the treadmill and to defibrillate him immediately.

6. What you should have done differently was paid more attention to Mr. Cameron's alarming change in blood pressure and his symptoms—cool clammy skin, dizziness, pallor, fatigue. He was in distress and the test should have been terminated.

# Glossary

**Absolute refractory period:** The period in which the cardiac cell will not respond to any stimulus, no matter how strong.

**Acetylcholine:** A hormone released as a result of parasympathetic stimulation.

**Action potential:** The depolarization and repolarization events that take place at the cell membrane. Also refers to the diagram associated with these polarity events.

**Acute:** Newly occurring.

**AED:** A defibrillator meant for use by the lay public.

**Age indeterminate:** A recent ST elevation MI, but can't be sure of the MI's exact age.

**Agonal rhythm:** A ventricular rhythm characterized by slow, irregular QRS complexes and absent P waves. Also called *dying heart.*

**AICD:** Automated implantable cardioverter-defibrillator. An implanted device that shocks the heart out of certain dangerous rhythms, such as V-Tach.

**Algorithm:** A flowchart.

**Amplifier:** An instrument that magnifies a signal.

**Amplitude:** The height of the waves and complexes on the EKG.

**Angina:** Chest pain caused by a decrease in myocardial blood flow.

**Anginal equivalent:** An individual's version of chest pain. May not involve pain at all—could be shortness of breath, fatigue, or other symptoms.

**Angiogram:** An invasive procedure in which dye is injected into blood vessels in order to determine their patency (openness).

**Antegrade:** In a forward direction.

**Anterior axillary line:** An imaginary line down from the front of the axilla (armpit).

**Anterior STEMI:** ST elevation MI affecting the anterior wall of the left ventricle.

**Anterior wall:** The front side of the left ventricle.

**Anteroseptal:** Pertaining to the anterior and septal walls of the left ventricle.

**Anteroseptal STEMI:** ST elevation MI affecting the septum and part or all of the anterior wall of the left ventricle.

**Antiarrhythmic:** Medications used to treat or prevent arrhythmias.

**Anticoagulants:** Medications used to prevent blood clot formation.

**Antihypertensives:** Medications used to treat hypertension.

**Antitachycardia pacing:** A special pacemaker function that interrupts tachycardias and helps convert the rhythm back to sinus rhythm.

**Aorta:** Largest artery in the body, into which the left ventricle empties.

**Aortic stenosis:** Narrowed opening to the aortic valve.

**Aortic valve:** Valve located between the left ventricle and aorta.

**Apex:** The pointy part of the heart where it rests on the diaphragm.

**Arrhythmia:** Abnormal heart rhythm.

**Arteriole:** A small artery that empties into a capillary bed.

**Artery:** A blood vessel that carries blood away from the heart to the tissues or the lungs.

**Artifact:** Unwanted jitter or interference on the EKG tracing.

**Asystole:** No heart beat. Characterized by a flat line on the EKG.

**Atrial kick:** The phase of diastole in which the atria contract to propel their blood into the ventricles.

**Atrial rate:** The heart rate of the P waves (or P wave alternatives such as flutter waves).

**Atrial tissue:** Tissue in the atria.

**Atrioventricular block:** Also called AV block. A block in impulse transmission from atrium to ventricle.

**Atrioventricular valves:** Also called AV valves. Heart valves located between atrium and ventricle.

**Atrium:** The upper, thin-walled receiving chambers of the heart.

**Augment:** Increase.

**Augmented leads:** Leads in which the EKG machine must increase (augment) the size of the waves and complexes. Includes aVR, aVL, and aVF.

**Automated implantable cardioverter-defibrillator (AICD):** See AICD.

**Automaticity:** The ability of cardiac cells to initiate an impulse without outside stimulation.

**Autonomic nervous system:** The nervous system controlling involuntary biological functions.

**AV blocks (atrioventricular blocks):** Disturbances in conduction in which some or all impulses from the sinus node are either delayed on their trip to the ventricles or do not reach the ventricle at all.

**AV dissociation (atrioventricular dissociation):** A condition in which the atria and ventricles depolarize and contract independently of each other.

**AV interval:** The interval between atrial and ventricular pacemaker spikes (It's an electronic PR interval).

**AV junction (atrioventricular junction):** Conductive tissue between the AV node and the atria.

**AV node (atrioventricular node):** The group of specialized cells in the conduction system that slows impulse transmission to allow atrial contraction to occur.

**Axillary:** Referring to the armpit.

**Axis:** The mean direction of the heart's current flow.

**Axis circle:** A circle that is formed by joining the ends of lead lines I, II, III, aVR, aVL, and aVF. This makes calculation of the electrical axis possible.

**Axis deviation:** An abnormal axis.

**Base:** The top of the heart; the area from which the great vessels emerge.

**Baseline:** The line from which the EKG waves and complexes take off. Also called the isoelectric line.

**Bayes's theorem:** The theorem that states that the predictive value of a test is based not only on the accuracy of the test itself but on the patient's probability of disease, as determined by a risk assessment done prior to the testing.

**Beta-blockers:** Class of cardiac medications that slows the heart rate, decreases blood pressure, and reduces cardiac workload.

**Beta-receptors:** Receptors that affect heart rate, contractility, and airway size.

**Bifascicular block:** A block of both fascicles of the left bundle branch, or a right bundle branch block plus a hemiblock.

**Bigeminy:** Every other beat is an abnormal beat.

**Bipolar:** Having a positive and a negative pole.

**Blood pressure:** The pressure exerted on the arterial walls by the circulating blood.

**Bradyarrhythmia:** An arrhythmia with a heart rate less than 60.

**Bradycardia:** Slow heart rate, usually less than 60.

**Bronchodilators:** Medications that dilate constricted airway passages in individuals with asthma, bronchitis, or emphysema.

**Bundle branch block:** A block in conduction through one of the bundle branches.

**Bundle branches:** Conduction pathways extending from the bundle of His in the lower right atrium to the Purkinje fibers in the ventricles. There is a right and a left bundle branch.

**Bundle of His:** A confluence of conduction fibers between the AV node and the bundle branches.

**Capillary bed:** The smallest blood vessels in the body; where nutrient and gas exchange occurs.

**Capture:** The depolarization of the atrium and/or ventricle as a result of a pacemaker's firing. Determined by the presence of a P wave and/or QRS after the pacemaker spike.

**Cardiac arrest:** An emergency in which the heart stops beating.

**Cardiac cycle:** The mechanical events that occur to pump blood. Consists of diastole and systole.

**Cardiac output:** The amount of blood expelled by the heart each minute. Measured as heart rate times stroke volume.

**Cardiogenic shock:** Shock induced by heart failure.

**Cardiologist:** A physician specializing in cardiac disease.

**Cardioversion:** Synchronized electrical shock to the heart to convert an abnormal rhythm back to sinus rhythm.

**Carotid sinus massage:** A method of slowing the heart rate by rubbing on the carotid artery in the neck.

**Catheter ablation:** A procedure in which a catheter is utilized to destroy the irritable heart tissue responsible for causing an arrhythmia.

**Chart speed:** EKG machine feature that regulates the speed of the paper printout.

**Chordae tendineae:** Tendinous cords that attach to the AV valves and prevent them from everting.

**Chronotropic incompetence:** Inability of the heart rate to increase with stress.

**Chronotropic reserve:** The ability of the heart rate to increase with exercise.

**Circumflex coronary artery:** The branch off the left main coronary artery that feeds oxygenated blood to the lateral wall of the left ventricle.

**Clockwise:** Moving in the direction of clock hands.

**Code:** Cardiac arrest.

**Complete compensatory pause:** Normally follows PVCs. Measures two R-R cycles from the beat preceding the PVC to the beat following the PVC.

**Conduction system:** A network of specialized cells whose job is to create and conduct the electrical impulses that control the cardiac cycle.

**Conduction system cells:** Cardiac cells whose job is to create and conduct electrical signals to trigger a heartbeat.

**Conductivity:** The ability of a cardiac cell to pass an impulse along to neighboring cells.

**Congestive heart failure (CHF):** Fluid buildup in the lungs as a result of the heart's inability to pump adequately.

**Contractile cells:** Cardiac cells whose job is to contract and cause blood to flow.

**Contractility:** The ability of a cardiac cell to contract and do work.

**Contraindications:** Reasons to avoid doing a test or procedure.

**Coronary arteries:** The arteries that feed oxygenated blood to the myocardium.

**Coronary vein:** Vein that returns deoxygenated blood from the heart tissues back to the right atrium.

**Counterclockwise:** In a direction opposite the way the clock hands move.

**Couplet:** A pair of beats.

**Coved ST segment:** Rounded ST segment elevation typical of an STEMI. Also called convex ST segment elevation.

**CPK:** Creatine phosphokinase. Chemical released by the heart during an MI.

**Critical rate:** The rate at which a bundle branch block appears or disappears.

**Decreased cardiac output:** Inadequate blood flow to meet the body's needs.

**Decreased diastolic filling time:** Caused by tachycardias. The decreased time between beats for the heart to fill up with blood.

**Defibrillation:** Asynchronous electrical shock to the heart, used to treat ventricular fibrillation and pulseless V-tach.

**Delta wave:** A slurred upstroke to the QRS complex, seen in Wolff-Parkinson-White Syndrome.

**Depolarization:** The wave of electrical current that changes the resting negatively charged cardiac cell to a positively charged one.

**Diaphoresis:** Sweating, usually a cold sweat. Also referred to as "cold and clammy."

**Diastasis:** The phase in diastole in which the atrial and ventricular pressures are equalizing.

**Diastole:** The phase of the cardiac cycle in which the ventricles fill with blood.

**Digital converter:** A device in an EKG machine that converts an analog signal to a digital one.

**Digitalis toxicity:** Overabundance of the medication digitalis in the bloodstream.

**Dissecting aneurysm:** The ballooning out of an artery into the wall of the artery itself.

**Dissociation:** The lack of relationship between two pacemaker sites in the heart.

**Diuretics:** Medications given to increase the urine output.

**Early repolarization:** Phases 1 and 2 of the action potential.

**Ectopic rhythms:** Rhythms originating in any pacemaker other than the sinus node.

**Einthoven's law:** The height of the QRS complexes in Lead I +Lead III = Lead II.

**Einthoven's triangle:** The triangle formed by joining Leads I, II, and III at the ends.

**Electrocardiogram:** The physical printout of the electrical signals generated by the heart.

**Electrocardiography:** The process of recording the heart's electrical signals.

**Electrodes:** Adhesive patches attached to the skin to receive the electrical signals from the heart.

**Electrolytes:** Blood chemicals.

**Embolus:** Blood clot that has broken off and is traveling through a blood vessel.

**Endocardium:** The innermost layer of the heart.

**Epicardium:** Outer layer of the heart.

**Erectile dysfunction medications:** Medications that treat erectile problems in males.

**Ergometer:** An arm bicycle used in stress testing.

**Escape:** A safety mechanism in which a lower pacemaker fires at its slower inherent rate when the faster, predominant pacemaker fails.

**Escaping:** A lower pacemaker taking over when a higher pacemaker fails.

**Event monitor:** A small device that can be used to determine if sporadic arrhythmias or ischemia are present.

**Evolution:** The gradual EKG changes that occur in an acute ST elevation MI.

**Excitability:** The ability of a cardiac cell to depolarize when stimulated.

**Extensive anterior STEMI:** A large ST elevation MI affecting the anterior and lateral walls of the left ventricle.

**Fascicle:** A branch.

**Fibrillation:** The wiggling or twitching of the atrium or ventricle.

**Firing:** The pacemaker's generation of an electrical impulse.

**Fixed-rate pacemaker:** An old-fashioned pacemaker that paced at a programmed rate with no regard to the patient's own intrinsic rhythm or beats.

**Foci:** Locations.

**Focus:** Location.

**Frontal leads:** Limb Leads I, II, III, aVR, aVL, and aVF. Leads located on the front of the body.

**Fusion beats:** A combination of a sinus beat and a PVC. Shape is intermediate between that of the sinus beat and the PVC.

**Gain:** EKG machine feature that regulates the height of the waves and complexes.

**Glaucoma medications:** Medications that decrease the eyeball pressure.

**Glottis:** The flap over the top of the windpipe.

**Heart rate:** The number of times the heart beats in one minute.

**Heart rhythm:** A pattern of successive heart beats.

**Hemiblock:** A block of one of the left bundle branch's fascicles.

**Hexiaxial diagram:** A diagram of the six frontal leads intersecting at the center; serves as the basis for the axis circle.

**Holter monitor:** A device used for 24-hour cardiac monitoring to check for arrhythmias or ST segment abnormalities.

**Hyperacute changes:** Those seen in the earliest stages of a disease or condition.

**Hypercalcemia:** Elevated blood calcium level.

**Hyperkalemia:** Elevated blood potassium level.

**Hypertension:** High blood pressure.

**Hypertrophic cardiomyopathy:** Heart disease caused by an overgrowth of the interventricular septum.

**Hypertrophy:** Overgrowth of myocardial tissue.

**Hyperventilating:** Breathing very rapidly.

**Hypocalcemia:** Low blood calcium level.

**Hypokalemia:** Low blood potassium level.

**Hypotension:** Low blood pressure.

**Hypoxia:** Low blood oxygen level.

**Indeterminate axis:** An axis that is between −90 and +−180 degrees.

**Indications:** Reasons to perform a test or procedure.

**Indicative changes:** EKG changes that indicate the presence of an MI.

**Infarction:** Death of tissue. A myocardial infarction (MI) is a heart attack.

**Inferior STEMI:** ST elevation MI involving the inferior wall of the left ventricle.

**Inferior vena cava (IVC):** Large vein that returns deoxygenated blood to the right atrium from the lower chest, abdomen, and legs.

**Inferior wall:** The bottom wall of the left ventricle.

**Inherent:** Preset.

**Injury:** Damage to tissue.

**Inotropic incompetence:** The inability of the blood pressure to increase with exercise.

**Inotropic reserve:** The ability of the blood pressure to increase with exercise.

**Interatrial septum:** The muscular band of tissue separating the right and left atria.

**Interatrial tracts:** The pathways that carry the electrical impulse from the sinus node through the atrial tissue.

**Intercostal spaces:** Spaces between the ribs.

**Internodal tracts:** Pathways that carry electrical impulses from the sinus node to the AV node.

**Intervals:** Measurements of time between EKG waves and complexes.

**Interventricular septum:** The muscular band of tissue separating right and left ventricles.

**Intrinsic:** The patient's own. Intrinsic beats are the patient's own beats.

**Inverted:** Upside down.

**Ions:** Electrically charged particles.

**Irritability:** Also called usurpation. The cardiac cell fires in prematurely, taking control away from the predominant pacemaker.

**Ischemia:** Oxygen deprivation in the tissues.

**Isoelectric:** As much above the baseline as below.

**Isoelectric line:** The flat line between the EKG waves and complexes. Also called the baseline.

**Isovolumetric:** Maintaining the same volume.

**Isovolumetric contraction:** The first phase of systole. The ventricles are contracting but no blood flow is occurring because all the valves are still closed.

**Isovolumetric relaxation:** The final phase of systole. The semilunar valves slam shut and blood flow from the ventricles stops.

**J point:** The point where the QRS complex and ST segment join together.

**Kent bundle:** The accessory pathway in WPW.

**Late potentials:** Electrical potentials that occur late in the QRS complex and can be a sign of ventricular irritability and impending ventricular arrhythmias.

**Lateral wall:** The left side wall of the left ventricle.

**Lateral wall STEMI:** ST elevation MI affecting the lateral wall of the left ventricle.

**Lead:** An electrocardiographic picture of the heart.

**Lead wires:** Wires that attach the electrode patches to the EKG machine.

**Leakage current:** Small amount of electrical current that escapes from an implanted device such as a pacemaker.

**Left anterior descending coronary artery:** A branch of the left main coronary artery. It feeds oxygenated blood to the anterior wall of the left ventricle.

**Left anterior hemiblock:** Block of the left anterior fascicle of the left bundle branch.

**Left axis deviation:** An axis between 0 and −90 degrees.

**Left bundle branch:** Conduction fibers that carry the cardiac impulses down the left side of the septum to the left ventricle.

**Left common bundle branch:** The part of the left bundle branch before it divides into its fascicles.

**Left main coronary artery:** The coronary artery that branches off into the circumflex and left anterior descending coronary arteries.

**Left posterior hemiblock:** Block of the left posterior fascicle of the left bundle branch.

**Limb leads:** Leads attached to the limbs. Includes I, II, III, aVR, aVL, and aVF.

**Low cardiac output:** Inadequate amount of blood pumped out by the heart every minute.

**Macroshock:** A large electrical shock caused by improper or faulty grounding of electrical equipment.

**Mean rate (mean heart rate):** The average heart rate.

**Mediastinum:** The cavity between the lungs, in which the heart is located.

**MET:** Metabolic equivalent, a measurement of oxygen consumption.

**Microshock:** A small electrical shock made possible by a conduit, such as a pacemaker, directly in the heart.

**Midaxillary line:** An imaginary line down from the middle of the axilla (armpit).

**Midclavicular line:** An imaginary line down from the middle of the clavicle (collarbone).

**Mitral:** Valve that separates the left atrium and left ventricle.

**Multifocal:** Coming from more than one location.

**Myocardial infarction:** Heart attack.

**Myocardium:** The muscular layer of the heart.

**Necroses:** Dies.

**Neuropathy:** Condition that causes a decrease in sensation, especially pain, in susceptible individuals.

**Nitrates:** Medications used to dilate coronary arteries and improve coronary blood flow.

**Nonconducted PAC:** A premature P wave not followed by a QRS complex.

**Norepinephrine:** The chemical released by the adrenal gland when stimulated by the sympathetic nervous system.

**Normal axis:** Axis between 0 and +90 degrees.

**NSTEMI:** Non-ST elevation MI.

**Occlusion:** Blockage.

**Oversensed:** Pacemaker sensed something it shouldn't have, such as a beat from another chamber.

**Oxygen:** An element inhaled from the atmosphere that is necessary for body function.

**Pacemaker:** The intrinsic or artificial focus that propagates or initiates the cardiac impulse.

**Pacing interval:** The programmed interval between paced beats.

**Papillary muscle:** The muscle to which the chordae tendineae are attached at the bottom.

**Parasympathetic nervous system:** The division of the autonomic nervous system that slows the heart rate, lowers blood pressure, stimulates digestion, and constricts pupils—all signs of the "rest-and-digest" response.

**Paroxysmal:** Occurring suddenly and stopping just as suddenly.

**PCI:** Percutaneous coronary intervention. A balloon procedure to open a blocked coronary artery.

**Perfusing:** Supplying blood to.

**Perfusion:** The supplying of blood and nutrients to tissues.

**Pericardial fluid:** Small amount of fluid found between the layers of the pericardial sac.

**Pericarditis:** An inflammation of the pericardium.

**Pericardium:** The sac that encloses the heart.

**Plateau phase:** The phase of the action potential in which the waveform levels off (flattens out). Phase 2 is the plateau phase.

**Platelet aggregation:** Clumping of platelets to form clots to stop bleeding.

**Platelets:** Cells responsible for blood clotting.

**Polarized:** Possessing an electrical charge.

**Polymorphic:** Possessing multiple shapes.

**Postangioplasty evaluation:** Evaluation of the patient's condition following a procedure to open up blocked coronary arteries.

**Posterior descending artery:** A branch off the right coronary artery that provides blood flow to the posterior wall of the left ventricle.

**Posterior MI:** MI affecting the posterior wall of the left ventricle.

**Posterior wall:** The back wall of the left ventricle.

**P-P interval:** The distance (interval) between consecutive P waves.

**Precordial:** Pertaining to the chest.

**Precordial leads:** The six leads on the chest (V1 through V6).

**Pre-excitation:** Depolarizing tissue earlier than normal.

**PR interval:** Measurement of time it takes the cardiac impulse to travel from atrium to ventricle.

**Protodiastole:** The phase of systole in which the blood flow out of the ventricles slows because of equalizing pressures between the ventricles and the aorta and pulmonary artery.

**PR segment:** Flat line between the P wave and the QRS complex.

**Pulmonary artery:** Large artery that takes deoxygenated blood from the right ventricle to the lungs. It is the ONLY artery that carries deoxygenated blood.

**Pulmonary embolus:** Blood clot in the lung.

**Pulmonary veins:** Four veins that return oxygenated blood from the lungs to the left atrium. They are the ONLY veins that carry oxygenated blood.

**Pulmonic valve:** Valve located between the right ventricle and the pulmonary artery.

**Purkinje fibers:** Fibers at the terminal ends of the bundle branches. Responsible for transmitting the impulses into the ventricular myocardium.

**P wave:** The EKG wave reflecting atrial depolarization.

**P wave asystole:** A type of asystole that still has P waves.

**QRS complex:** The EKG complex representing ventricular depolarization.

**QRS interval:** The spiked wave on the EKG. Represents ventricular depolarization.

**QS wave:** A QRS complex with only a downward wave—no upward wave(s).

**QT interval:** Measures ventricular depolarization and repolarization time.

**Quadrigeminy:** Every fourth beat is abnormal.

**Q wave:** A downward wave preceding an R wave in the QRS complex. If a Q wave is present, it is ALWAYS the first wave of the QRS complex.

**R´** Pronounced "R prime." Is the second R wave in a QRS complex.

**Rapid-filling phase:** The first phase of diastole in which the ventricles rapidly fill with blood from the atria.

**Rapid repolarization:** Phase 3 of the action potential.

**Rate-related bundle branch blocks:** Bundle branch blocks that appear only at certain heart rates.

**Reciprocal changes:** EKG changes (ST depression) seen in the area electrically opposite the infarcted area.

**Refractory:** Resistant to.

**Regularity:** Spacing of the P waves or QRS complexes.

**Relative refractory period:** The period in which only a strong stimulus will cause depolarization of the cardiac cell.

**Reperfusion arrhythmia:** A rhythm, usually AIVR, that was thought to result from the return of blood and oxygen supply to tissues that have been deprived for a period of time.

**Repolarization:** The wave of electrical current that returns the cardiac cell to its resting, electrically negative state.

**Resuscitation:** Restoring respirations and/or pulse by way of artificial respiration and cardiac compressions.

**Retrograde:** In a backward direction.

**Rhythm strip:** A printout of one or two leads at a time, done on special rolls of paper.

**Right axis deviation:** An axis between +90 to +−80 degrees.

**Right bundle branch:** Conduction fibers that carry the cardiac impulses down the right side of the septum to the right ventricle.

**Right coronary artery (RCA):** The coronary artery that feeds oxygenated blood to the right ventricle and the inferior wall of the left ventricle.

**R-on-T phenomenon:** The PVC that falls on the T wave of the preceding beat. Predisposes to rapid arrhythmias.

**R-R interval:** The distance (interval) between consecutive QRS complexes. Usually measured at the peaks of the R waves.

**R wave:** An upward wave in the QRS complex.

**Scooping ST segment:** Rounded ST segment seen with digitalis effect.

**Segment:** The flat line between EKG waves and complexes.

**Semilunar valves:** Half-moon-shaped. Refers to the aortic and pulmonic valves.

**Sensing:** The ability of an artificial pacemaker to "see" the intrinsic rhythm in order to determine whether the pacemaker needs to fire.

**Sensitivity:** The ability of a test to pick out the people who are truly diseased.

**Septum:** The fibrous tissue that separates the heart into right and left sides.

**Sinus node:** The normal pacemaker of the heart.

**Sleep apnea:** Temporary, often repetitive cessation of breathing during sleep.

**Sodium-potassium pump:** The active transport system that returns the cardiac cell to its resting, electrically negative state following depolarization.

**Somatic:** Referring to the body.

**Specificity:** The ability of a test to exclude those who are not diseased.

**STEMI:** ST elevation MI.

**Stenosis:** Narrowed opening.

**Stenotic:** Pertaining to stenosis.

**Stent:** A wire mesh inserted into a coronary artery to hold it open following PCI.

**Sternum:** Breastbone.

**Stress test:** A test done to determine the presence of coronary artery disease. Can be done using exercise or medications to stress the heart.

**Stress testing:** A method of utilizing a bicycle or treadmill to stress the heart and determine if coronary disease is present.

**ST segment:** The flat line between the QRS complex and the T wave.

**Subendocardial:** Referring to the myocardial layer just beneath the endocardium.

**Submaximal test:** A stress test that is concluded when 70% of the target heart rate is reached.

**Superior vena cava (SVC):** Large vein that returns deoxygenated blood to the right atrium from the head, neck, upper chest, and arms.

**Supernormal period:** The period in which the cardiac cell is "hyper" and will respond to a very weak stimulus.

**Supine:** Back-lying.

**Supraventricular:** Originating in a pacemaker above the ventricle.

**S wave:** A negative wave that follows an R wave in the QRS complex.

**Sympathetic nervous system:** The division of the autonomic nervous system that regulates the "fight-or-flight" response, causing the heart rate and blood pressure to rise, digestion to slow, and pupils to dilate.

**Syncope:** Fainting spell.

**Systole:** The phase of the cardiac cycle in which the ventricle contracts and expels its blood.

**Tachycardia:** Fast heart rate, greater than 100.

**T$_a$ wave:** The rarely-seen wave that follows the P wave and represents repolarization of the atria.

**Telemetry:** A method of monitoring a patient's rhythm remotely. The patient carries a small transmitter that relays his or her cardiac rhythm to a receiver located at another location.

**Thallium-201:** A radioactive medication used to enable special x-ray images to be done following a stress test.

**Therapeutic hypothermia:** Cooling the post-cardiac arrest patient's body temperature down to 90 to 93 degrees Fahrenheit in order to decrease brain damage and improve brain function.

**Thoracic:** Referring to the chest cavity.

**Thoracic cavity:** Chest cavity.

**Three-channel recorder:** An EKG recorder that prints out 3 leads simultaneously.

**Thrombolysis:** The act of dissolving a blood clot.

**Thrombolytics:** Medications used to dissolve the clot causing an MI or a stroke.

**Thyrotoxicosis:** Also called thyroid storm. A condition in which the thyroid gland so overproduces thyroid hormones that the body's metabolic rate is accelerated to a catastrophic degree. The body temperature, heart rate, and blood pressure rise to extreme levels.

**Trachea:** Windpipe.

**Transcutaneous:** By way of the skin.

**Transmembrane potential:** The electrical charge at the cell membrane.

**Transmural:** Through the full thickness of the wall at that location.

**Transvenous:** By way of a vein.

**Triaxial diagram:** The diagram of Leads I, II, and III joined at the center or of aVR, aVL, and aVF joined at the center.

**Tricuspid:** Having three cusps.

**Tricuspid valve:** Valve that separates the right atrium and right ventricle.

**Tricyclic antidepressants (TCA):** A kind of medication used for the treatment of depression.

**Trigeminy:** Every third beat is abnormal.

**Troponin:** A chemical released by the heart during an MI.

**Troubleshooting:** Determining and correcting the cause of artifact and recording errors.

**Unifocal:** Coming from one location.

**Unipolar:** A lead consisting of only a positive pole.

**Unipolar leads:** Leads having only a positive pole. Unipolar leads include aVR, aVL, aVF, V1, V2, V3, V4, V5, and V6.

**Unstable angina:** Chest pain that is increasing in intensity and/or frequency.

**Usurpation:** The act of a lower pacemaker stealing control from the predominant pacemaker; results in a faster heart rate than before. Also called irritability.

**U wave:** A small wave sometimes seen on the EKG. It follows the T wave and reflects late repolarization.

**Vagus nerve:** The nerve that is part of the parasympathetic nervous system. Causes the heart rate to slow when stimulated.

**Valve:** A structure in the heart that prevents backflow of blood.

**Vasoconstrict:** To make a blood vessel's walls squeeze down, narrowing the vessel's lumen.

**Vasodilate:** To make the blood vessel's walls relax, thus widening the blood vessel.

**Vasodilators:** Medications that relax blood vessel walls.

**Vector:** An arrow depicting the direction of electrical current flow in the heart.

**Vein:** A blood vessel that transports deoxygenated blood away from the tissues.

**Vena cava:** The largest vein in the body; returns deoxygenated blood to the heart.

**Ventricles:** The lower pumping chambers of the heart.

**Ventricular asystole:** Another name for P wave asystole. There are P waves but no QRS complexes.

**Ventricular dilatation:** Stretching of the myocardial fibers from overfilling or inadequate pumping of blood from the ventricles. Results in a weakened pumping efficiency.

**Ventricular ejection:** The phase of systole in which the semilunar valves pop open and blood pours out of the ventricles.

**Venule:** A small vein that drains blood away from a capillary bed.

# Index